Therapeutic Protein Targets for Drug Discovery and Clinical Evaluation

Bio-Crystallography and Drug Design

Therapeutic Protein Targets for Drug Discovery and Clinical Evaluation

Bio-Crystallography and Drug Design

Editors

D Velmurugan
AMET University, India

Atanu Bhattacharjee
North Eastern Hill University, India

D Gayathri
University Of Madras, India

World Scientific

NEW JERSEY • LONDON • SINGAPORE • BEIJING • SHANGHAI • HONG KONG • TAIPEI • CHENNAI • TOKYO

Published by

World Scientific Publishing Co. Pte. Ltd.
5 Toh Tuck Link, Singapore 596224
USA office: 27 Warren Street, Suite 401-402, Hackensack, NJ 07601
UK office: 57 Shelton Street, Covent Garden, London WC2H 9HE

British Library Cataloguing-in-Publication Data
A catalogue record for this book is available from the British Library.

THERAPEUTIC PROTEIN TARGETS FOR DRUG DISCOVERY AND CLINICAL EVALUATION
Bio-Crystallography and Drug Design

ISBN 978-981-125-478-9 (hardcover)
ISBN 978-981-125-479-6 (ebook for institutions)
ISBN 978-981-125-480-2 (ebook for individuals)

For any available supplementary material, please visit
https://www.worldscientific.com/worldscibooks/10.1142/12791#t=suppl

Typeset by Stallion Press
Email: enquiries@stallionpress.com

https://doi.org/10.1142/9789811254796_fmatter

Contents

Preface

The need for innovative therapeutic drug molecules with pharmacological indications is quickly expanding in today's world in order to cure life-threatening diseases, reduce unpleasant side effects and promote patient care and public health. The combination of current methodologies and recent discoveries from diverse research disciplines is required for the creation of a novel medication to cure the present untreatable diseases. This book presents an overview of several state-of-the-art methodologies for evidence-based validation, phytochemical analysis and pharmacological evaluation from researchers across the world working on the latest areas of traditional medicine. This book allows the researchers to understand the efficacy of traditional medicine in drug development and also to understand the viral infection pathways. Drug discovery has benefited greatly from technological advancements. Artificial Intelligence and Machine Learning can help in structure-based drug discovery by predicting the 3D protein structure, which can help to assess the influence of a compound on the target as well as safety considerations before it is synthesised or commercially produced.

The first chapter of this book introduces the structural and functional aspects on the macrolide efflux transporter. The second chapter focuses on the catalytic mechanism of secretory phospholipase A2 and its inflammatory action. The third chapter examines the shock and kill strategy for controlling HIV-1 viral transcription via TAT. The fourth chapter of this book describes how machine learning is being used to identify protein targets and structure-based drug discovery in the early stages of structure-based drug design. With a structure-based viewpoint, the fifth chapter discusses current advances in the usage of protease and protease inhibitor therapeutic targets. The sixth chapter explores the antimicrobial resistance pathogen. The seventh chapter outlines all of the therapeutic protein targets that can be used to help with drug development. The natural peptide having antiviral activity is discussed in the eighth chapter. The invention of a multi-epitope peptide-based vaccination for human influenza A/H1N1 virus is discussed in the ninth chapter. The tenth chapter discusses certain medicinal plants as well as a nanoparticle formulation for cancer treatment with minimal side effects. The eleventh chapter deals with the molecular dynamics simulations, majorly focussing on the mutation in R233 to H233, which leads to the renal cell cancer. The last chapter discusses about the phytochemicals present in the *Indigofera aspalathoides* oil, which may help in treating the various diseases. This book thus provides a detailed coverage of various drug targets and also about the treatment of a variety of diseases. I am sure the readers will benefit a lot from the above.

Prof. D. Velmurugan

Acknowledgments

I wish to acknowledge the hard work and dedication of all the contributors of various chapters in this book. I would also like to thank the co-editors Drs. Atanu Bhatacharjee and D. Gayathri for their timely help.

I have to thank my collaborator Dr. Pachaiappan Raman from SRM Institute of Science and Technology, Kattankulathur, Chennai, his Ph.D. scholars Mrs. Nagasathya and Ms. Pinki Singh, and his M.Tech student Ms. Vinduja for going through the chapters.

My sincere thanks to Prof. T.P. Singh, DBT-SERB Distinguished Professor, Department of Biophysics, All India Institute of Medical Sciences, New Delhi for writing the foreword.

I whole heartedly thank World Scientific Publishers for their patience and kindness to me, particularly Ms. Sandhya Devi for immediately answering my frequent mails.

I am sure that this book will definitely be of interest to not only the structural biologists but also to scientists and research scholars interested in natural products research for disease prevention and treatment.

Prof. D. Velmurugan

Foreword

Drug discovery is the process of identifying possible novel therapeutic agents by bringing together a variety of scientific fields such as biology, chemistry and pharmacology. Protein targets must be identified in order to better understand the mechanisms of action and create therapeutic drugs. Target selection and validation include assay developments, lead optimization, and the identification of a candidate for further development of the discovery process. A preclinical drug discovery program's purpose is to generate one or more clinical candidate molecules that have enough evidence of biological action at a disease-relevant target, as well as adequate safety and drug-like qualities, efficacy to be tested in humans. When looking for a novel drug to treat a specific disease, high-throughput screening is used, in which enormous libraries of compounds are examined for their capacity to change the target. Drug development is a time-consuming process due to the five critical phases: (a) Discovery and development (b) Preclinical research (c) Clinical development (d) Food and drug administration review and (e) post-market monitoring. Improvements in drug development have been aided by technological advances. Because the design is in accordance with the chemical environment of the target protein site, artificial intelligence can assist in structure-based drug discovery by predicting the 3D protein structure, which can help to predict the effect of a compound on the targets as well as safety considerations prior to its synthesis or production. The demand for novel treatments to treat a variety of deadly diseases has prompted substantial drug development. It is critical to gather such study findings together, so that researchers may learn about their significance and the most recent developments in the area. The book entitled "Therapeutic Protein Targets for Drug Discovery and Clinical Evaluation: Bio-Crystallography and Drug Design" is one such book edited by Prof. D. Velmurugan, one of India's leading crystallographer and his colleagues.

This book examines recent advances in innovative technologies and speculates on the future prospects for identifying therapeutic protein targets for the treatment of dreadful diseases such as cancer, human influenza and HIV-AIDS, etc. This book also covers the molecular mechanisms of plant-based compounds which interact with various proteases. This book is enlightening the current state of knowledge in the field of drug development. An important element is a new way of illustrating the plant's function and the potential of phytoconstituents as anti-cancer and anti-HIV. Overall, this book provides readers with a comprehensive overview of the dynamic subject of drug development research. I commend the authors for providing researchers with a comprehensive view of the subject and effectively stimulating excitement for developing a new strategy to address the ever-increasing demands in the field of drug development. I wish this book a great success and broad circulation.

Department of Biophysics
ALL INDIA INSTITUTE
OF MEDICAL SCIENCES
Ansari Nagar, New Delhi-110 029, India

Prof. T. P. Singh Ph.D., D.Sc. (*hc*)
FTWAS, FNA, FASc, FNASc, FBRS
DST-SERB Distinguished Fellow
Honorary Distinguished Professor (UOM)
Honorary Visiting Professor (INST)
June 2, 2022

T.P. Singh

https://doi.org/10.1142/9789811254796_0001

1 Structural and Functional Aspects of the Macrolide Efflux Transporter, MacB — A Tripartite ABC Transporter

Ui Okada and Satoshi Murakami*

Department of Life Science, Tokyo Institute of Technology, 4259-J2-17, Nagatsuta, Midori-ku, Yokohama, 226-8501, Japan.

Abstract

The macrolide efflux transporter MacB is a member of ATP-binding cassette (ABC) transporters. Recent structural analyses of MacB revealed their unique structures compared with canonical ABC transporters, and a novel substrate translocation model has been proposed. In this chapter, we introduce the structural and functional aspects on the macrolide efflux transporter MacB.

1. Introduction

1.1. Tripartite Efflux Transporter

Multidrug-resistant Gram negative pathogens such as *Escherichia coli*, *Acinetobacter baumannii*, and *Pseudomonas aeruginosa* are a serious public health threat. The drug resistance of these pathogens is mediated by several mechanisms, for example, the active efflux of drugs, enzymatic inactivation of drugs, membrane permeability

*Corresponding author: e-mail: murakami@bio.titech.ac.jp

barrier, and alteration of drug target (Munita & Arias, 2016). Among them, the active efflux from the cell plays an important role in multidrug resistance. In Gram-negative bacteria, tripartite efflux transporters, also called as "tripartite efflux pumps," are used to export various substrates across both inner and outer membranes. Tripartite efflux transporter is composed of three proteins, inner membrane (IM) transporter, periplasmic adaptor protein (PAP) which

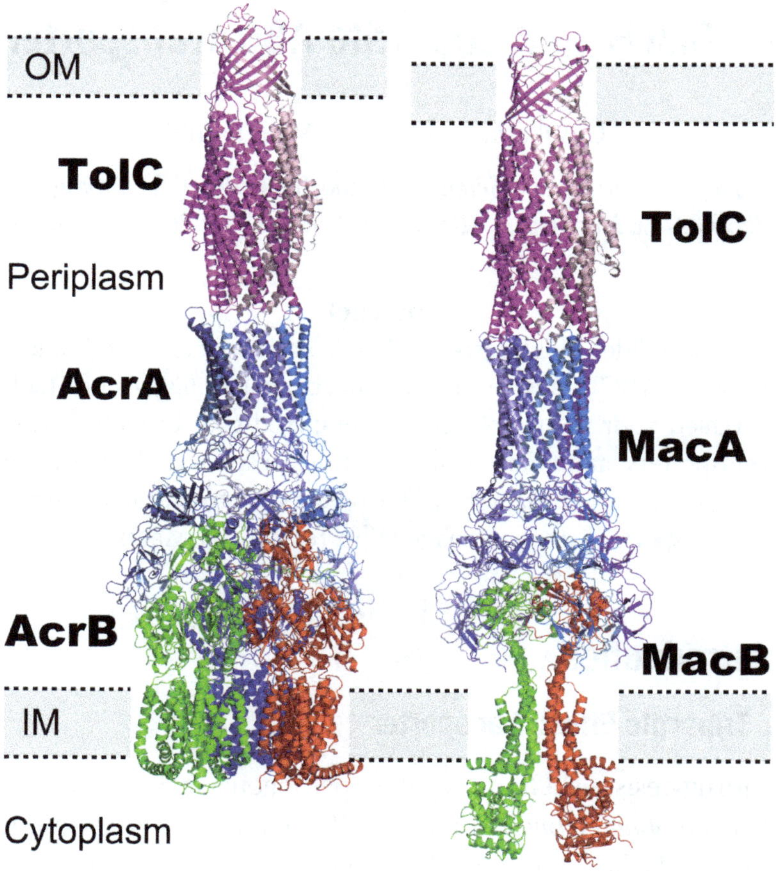

Fig. 1 Cryo-EM structure of tripartite efflux transporters. (Left) AcrAB-TolC complex (Protein Data Bank (PDB) ID: 5V5S) and (right) MacAB-TolC complex (PDB ID: 5NIL). Dotted lines indicate estimated membrane boundaries. Each protomer of trimeric TolC is colored in magenta, light pink, and dark pink. Each protomer of hexameric AcrA or MacA is colored in sky blue, purple blue, deep blue, marine blue, slate blue, and light blue. Each protomer of trimeric AcrB is colored in green, red, and blue. Each protomer of dimeric MacB is colored in green and red.

is also known as membrane fusion protein, and outer membrane channel (OMC). One of the well-studied tripartite efflux transporters is AcrA-AcrB-TolC complex, which confers multidrug resistance in *E. coli* (**Fig. 1**, left). The tripartite complex contains AcrB homotrimer, AcrA homohexamer, and TolC homotrimer. AcrB as IM transporter is a member of resistance-nodulation-cell division (RND) transporter, which is driven by the proton motive force. AcrB pumps out various substrates from the outer leaflet of the IM or the periplasm to funnel-like AcrA hexamer. AcrA as PAP covers periplasmic domain (PLD) of AcrB, and connects to TolC as OMC. TolC trimer forms duct-like substrate translocation pathway composed of periplasmic α-helical barrel and β-barrel across the OM. Structural analyses of three protein components by X-ray crystallography and tripartite AcrAB-TolC complex by cryo-electron microscopy (cryo-EM) revealed the molecular mechanism of the substrate translocation (Du *et al.*, 2014; Koronakis *et al.*, 2000; Mikolosko *et al.*, 2006; Murakami *et al.*, 2002, 2006; Wang *et al.*, 2017).

Incidentally, some major facilitator superfamily (MFS) transporters such as EmrB form tripartite efflux complex as IM transporters. However, structural information of tripartite complex which contains MFS transporter has not been reported. So it is unclear how the MFS-type tripartite complex exports substrates.

As IM transporter, ABC transporter MacB also assembles into tripartite efflux transporter spanning the inner and outer membranes (**Fig. 1**, right). This is the most distinctive feature of MacB in comparison with many other ABC transporters which transport solely in IM. Cryo-EM structure of MacAB-TolC tripartite complex was reported in 2017, in which MacA is PAP and TolC is OMC (Fitzpatrick *et al.*, 2017). The details of this tripartite complex will be discussed in the later section.

1.2. ABC Transporter

ABC transporters are one of the largest superfamilies found in all three domains of life. These transporters use the binding and hydrolysis of ATP to import or export various substrates, such

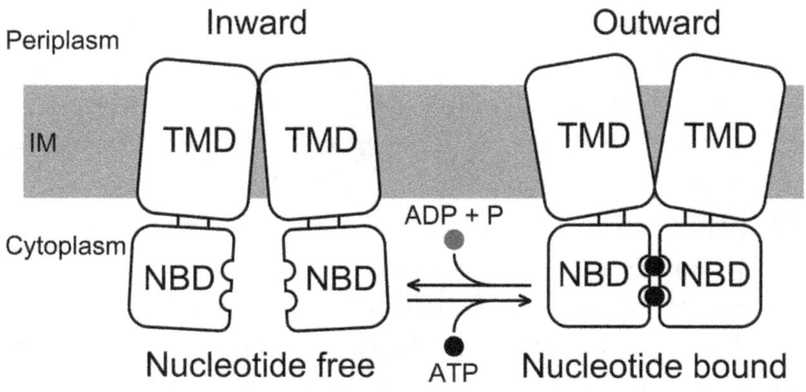

Fig. 2 Architecture of ABC transporter.

as ions, sugars, amino acids, peptides, proteins, drugs, or lipids (Davidson *et al.*, 2008). The functional unit of ABC transporter consists of four domains: two transmembrane domains (TMDs) that are buried in the IM and contains the substrate binding site, and two nucleotide binding domains (NBDs) that catalyze ATP hydrolysis in the cytoplasm (**Fig. 2**). The transporter that contains all four domains, TMD1, NBD1, TMD2, and NBD2 in the single polypeptide chain, typically ordered from amino- to carboxyl-terminus, is called “full transporter”. On the other hand, “half transporter” that contains one TMD and one NBD in the single chain, forms the functional unit by the dimerization. The amino acid sequences and the three-dimensional structures of NBDs are highly conserved. By contrast, those of TMDs are highly divergent, reflecting the chemical and structural varieties of the transported substrates.

The mechanism of the substrate translocation by ABC transporter has been explained by the alternating access model (Jardetzky, 1966). The model is illustrated in **Fig. 2**. In this model, ABC transporter adopts mainly two conformations: one is the inward-facing conformation in which the substrate binding site, normally positioned at the middle of the interface between two TMDs, can be accessed from the inside of the membrane via the cytoplasmic gate, but not be accessed from the periplasmic side

(**Fig. 2**, left); and the other is the outward-facing conformation in which the periplasmic gate is opened and cytoplasmic gate is closed (**Fig. 2**, right). In the case of the ABC exporter, inward-facing conformation facilitates that the substrate binds to the substrate binding site from the cytoplasm, and then the conformational change to the outward-facing conformation leads to release of the substrate toward the periplasmic space. As a consequence, the substrates are transported from the cytoplasm to the periplasm. The conformational changes between the inward- and outward-facing conformations are induced by the binding and hydrolysis of ATP at the NBDs. ATP binding induces a tight association of two NBDs. On the contrary, ATP hydrolysis induces a dissociation of NBDs. These conformational changes of NBDs transmit to the TMDs; ABC transporters switch between the outward- and inward-facing conformations.

As mentioned previously, MacB is a member of the ABC transporters. The amino acid sequence and the membrane topology analysis of MacB indicated that MacB monomer has one N-terminal NBD and one C-terminal TMD composed of four transmembrane (TM) helices. Additionally, unlike many other ABC transporters that work solely, MacB has a large PLD of about 200 residues between TM helix 1 and 2 (Kobayashi *et al.*, 2003).

In 2020, new classification of ABC transporters were suggested (Thomas *et al.*, 2020). ABC transporters were classified into seven types according to their structural homology in the TMDs (**Fig. 3**). Types I– III contain importers and types IV–VII contain mainly exporters. Type IV also contains channels and some importers, and type V contains some importers. MacB belongs to type VII, which was the newly defined type according to the unique structure of TMD of MacB.

2. Substrates of MacAB-TolC System

In 2001, Kobayashi *et al.* revealed that in the putative PAP gene *ybjY* and the putative ABC transporter gene *ybjZ* in *E. coli*

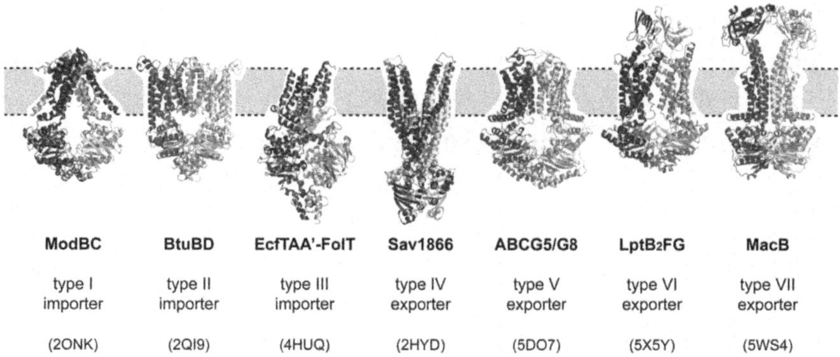

Fig. 3 Seven types of ABC transporter. Each half transporter is colored in dark gray or light gray, respectively. PDB IDs are shown in parentheses. Dotted lines indicate estimated membrane boundaries.

chromosome, the open reading frames (ORFs) of these genes partially overlap and are organized in one operon, influencing the macrolide susceptibility (Kobayashi *et al.*, 2001). Overexpression of *ybjYZ* gene products increases the resistance against macrolide antibiotics, including erythromycin (EM, **Fig. 4a**), clarithromycin (CAM), oleandomycin (OLM), and azithromycin (AZM), in an *E. coli* strain KAM3 which lacks constitutive multidrug transporter AcrAB. The reason why they utilized KAM3 is to avoid the masking of the effect of overexpression of the target genes with powerful efflux of drugs by the RND-type tripartite complex AcrAB-TolC. These results were obtained by the measurements of the minimum inhibitory concentration (MIC) values. The details of MIC measurement are described in Appendix of this chapter. Therefore, *ybjY* and *ybjZ* were renamed *macA* and *macB*, respectively (macrolide-specific ABC-type efflux carrier). In addition, they showed MacA and MacB require TolC as OMC for the resistance against macrolide antibiotics.

Since first identification of MacAB in *E. coli*, several substrates that can be effluxed by the MacAB-TolC system have been

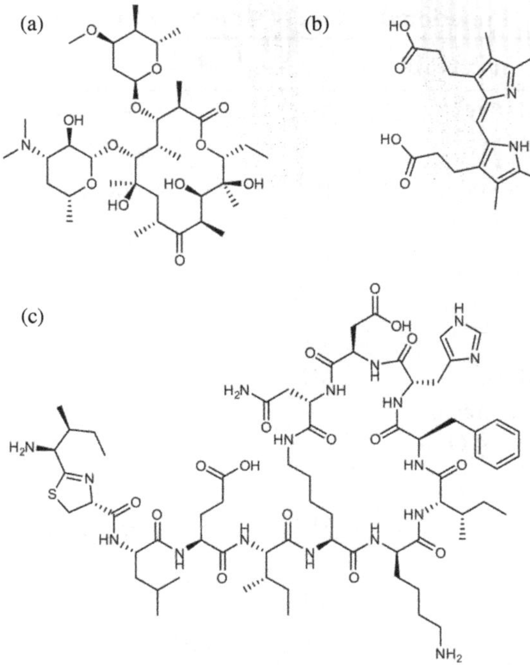

Fig. 4 Substrates of MacAB-TolC complex: (a) erythromycin, (b) protoporphyrin IX, and (c) bacitracin.

reported in various bacteria (**Fig. 4**). These are summarized in **Table 1**. Some examples are presented as follows.

Turlin *et al.* (2014) showed the overproduction of protoporphyrin IX (PPIX, **Fig. 4b**), which is the heme precursor. This reduced the MIC value of EM in the *E. coli* strain overexpressing MacAB, although that did not influence in the strains overexpressing other drug efflux transporters such as AcrAB or EmrAB. These results suggested that PPIX is a substrate or an inhibitor of MacAB. To determine whether PPIX is a substrate or an inhibitor for MacAB, the *macAB*-deletion mutation was introduced into the PPIX overproduction strain. The deletion of *macAB* increased the cellular accumulation of PPIX in comparison with the WT strain. These results indicate that PPIX is a translocation substrate of MacAB system.

Table 1 Functional assays of MacAB-TolC system.

Organism	Substrate	Method	Reference
Escherichia coli	EM, CAM, OLM, AZM	MIC	Kobayashi *et al.* (2001)
	Heat-stable enterotoxin II	Pulse-chase analysis	Yamanaka *et al.* (2008)
	Protoporphyrin IX	MIC, accumulation of substrate	Turlin *et al.* (2014)
	EM, colistin, bacitracin	MIC	Crow *et al.* (2017)
Neisseria gonorrhoeae	EM, AZM	MIC	Rouquette-Loughlin *et al.* (2005)
	AZM	MIC	Golparian *et al.* (2014)
Salmonella enterica	EM	MIC	Nishino *et al.* (2006)
	Virulence factor	Survival of mice	
Pseudomonas aeruginosa	Siderophore pyoverdine	Accumulation of substrate	Imperi *et al.* (2009)
Acinetobacter baumannii	Tigecycline	qRT-PCR of clinical isolate	Lin *et al.* (2015)
	EM, CAM, RXM, AZM, SPM, LM	MIC	Okada *et al.* (2017)
Klebsiella pneumoniae	Eravacycline, tigecycline	qRT-PCR of clinical isolate, MIC	Zheng *et al.* (2018)
Streptococcus pneumoniae	LL-37 (antimicrobial peptide)	MIC	Yang *et al.* (2018)
Agrobacterium tumefaciens	EM, penicillin G, ampicillin, Oxacillin	MIC	Shi *et al.* (2019)
	As(III)	Bacterial growth, accumulation of substrate	

Nishino *et al.* (2006) showed that there are obvious differences in survival ratio of mice inoculated wild type or deletion mutant of *macAB* gene of *Salmonella enterica*. The results suggest that MacAB contributes to the efflux of *Salmonella* virulence factor.

Yamanaka *et al.* (2008) showed heat-stable enterotoxin (ST) II, which is a peptide toxin produced by enterotoxigenic *E. coli*, is exported by MacAB-TolC system. Compared with wild-type *E. coli*, *macAB*-disrupted mutant caused a periplasmic accumulation of ^{35}S isotope-labeled ST II. Furthermore, the introduction of the plasmid containing *macAB* into the disrupted mutant completely restores the extracellular secretion of ST II. These results indicated that MacAB plays an important role in the translocation of ST II from the periplasm to the outside of the cell.

In summary, MacAB-TolC can export various compounds such as macrolide antibiotics and peptide toxins.

3. Structure

3.1. Crystal Structure of MacB

In 2009, the crystal structure of PLD of MacB from Gram-negative pathogen *Actinobacillus actinomycetemcomitans* was determined (Xu *et al.*, 2009). Parts of MacB PLD have structural similarity to the porter domain of RND-type transporter AcrB. However, due to the lack of information such as structure of NBD and TMD, oligomeric state, and connections among the three domains, it was difficult to understand the molecular mechanism of substrate translocation by MacB.

In 2017–2018, crystal structures of full-length MacB from three different source organisms were determined by three groups (Crow *et al.*, 2017; Okada *et al.*, 2017; Yang *et al.*, 2018). *A. baumannii* and *A. actinomycetemcomitans* are Gram-negative pathogens, and *Streptococcus pneumoniae* is a Gram-positive pathogen. In *S. pneumoniae*, MacB is encoded by two divided ORFs: *spr0694*

Table 2 List of MacB structures determined by X-ray crystallography.

PDB ID	Organism	Resolution (Å)	Nucleotide	Note	Reference
5GKO	*Acinetobacter baumannii*	3.39	—	Se-Met-labeled	Okada *et al.* (2017)
5WS4		3.4	ADPβS		
5LIL	*Actinobacillus actinomycetem-comitans*	3.35	ATPγS	Form 1 ($P2_1$)	Crow *et al.* (2017)
5LJ6		3.9	ATPγS	Form 2 ($P6_522$)	
5LJ7		3.25	ATP		
5XU1	*Streptococcus pneumoniae*	3.3	—		Yang *et al.* (2018)

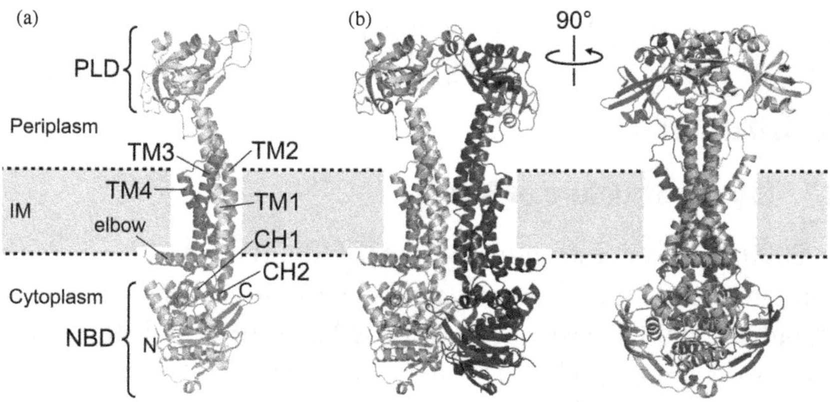

Fig. 5 Crystal structure of AbMacB. (a) Monomer structure. Dotted lines indicate estimated membrane boundaries. (b) Dimer structures in two orientations. Each protomer is colored in dark gray or light gray, respectively.

which encodes NBD and *spr0695* which encodes TMD and PLD. These are summarized in **Table 2**. These structures are different in detail, but they have almost the same structural features. **Figure 5a** shows the monomer structure of MacB from *A. baumannii* (AbMacB). AbMacB monomer is "half transporter" which has one

NBD and one TMD. Like many other ABC transporters, AbMacB monomers related by pseudo twofold symmetry form a dimer as a functional unit (**Fig. 5b**). The structure of NBD was highly conserved with other ABC transporters. Following N-terminal NBD, at the cytoplasmic side of TM 1, an elbow helix (or amphipathic helix) was observed in parallel to the membrane plane. This helix was observed in the solved structures of MacB from the other organisms.

TMD of MacB has four TM helices in monomer. As a result of the dimerization, eight helices span across the IM (**Fig. 5**). This is the smallest number of TM helices among the ABC transporters (**Fig. 3**). In general, most ABC importers have 10–20 TM helices, and exporters have 12 TM helices as a functional unit. In many other ABC exporters, especially in type IV transporters (previously called type I exporter), TMD is constructed with domain swapping. To put it more concretely, TM 1 and 2 from one protomer and TM 3–6 from the symmetric counter protomer (TM 3′-6′) form a six-helix bundle (**Fig. 6b**). On the other hand, TMD of

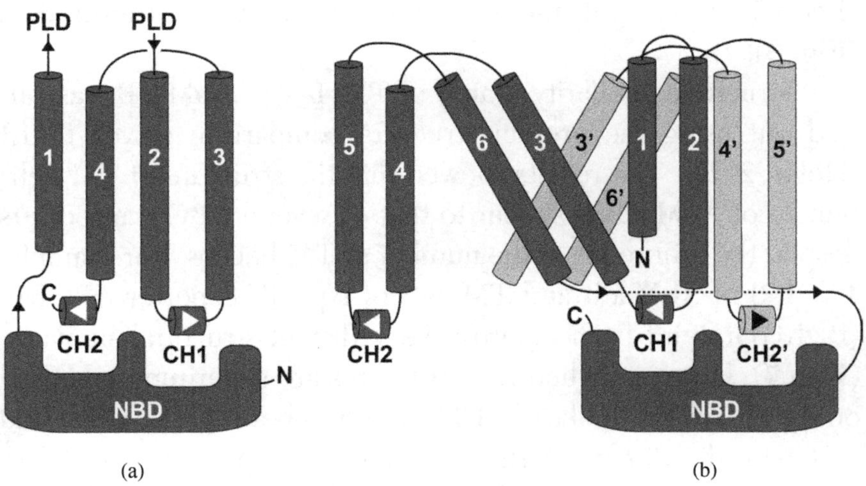

Fig. 6 Topological comparison of CHs and TM helices between MacB and type IV ABC exporter. Topological diagrams of (a) MacB and (b) type IV ABC exporter. One protomer (or half transporter) is colored in dark gray, and the counter protomer is colored in light gray. Long cylinders are TM helices, and short cylinders are CHs.

MacB is composed with four TM helices from one protomer, so domain swapping does not occur (**Fig. 6a**).

TMD of ABC transporters has two short helices that are called coupling helices (CHs) in parallel to the membrane plane on the cytoplasmic side. CH binds in a groove of NBD and transmits the conformational change of NDBs caused by ATP hydrolysis to TMDs. Like many other ABC exporters, MacB also has two CHs (CH 1 and CH 2) in a TMD. CH 1 is located between TM 2 and TM 3, and CH 2 is located at the C-terminal of TMD, despite MacB has only one cytoplasmic loop in a TMD due to the smallest number of TM helices. Both CH 1 and CH 2 interact with NBD of the same protomer (**Fig. 6a**). In the case of type IV exporter, CH 1 and CH 2′ from the counter protomer interact with one NBD from the protomer which has CH 1 (**Fig. 6b**). This is a difference of the structural feature between MacB and other ABC exporters.

TM 1 and 2 connecting to the PLD are elongated about 25 Å from the periplasmic side of IM to the periplasm, while TM 3 and 4 are fully buried in IM (**Fig. 5**). The PLDs and these elongated parts of TM 1 and 2 form a large periplasmic architecture with almost 50 Å in height, and it is not seen in other ABC transporters (**Fig. 3**).

Structural similarity search of TM 1–4 of AbMacB was carried out using the protein structure comparison server DALI (Holm, 2020). The results showed that the structure of TM helix bundle of AbMacB is similar to that of several ABC transporters despite the difference in the number of TM helices. For example, TM 1–3 of AbMacB and TM 1–3 of type IV exporter ABCB1a (P-glycoprotein) from mouse have sufficient structural similarity (**Fig. 7**). However, when two structures are superimposed based on the structural similarity of TM bundles between AbMacB and ABCB1a, the dimer interface of AbMacB appears in the different orientation from that of ABCB1a. This means that in the case of AbMacB, the corresponding part of the substrate translocation pathway of ABCB1a located between the dimer interface is positioned at the outside of the dimer and not in the dimer interface.

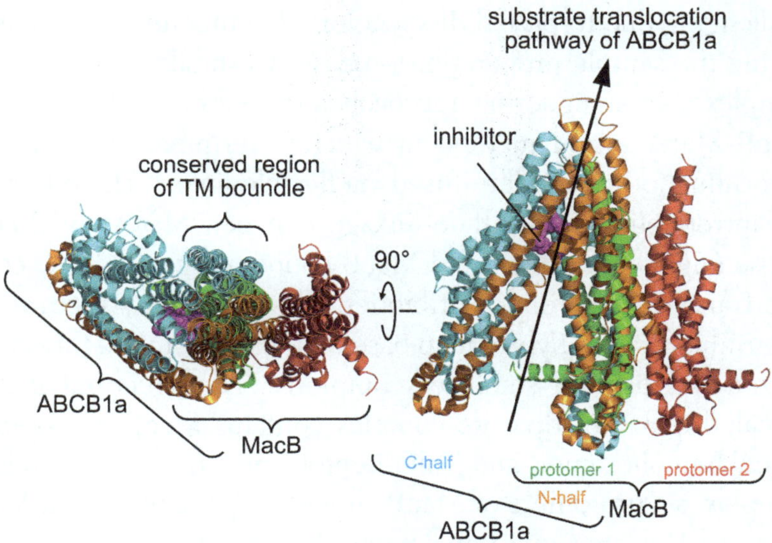

Fig. 7 Superposition of TMDs of AbMacB and ABCB1a. TMDs of AbMacB and ABCB1a from mouse (PDB ID: 4M2S) are superimposed, and shown in two orientations. Protomers of MacB are colored in green and red. Half-transporters of ABCB1a are colored in orange and cyan. The bound inhibitor of ABCB1a is colored in magenta. The substrate translocation pathway of ABCB1a is shown by a black arrow.

On the other hand, the structural comparison between AbMacB and type V exporter ABCG2 in the same way as ABCB1a shows that the dimer interfaces of AbMacB and ABCG2 are located at the same orientation. As has been noted, the TM helix bundle of MacB is structurally conserved between ABC exporters; however, overall structure of the functional unit of MacB is different from other ABC exporters.

As mentioned above, MacB has several characteristic structural features in comparison with many other ABC transporters.

3.2. Cryo-EM Structure of MacAB-TolC Tripartite Complex

In 2017, the three-dimensional structure of MacAB-TolC tripartite complex from *E. coli* was determined by cryo-EM (**Fig. 1**, right) (Fitzpatrick *et al.*, 2017). Structural analysis of protein complex is challenging due to partial dissociation of components of complex during the sample preparation process. To stabilize the tripartite complex, two engineering approaches were applied. One was the MacB-MacA fusion method in which C-terminal of MacB and N-terminal of MacA were fused via flexible linker. The other was the introduction of disulfide-linkage between MacA and MacB. Those engineered MacA and MacB cooperating with TolC could also transport macrolide antibiotics. The cryo-EM structure was determined with a hybrid map based on maps from the fusion-stabilized and disulfide-stabilized complexes. The structural analysis revealed that the tripartite complex contains MacB homodimer, MacA homohexamer, and TolC homotrimer. In fusion-stabilized complex, six protomers of MacB should be presented with MacA hexamer. However, only one dimer of MacB, that is two protomers, was observed in a density map from fusion-stabilized complex. The remaining four MacB protomers might be flexible toward the core of the tripartite complex, and it is not observed in the map because density of those protomers was diffused during the image processing. The map from the disulfide-stabilized complex also showed that MacB dimer and MacA hexamer form the complex.

The N-terminal TM helix of MacA is not observed in either the maps from the fusion- or disulfide-stabilized complexes. In addition, all crystal structures of MacA from *E. coli*, *A. actinomycetemcomitans*, and *S. pneumoniae* were determined with the construct omitting the N-terminal TM helix (Xu *et al.*, 2012; Yang *et al.*, 2018; Yum *et al.*, 2009). Thus, there is no structural information about the TM helix. However, functional assays showed the importance of the N-terminal TM helix of MacA. MacA binding to MacB stimulates ATPase activity of MacB, but MacA lacking the N-terminal TM helix does not stimulate those activity. Furthermore, the TM helix of MacA is essential for the macrolide efflux by MacAB-TolC complex (Tikhonova *et al.*, 2007). Further research is needed to elucidate the function and molecular mechanism of the TM helix of MacA.

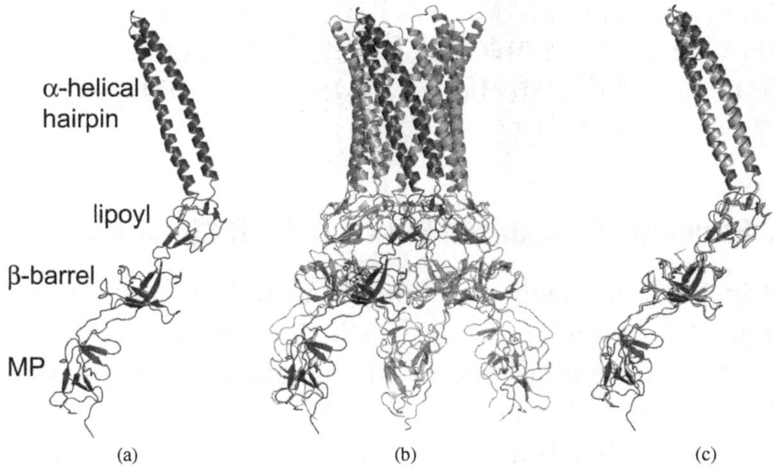

Fig. 8 Structure of MacA: (a) Monomer and (b) hexameric structure of MacA from *E. coli* determined by cryo-EM (PDB ID: 5NIK). One protomer is colored in dark gray, and the other protomers are colored in light gray in hexamer. (c) Superposition of MacA structures determined by cryo-EM (dark gray) and X-ray crystallography (PDB ID: 4DK0, light gray, from *Actinobacillus actinomycetemcomitans*).

MacA structure consists of four subdomains: α-helical hairpin, lipoyl, β-barrel, and membrane proximal (MP) domains (**Fig. 8a**). MacA forms hexamer similarly to AcrA in the AcrAB-TolC tripartite complex (**Figs. 1 and 8b**). All MacA structures determined by cryo-EM and X-ray crystallography are highly conserved except for the following point (**Fig. 8c**). In cryo-EM structure, six glutamine residues (Q209) on the loops of lipoyl domains from each protomer form inter-protomer hydrogen bonds. This glutamine gating ring was not observed in crystal structures of MacA. This glutamine residue is highly conserved among MacA homologs. However, alanine substitution at the glutamine residue did not affect macrolide resistance. In the cryo-EM map, this ring is too narrow to pass the substrates. Molecular dynamics simulations suggested that erythromycin partially disrupts the hydrogen bond network of the gating ring, and then the substrate can pass through the gating ring. This glutamine gating ring is the unique structural feature in MacA of the MacAB-TolC tripartite complex, not seen in AcrA of the AcrAB-TolC complex. It might operate as a one-way valve to control the direction of substrates flow (Fitzpatrick *et al.*, 2017).

3.3. Structural Comparison Between MacB Structures

In **Fig. 9**, four MacB structures from different organisms are described for comparison, in which three structures are determined by X-ray crystallography and the other is a part of MacAB-TolC complex determined by cryo-EM.

AbMacB, MacB from *A. actinomycetemcomitans* (AaMacB) and MacB from *S. pneumoniae* (SpMacB) were crystallized in the presence of ATP or ADP analogs. In the crystal structures of AaMacB and AbMacB, electron density maps of those nucleotides were observed in the nucleotide binding pockets that are positioned at the dimer interface of NBDs, and the nucleotide-bound

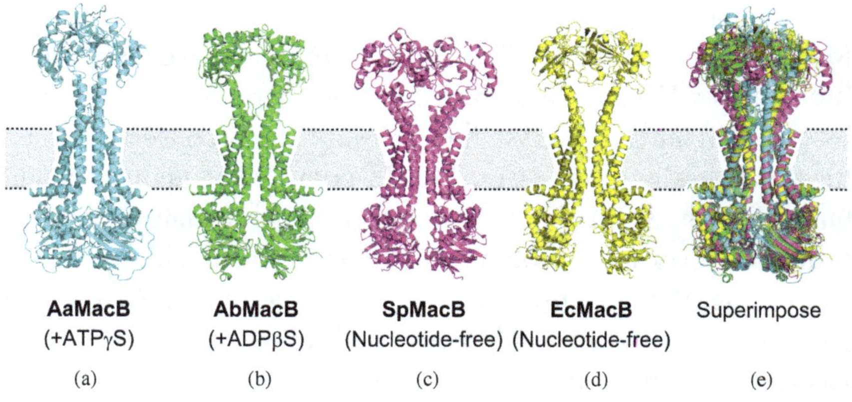

Fig. 9 Structural comparison between the MacB structures. MacB structures determined by X-ray structures, (a) ATPgS bound AaMacB (PDB ID: 5LIL, cyan), (b) ADPβS bound AbMacB (PDB ID: 5WS4, green), (c) nucleotide-free state of SpMacB (PDB ID: 5XU1, magenta), (d) EcMacB part of tripartite complex structure determined by cryo-EM (PDB ID: 5NIL, chain J and L, yellow), and (e) superposition of these MacB structures.

NBDs are tightly packed and form closed conformations (Crow *et al.*, 2017; Okada *et al.*, 2017), whereas, in the crystal structure of SpMacB, the electron density map of the nucleotide was not observed in the nucleotide binding pocket (Yang *et al.*, 2018). The crystal structure of SpMacB should be the nucleotide-free state, but two NBDs of SpMacB are slightly separated and the overall fold of NBDs is almost the same with that of nucleotide-bound AaMacB or AbMacB structures. NBDs of MacB from *E. coli* (EcMacB) determined by cryo-EM are separated (Fitzpatrick *et al.*, 2017). Further structural information is needed to establish the molecular model about the conformational change caused by the binding or hydrolysis of nucleotide to the NBDs of MacB.

In MacB structure, TM 1 and 2 connecting to the PLD are elongated toward the periplasm. These periplasmic parts of TM 1 and 2, and the orientation of connecting PLDs are most different between MacB structures from four organisms (**Fig. 9**). TM 1 and 2 of AaMacB are approximately straight and tightly packed between two protomers from the parts buried in IM to the periplasmic region. On the contrary, those of SpMacB are bent at the outer surface of the plasma membrane, and they form a V-shaped cavity located outside the membrane. TM 1 and 2 of AbMacB and EcMacB are also bent with a moderate bent angle between SpMacB and AaMacB. The structural variation of the periplasmic region of TM 1 and TM 2 causes the differences in the orientations of connecting PLDs between AaMacB, AbMacB, EcMacB, and SpMacB. These results might indicate that TM 1 and 2 of MacB could bend at the outer surface of the IM, and the conformational change of PLDs and periplasmic parts of TM 1 and 2 could occur during the substrate translocation cycle.

On the other hand, folds of TMDs buried in the membrane are highly conserved between MacB structures (**Fig. 9e**). TM 1 and 2 from each protomer form tightly packed helix bundle, and there is no significant space that substrates could pass through, regardless of the presence or absence of nucleotides.

4. Molecular Mechanism of Substrate Translocation

Canonical ABC transporters mediate substrate translocation across the IM via the translocation pathway at the interface between two TMDs. However, structural analyses of MacB revealed that MacB does not have substrate translocation pathway at the part of TMD buried in the IM. Furthermore, peptide toxin ST II is exported from the periplasm by MacAB-TolC complex (Yamanaka *et al.*, 2008). Lipoprotein transporter LolCDE from *E. coli*, that is one of the close homologs of MacB, collects substrates from the outer leaflet of the IM (Narita & Tokuda, 2017). These structural and functional analyses suggest that MacB does not transport substrates across the IM, but they capture substrates at the outer leaflet of the IM or the periplasmic space. This is the same way with RND-type tripartite efflux transporter. RND-type tripartite complex such as AcrAB-TolC complex translocates substrates from the outer leaflet of the IM or the periplasmic space to the extracellular space. The substrate binding site might be in the periplasmic part of MacB. TM 1 and 2 transmit the conformational change of NBDs to the PLD like a string puppet. So type VII ABC transporters including MacB are also called "mechanotransmitter" (Crow *et al.*, 2017; Thomas *et al.*, 2020). Several models that explain the substrate translocation by MacB were proposed, such as "fireplace bellows mechanism" or "periplasmic alternating-access mechanism" (Greene *et al.*, 2018; Murakami *et al.*, 2020).

Recent structural and functional analyses of MacB and related proteins provide a new concept called "mechanotransmitter" to the ABC transporter superfamily. However, there is little information about how MacB recognizes substrates due to the lack of structural information about substrate-bound state of MacB. Further research is necessary to completely understand the molecular mechanism of the substrate translocation by the ABC-type tripartite efflux transporter.

Appendix Measurement of MIC

Determination of MIC values is one of the major methods for the functional analyses of transporters. MIC is the minimum concentration of the substrate when the host organism expressing the target gene could not grow. For example, if *E. coli* strain expressing some drug exporter can grow in the media with 5 μg/mL antibiotics, but not in 10 μg/mL antibiotics, then MIC is 10 μg/mL antibiotics. MIC value is determined only in the steps of concentrations that were tested. It is not clear whether this strain can grow in the media with 7 μg/mL antibiotics. In many case, twofold dilution series are used for the substrate concentrations. It must be noted that MIC is not an absolute value, and it is essential to compare with MICs from the same experimental system, because MICs could be shifted by the difference of experimental conditions such as host strain, expression level of the target protein, incubation media, or temperature. Normally, MICs are compared between wild-type strain and knockout mutant of the target transporter, or strain harboring the empty vector and strain harboring the overexpression vector of the target transporter. If MICs are different between these strains, it indicates that the transporter can transport the substrate. Furthermore, it is necessary to keep in mind that MIC study is only applicable in the case where the substrate is toxic to survive for the host, so if the substrate is not toxic, other methods are required.

As mentioned above, many MIC studies against MacAB-TolC system have been reported. For example, we would like to introduce the determination of MICs of macrolide antibiotic roxithromycin (RXM) about MacAB-TolC from Gram-negative pathogen *A. baumannii* (**Fig. 10**, **Table 3**) (Okada *et al.*, 2017). The *macA-macB-tolC* operon from *A. baumannii* was introduced into the expression vector. Deletion mutants lacking *macA*, *macB*, or *tolC* gene from the operon, and *macA-macB-tolC* with nonfunctional mutation in *macB* (*macA-macB* (E172Q)-*tolC*) were also cloned. The empty vector and these expression vectors were transformed

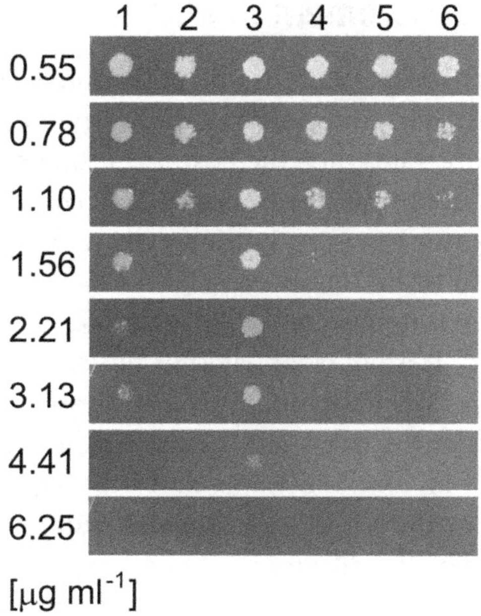

Fig. 10 Example of MIC measurement: Growth of *E. coli* expressing MacA-MacB-TolC from *A. baumannii*, or combinations of components and mutant in the presence of various concentrations of RXM. Lane 1, empty vector; lane 2, MacA-MacB (E172Q)-TolC; lane 3, MacA-MacB-TolC; lane 4, MacA-MacB; lane 5, MacA-TolC; lane 6, MacB-TolC.

Table 3 MIC values of MacAB-TolC from *Acinetobacter baumannii* against RXM.

	Components Expressed	MIC (μg/mL)
1	None (empty vector)	4.41
2	MacA-MacB(E172Q)-TolC	1.56
3	MacA-MacB-TolC	6.25
4	MacA-MacB	1.56
5	MacA-TolC	1.56
6	MacB-TolC	1.56

into *E. coli*, and growth of each strain on the agar media containing various concentration of RXM was tested. The difference of MICs between empty vector (**Fig. 10**, lane 1) and MacAB-TolC (**Fig. 10**, lane 3) was only marginal. The reason could be the influence of the overexpression of heterogeneous integral membrane proteins MacB and/or TolC from *A. baumannii* on the growth of *E. coli*. To exclude this effect, when compared with nonfunctional and functional MacAB-TolC (**Fig. 10**, lanes 2 and 3), both those strains overexpressed heterogeneous membrane proteins and there is an obvious difference of the susceptibility of RXM. The results indicated that MacAB-TolC from *A. baumannii* efflux RXM. Comparison between the full MacAB-TolC and deletion mutants (**Fig. 10**, lanes 3–6) reveals that all components are essential for the efflux of RXM.

In conclusion, as has been noted, when one validates MIC studies, the details of experimental conditions should be confirmed, and comparison of MIC values should be done relatively between the comparable conditions only.

References

Crow, A., *et al.* (2017). Structure and mechanotransmission mechanism of the MacB ABC transporter superfamily. *Proceedings of the National Academy of Sciences of the United States of America, 114*, 12572–12577.

Davidson, A. L., *et al.* (2008). Structure, function, and evolution of bacterial ATP-binding cassette systems, *Microbiology and Molecular Biology Reviews*, *72*, 317–364.

Du, D., *et al.* (2014). Structure of the AcrAB-TolC multidrug efflux pump. *Nature*, *509*, 512–515.

Fitzpatrick, A. W. P., *et al.* (2017). Structure of the MacAB-TolC ABC-type tripartite multidrug efflux pump. *Nature Microbiology*, *2*, 17070.

Golparian, D., *et al.* (2014). Importance of multidrug efflux pumps in the antimicrobial resistance property of clinical multidrug-resistant isolates of *Neisseria gonorrhoeae*. *Antimicrobial Agents and Chemotherapy*, *58*, 3556–3559.

Greene, N. P., *et al.* (2018). Antibiotic resistance mediated by the MacB ABC transporter family: A structural and functional perspective. *Frontiers in Microbiology*, *9*, 950.

Holm, L. (2020). DALI and the persistence of protein shape. *Protein Science*, *29*, 128–140.

Imperi, F., *et al.* (2009). Molecular basis of pyoverdine siderophore recycling in *Pseudomonas aeruginosa*. *Proceedings of the National Academy of Sciences of the United States of America*, *105*, 20440–20445.

Jardetzky, O. (1966). Simple allosteric model for membrane pumps. *Nature*, *211*, 969–970.

Kobayashi, N., *et al.* (2001). Novel macrolide-specific ABC-type efflux transporter in *Escherichia coli*. *Journal of Bacteriology*, *183*, 5639–5644.

Kobayashi, N., *et al.* (2003). Membrane topology of ABC-type macrolide antibiotic exporter MacB in *Escherichia coli*. *FEBS Letters*, *546*, 241–246.

Koronakis, V., *et al.* (2000). Crystal structure of the bacterial membrane protein TolC central to multidrug efflux and protein export. *Nature*, *405*, 914–919.

Lin, M. F., *et al.* (2015). The role of the two-component system BaeSR in disposing chemicals through regulating transporter systems in *Acinetobacter baumannii*. *PLoS One*, *10*, e0132843.

Mikolosko, J., *et al.* (2006). Conformational flexibility in the multidrug efflux system protein AcrA. *Structure*, *14*, 577–587.

Munita, J. M. & Arias, C. A. (2016). Mechanisms of antibiotic resistance. *Microbiology Spectrum*, 4:2.

Murakami, S., *et al.* (2002). Crystal structure of bacterial multidrug efflux transporter AcrB. *Nature*, *419*, 587–593.

Murakami, S., *et al.* (2006). Crystal structures of a multidrug transporter reveal a functionally rotating mechanism. *Nature*, *443*, 173–179.

Murakami, S., *et al.* (2020). Tripartite transporters as mechanotransmitters in periplasmic alternating⊠access mechanisms. *FEBS Letters*, *594*, 3908–3919.

Narita, S., & Tokuda, H. (2017). Bacterial lipoproteins; biogenesis, sorting and quality control. *Biochimica et Biophysica Acta*, *1862*, 1414–1423.

Nishino, K., *et al.* (2006). Virulence and drug resistance roles of multidrug efflux systems of *Salmonella enterica* serovar Typhimurium. *Molecular Microbiology*, *59*, 126–141.

Okada, U., *et al.* (2017). Crystal structure of tripartite-type ABC transporter MacB from *Acinetobacter baumannii*. *Nature Communications*, *8*, 1336.

Rouquette-Loughlin, C. E., *et al.* (2005). Characterization of the MacA-MacB efflux system in *Neisseria gonorrhoeae*. *Journal of Antimicrobial Chemotherapy*, *56*, 856–860.

Shi, K., *et al.* (2019). Efflux proteins MacAB confer resistance to arsenite and penicillin/macrolide-type antibiotics in *Agrobacterium tumefaciens* 5A. *World Journal of Microbiology and Biotechnology*, *35*, 115.

Thomas, C., *et al.* (2020). Structural and functional diversity calls for a new classification of ABC transporters. *FEBS Letters*, *594*, 3767–3775.

Tikhonova, E. B., *et al.* (2007). Reconstitution of the *Escherichia coli* macrolide transporter: The periplasmic membrane fusion protein MacA stimulates the ATPase activity of MacB. *Molecular Microbiology*, *63*, 895–910.

Turlin, E., *et al.* (2014). Protoporphyrin (PPIX) efflux by the MacAB-TolC pump in *Escherichia coli*. *MicrobiologyOpen*, *3*, 849–859.

Wang, Z., *et al.* (2017). An allosteric transport mechanism for the AcrAB-TolC multidrug efflux pump, *eLife*, *6*, e24905.

Xu, Y., *et al.* (2009). Crystal structure of the periplasmic region of MacB, a noncanonic ABC transporter. *Biochemistry*, *48*, 5218–5225.

Xu, Y., *et al.* (2012). Assembly and channel opening of outer membrane protein in tripartite drug efflux pumps of Gram-negative bacteria. *Journal of Biological Chemistry*, *287*, 11740–11750.

Yamanaka, H., *et al.* (2008). MacAB is involved in the secretion of *Escherichia coli* heat-stable enterotoxin II. *Journal of Bacteriology*, *190*, 7693–7698.

Yang, H. B., *et al.* (2018). Structure of a MacAB-like efflux pump from *Streptococcus pneumoniae*. *Nature Communications*, 9, 196.

Yum, S., *et al.* (2009). Crystal structure of the periplasmic component of a tripartite macrolide-specific efflux pump. *Journal of Molecular Biology*, *387*, 1286–1297.

Zheng, J. X., *et al.* (2018). Overexpression of OqxAB and MacAB efflux pumps contributes to eravacycline resistance and heteroresistance in clinical isolates of *Klebsiella pneumoniae*. *Emerging Microbes & Infections*, 7, 139.

https://doi.org/10.1142/9789811254796_0002

2 Pro-inflammatory Secretory Phospholipase A_2 Enzyme: Evaluation of Hydrophobic and Antioxidant Properties of Inhibitors

M.D. Milan Gowda,
K. Jayachandra, Noor Mohamed Jameel*
and Bannikuppe S. Vishwanath*

Department of Studies in Biochemistry, University of Mysore, Manasagangotri, Mysore, Karnataka, India

Abstract

Secretory phospholipase A_2 (sPLA$_2$, EC 3.1.1.4) enzymes cleave membrane phospholipids preferentially at the *sn-2* position, thereby liberating free fatty acids and lysophospholipids. Excessive release of free fatty acids by sPLA$_2$ elevates the activity of downstream enzymes cyclooxygenase and lipoxygenase in the synthesis of pro-inflammatory eicosanoids, resulting in enhanced formation of free radicals which aggravates inflammation further. Several sPLA$_2$ inhibitors with antioxidant potential are known to exhibit potent anti-inflammatory activity. Studies have shown that hydrophobicity of a molecule is vital for sPLA$_2$ inhibitor. In-depth knowledge of such molecules and sPLA$_2$ enzyme is essential to develop novel potent anti-inflammatory drugs. This

*Corresponding authors: e-mail: jameel.nm@gmail.com; vishmy@biochemistry.uni-mysore.ac.in

chapter focuses on understanding the structure of $sPLA_2$, catalytic mechanism, assay methods and its role in inflammatory diseases. The significance of antioxidant hydrophobic small molecules as $sPLA_2$ inhibitors may perhaps develop into potent anti-inflammatory drug is also discussed.

1. Introduction

Enzymes are considered to be one of the important drug targets in developing therapeutic molecules against various pathophysiological events. Small-molecule-based enzyme inhibitors have revolutionized the field of medicine, and it is estimated to have about one-third of all marketed drugs (Nikolaou *et al.*, 2019). Among them the importance of targeting bioactive lipids has been recognized and a great attention has been given to enzymes associated with lipid metabolism (Chiurchiù & Maccarrone, 2016). One of the important enzymes to be considered is phospholipase A_2 (PLA_2s) enzyme. These enzymes known to be involved in the development and progression of various inflammatory diseases attracted a great number of academicians and pharmaceutical companies to develop many small molecules as inhibitors (Jameel *et al.*, 2005; Joshi, Umashankara, *et al.*, 2016; Nanda *et al.*, 2007; Pérez-Jeldres *et al.*, 2019). PLA_2 enzymes belong to esterases family that catalyzes the hydrolysis of membrane glycerophospholipids at the *sn-2* position to release free fatty acids including arachidonic acid. In this way, PLA_2s initiates the downstream cascade by supplying free fatty acids to enzymes such as cyclooxygenases (COXs), lipoxygenases (LOXs), and cytochrome P450, which in turn produce various pro-inflammatory mediators; prostaglandins, prostacyclins, leukotrienes, and thromboxanes. Depending on physical characteristics, biological location, calcium dependency, and catalytic mechanism, these enzymes can be categorized into different classes. PLA_2 superfamily consists of six types of diverse enzymes: several groups of secreted PLA_2 ($sPLA_2$), cytosolic calcium-dependent PLA_2

($cPLA_2$), calcium-independent PLA_2 ($iPLA_2$), two groups of platelet-activating factor-acetylhydrolases (PAF-AHs) PLA_2, lysosomal PLA_2, and adipose PLA_2. The nomenclature and history of the PLA_2 superfamily are well described in a review article by Dennis (1994). Among these classes of PLA_2 enzymes, the role of secretory PLA_2 ($sPLA_2$) in the regulation of inflammatory reactions is well established.

In this chapter, we discuss the inhibitors targeting pro-inflammatory $sPLA_2$ enzymes. We present the most important small-molecule $sPLA_2$ inhibitors developed and studied recently in our laboratory along with few other molecules focusing on their recent studies and their therapeutic potential. Computational studies aiming at understanding in-depth enzyme-inhibitor interactions as well as recent advances in assaying the activity of $sPLA_2$s are discussed. Inhibitors that reached clinical trials are also summarized, although only few of them entered the clinical market yet. Apart from their importance as new potential therapeutics to treat inflammatory diseases, small-molecule $sPLA_2$ inhibitors are excellent tools to unveil the role that each $sPLA_2$ type plays in cells and *in vivo*.

2. Structure of $sPLA_2$ Enzyme

Secreted PLA_2s ($sPLA_2$s) are a group of PLA_2 enzymes that are secreted extra-cellularly. These enzymes have 13–19 kDa low-molecular-weight compared to other PLA_2s, and require Ca^{2+} in millimolar concentration for their catalytic activity (Piomelli & Greengard, 1991). Structures of several $sPLA_2$ enzymes have been elucidated; they share a common protein secondary structure and three-dimensional fold. These enzymes contain three long α-helices and two stranded β-sheets referred to as β-wings. The plant $sPLA_2$ has been shown to lack β-wings and prokaryotic $sPLA_2$ have all α-helical protein folding. $sPLA_2$ enzymes are shown to possess six conserved disulfide bonds with one or two variable disulfide bonds. Across all the $sPLA_2$ enzymes subtypes, an active site sequence (Asp-Xxx-Cys-Cys-Xxx-Xxx-His-Asp) and a calcium binding loop (Xxx-Cys-Gly-Xxx-Gly-Gly) are highly conserved. The histidine in the active site (His48) forms a catalytic dyad with an aspartate present remotely in the sequence (Asp99) and is also conserved across the subtypes of $sPLA_2$. This active site structure is deeply buried inside the enzyme at the cavity and present in close proximity to calcium ion which is bound to the calcium binding loop. One more common structural feature of $sPLA_2$s is the presence of ~15 Å deep active site slot where a single phospholipid molecule binds to position the enzyme-susceptible ester next to the catalytic residues. The part of $sPLA_2$ enzymes involved in direct binding to the phospholipid substrate forms a structure called the interfacial binding surface (i-face). The i-face is in direct contact with the membrane when the enzyme transfers from the aqueous phase to the membrane surface. The i-face exerts strong hydrophobic interactions due to the presence of mostly hydrophobic amino acids, but may also contain some cationic amino acid residues that can form hydrogen bonds with anionic substances. Within the i-face there are amino acids that form the entrance to the active site, and that also play an important role in interacting with the substrate or inhibitors. These amino acids are mostly hydrophobic as well, but also form a relatively planar surface to the external surroundings. The entrance is a region where the single phospholipid molecule (substrate) or inhibitors can enter and penetrate through the active site to reach a catalytic dyad which is located at the end of the cavity (Kim *et al.*, 2020; Tessmer *et al.*, 2017) (**Fig. 1**).

3. Catalytic Mechanism

The catalytic mechanism originally projected for hydrolysis of phospholipids by $sPLA_2$s is based on high-resolution X-ray structures of different $sPLA_2$s containing a bound phosphonate-phospholipid analog, a transition state analog inhibitor, and presence

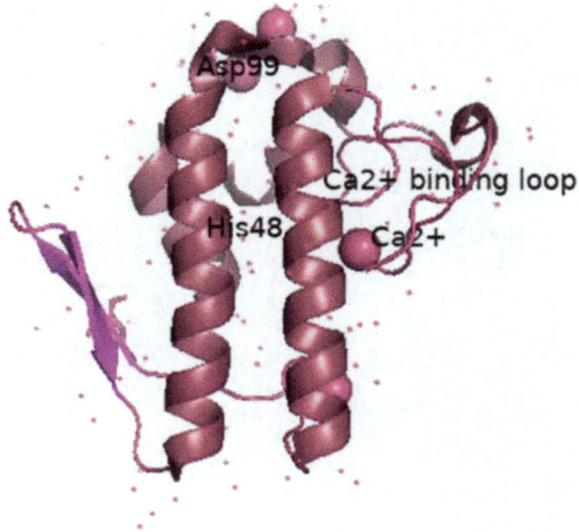

Fig. 1 Structure of i-phase of $sPLA_2$enzyme.

of conservation structural features of the active sites. The highly conserved catalytic dyad consists of charged molecules, histidine and an aspartate, utilized for substrate hydrolysis. Since one amino acid being basic and the other being acidic, there is an electrostatic interaction between the nitrogen atom of the histidine ring (N-2) and carboxyl oxygen atom (O-1) of the aspartate. There are two models proposed to explain the catalytic mechanism of $sPLA_2$ enzyme. The earliest proposed model is the triad model (**Fig. 2a**). According to this model, water molecule that binds to N-1 atom of the active site histidine acts as a nucleophile. The catalytic mechanism may originate from a dyad of histidine and aspartic acid; the water molecule becomes polarized by the N-1 atom of His and attacks the carbonyl group of the phospholipid substrate. This reaction is partially aided by the presence of aspartate at the catalytic dyad, making the N-1 atom more electrophilic by direct electrostatic interaction with the histidine N-2 atoms. Among two commonly observed calciums in the structures, calcium closest to the active site plays a vital role in this mechanism. This calcium ion interacts with the conserved Asp49 next to the active site histidine

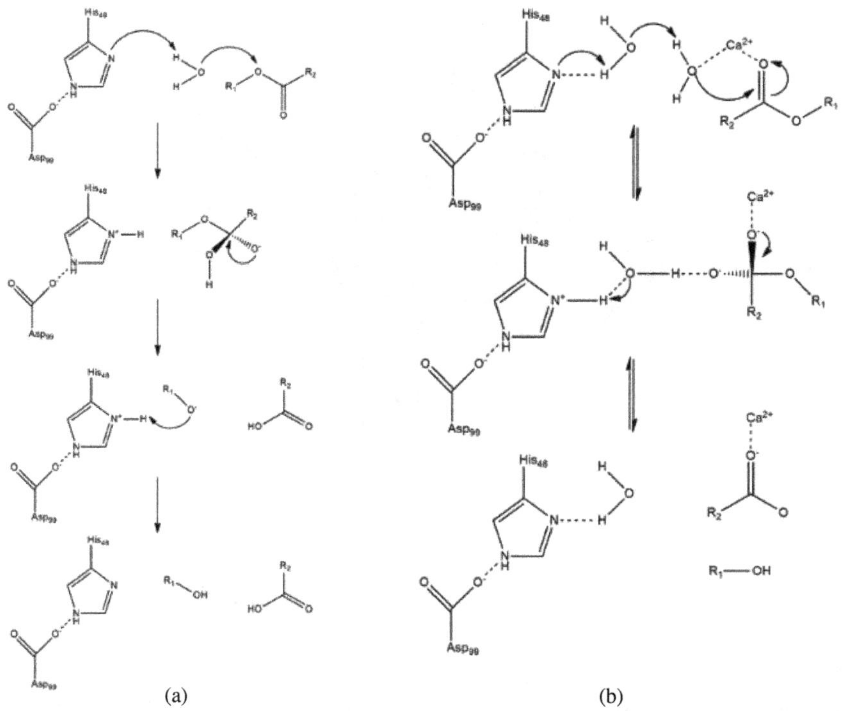

Fig. 2 Catalytic mechanism of sPLA$_2$: (a) triad model and (b) calcium-coordinated oxyanion model.

and coordinated by three carbonyl backbone oxygen atoms from His28, Gly30, and Gly32 on the calcium binding loop and both the carboxyl oxygens from the side chain of Asp49. The calcium ion stabilizes the intermediate by coordinating the carbonyl group of the phospholipid substrate and the negative charge from the phosphate oxygen.

An alternative mechanism known as oxyanion mechanism, addition to the water molecule discussed in previous mechanism, another water molecule is also involved in the catalysis (Verheij *et al.*, 1981). According to this model, a second water molecule is coordinated to the calcium ion and indirectly interacts with the histidine N-1 atom by forming a hydrogen bond with another water molecule which then makes a connection to the N-1 atom. As a result, when the N-1 atom becomes protonated, the water molecule becomes polarized and may act as a nucleophile. The nucleophile polarized water attacks the substrate carbonyl group to form an oxyanion, which coordinates the calcium ion. The advantage of this mechanism compared to first mechanism is that the second water molecule lowers the activation energy required for tetrahedral formation that protonates the N-1 atom. In both mechanisms, the involvement of calcium ion is clear, and it acts as an important cofactor in the hydrolysis process, which is evidenced by experimental conditions where millimolar concentrations of calcium is desirable for the $sPLA_2$ catalytic activity (Scott & Sigler, 1994).

The oxyanion mechanism is more consistent since in order for the hydrolysis to occur, the enzyme must initially bind with the phospholipid substrate which is micelle/bilayer form, rather than as discrete molecules. Hence, binding to the substrate involves adsorption of the enzyme to the substrate surface. To explain the behavior of $sPLA_2$ once it is adsorbed to the substrate surface, two models of the kinetics have been suggested. In the "hopping mode" model, the $sPLA_2$ enzyme would hydrolyze only a single substrate molecule after adsorbing to the surface of substrate, and then detach from the surface before it finds the next substrate molecule. In the "scooting mode" model, the enzyme hydrolyzes multiple substrate molecules without desorbing from the substrate surface (**Fig. 2b**). In both mechanisms, it is essential for the free enzyme to form a surface-bound form before it proceeds with classical Michaelis–Menten kinetics.

4. $sPLA_2$ Enzyme Assay

Various efforts have been made to design and develop a sensitive assay for the determination of catalytic activity of $sPLA_2$ enzyme. The preference of a detection method depends partly on the purpose of a particular experiment with the most important factor to be consideration in the choice of assay is the sensitivity required. The sensitivity of an assay is influenced by a number of factors, the most important of which is the detection limit such as the absorbance coefficient of a chromophore or the physical limitations of the instrumentation and also purity of $sPLA_2$ enzyme. Some assays are based on artificial substrates such as liposomes or micelles, and other assays use labeled membranes; synthetic substrate has also been considered recently. The photometric micelle assay developed by G. E. Hoffmann, which is commercially available, is also a choice of assay (Hoffmann *et al.*, 1986). The labeled *Escherichia coli* membrane assay method combines the advantage of the sensitivity of a radiometric assay based on a natural substrate, with the determination of the true and total activity of $sPLA_2$. The most common $sPLA_2$ assay methods adopted in our laboratory along with other assays is described in **Table 1**.

5. $sPLA_2$s as Mediators of Inflammation

Inflammation is a comprehensive array of physiological response that can arise in any tissue in response to traumatic, infectious (virus and bacterial), post-ischemic, toxic, or autoimmune injury (Kotas & Medzhitov, 2015). Inflammations are mainly divided into acute and chronic inflammation depending on various inflammatory processes and cellular mechanisms (Medzhitov, 2008). Endogenous lipids are arguably the most important mediators to be implicated in all phases of inflammation (Chiurchiù *et al.*, 2018). These bioactive lipids collectively termed as eicosanoids, represent a huge array of molecules that have the ω-6 poly unsaturated fatty acid (PUFA) arachidonic acid as their common biosynthetic precursor released from membrane phospholipids by an enzyme PLA_2 (specifically, $sPLA_2$) (Fonteh *et al.*, 1994). The released arachidonic acid is primarily acted upon by three enzymatic oxygenation pathways, each involving a distinct family of enzymes: COXs, epoxygenases, and LXOs (Davies *et al.*, 1984; Kuehl & Egan, 1980). At the cellular level, the activity of these enzymes is regulated by induction with various pro-inflammatory signaling molecules such as interleukin-1 (Dinarello & Wolff, 1993), interleukin-6 (Naugler & Karin, 2008),

Table 1 Different assay methods to determine the sPLA$_2$ activity.

S. No.	sPLA2 Assay	Brief Procedure	References
1.	**Titrimetric method**	In a volume of 15 ml containing lecithin emulsion, added sPLA$_2$ and adjusted the pH to 8.9. The titrant volume required to maintain consistent pH was recorded. Volume of titrant consumed by sample was also determined. Blank value was determined by titrating the 15 ml of lecithin emulsion against alkali. One unit of an enzyme releases 1 μM of fatty acid/min from lecithin emulsion at pH 8.9 and 25°C.	Nair *et al.* (1976)
2.	**Colorimetric method:** Bhat and Gowda method	Reaction mixture: sPLA$_2$, 1 μM PC, 300 μl of ether, 500 μl of Tris-HCl buffer, and calcium chloride. The mixture was thoroughly mixed and incubated at 37°C for 60 min. Dole's reagent was added to the reaction mixture, followed by the addition of petroleum ether, and mixed the content for 1 min. Then the tubes were centrifuged at 500 g for 5 min. 0.8 ml of chloroform: petroleum ether (5:1, v/v) and 0.5 ml of freshly prepared cobalt reagent were added to the 0.8 ml of supernatant containing lipid extract. Again tubes were thoroughly mixed and centrifuged at 1200·g for 10 min. The soap was formed and carefully transferred to a tube containing 0.75 ml nitroso-2-naphthol, indicator solution. From the result, color intensity formed was directly proportional to the cobalt content. 2.0 ml of 96% ethanol was added to dilute the .content and the absorbance was measured at 500 nm. The values obtained by linoleic acid were used as the standard. The sPLA$_2$ activity was determined by the amount of fatty acids released per min/mg of protein.	Bhat and Gowda (1989)

(*Continued*)

Table 1 (*Continued*)

S. No.	sPLA2 Assay	Brief Procedure	References
i.	Continuous spectrophotometric assay	The activity of $sPLA_2$ enzyme was determined by using a substrate; dilinoleoylphosphatidylcholine and LOX as a coupling enzyme. The released product by the action of $sPLA_2$ enzyme activity was further oxidized by LOX enzyme, and the hydroperoxide derivatives were formed. The standard reaction mixture containing 50 mM Tris buffer, pH 8.5, containing 3 mM deoxycholate, 65 μM of dilinoleoylphosphatidylcholine, and 0.23 μl of lipoxygenase in a total volume of 1 ml. To the reaction mixture 0.25 μl/ml $sPLA_2$ was added to initiate the reaction. The above-mentioned reaction mixture without enzymes served as a blank. The intensity of color was increased due to the formation of hydroperoxide (ε_{234} = 25,000 M/cm). The increase in absorbance due to was measured at 234 nm.	Jimenez *et al.* (2003)
iii.	4-Nitro-3-octanoyloxy-benzoic acid (NOB) method.	The standard reaction mixture of 260 μl contained 200 μl assay buffer (10 mM Tris-HCl, 10 mM $CaCl_2$, 100 mM NaCl, pH 7.8), 20 μl of distilled water, 20 μl $sPLA_2$ (30 μg), and 20 μl NOB used as a substrate. After the addition of substrate, the mixture was incubated for up to 40 min at 37°C, and its absorbance at 425 nm was read at 10 min intervals. The increase in absorbance after 20 min interval was used to determine the $sPLA_2$ activity.	Lee *et al.* (1999)
iv.	Indirect hemolytic assay	1 μg $sPLA_2$ was added to the reaction containing 200 μmol of Tris-maleic acid buffer (pH 7.5), 0.1 μmol of 2-hexadecanoylthio-l-ethyl-phosphocholine, 100 nmol, 0.6 μmol of EDTA, 1 μmol DTNB, and 100 μmol of Ca^{2+}. The increase in absorbance was recorded at 412 nm.	Magee and Thompson (1960)

3.	**Radiometric method:**		
	i. ^{14}C and HPLC coupled method	$sPLA_2$ activity was determined by using [^{14}C] oleate-labeled lyophilized *Escherichia coli* membrane as a substrate. To the 150 μl of reaction mixture containing 18 nmol of substrate, 0.1 M Tris HC1 (pH 8.0), 5 mM $CaC1_2$, and 0.2% fatty acid-free bovine serum albumin (BSA) were added. The mixture was incubated at 37°C for 15 min after addition of 20 μg of PLA_2. The reaction was terminated by adding 10 μl of 0.03 M of EDTA. The lipids were extracted in 1.25 ml of modified Dole's reagent. 0.75 ml distilled water and 0.2 ml of n-heptane were added. The extract was subjected to phase separation by passing through aminopropyl solid phase column. The hydrolyzed product of [^{14}C] oleic acid was eluted into scintillation vial. Blank value was measured by using unincorporated [^{14}C] oleate. The enzyme activity was calculated by released fatty acids, determined from the ratio between counted radioactivity and total liberated fatty acids as determined by HPLC.	Aufenanger *et al.* (1993)
	ii. ^{14}C method	The standard reaction mixture of 350 μl containing 100 mM Tris-HCl buffer with pH 7.4 containing 5 mM $CaCl_2$ was incubated for 60 min at 37°C with a substrate ^{14}C oleate-labeled *E. coli* (3.18×10^9 cells, which corresponds to 60 nmoles of phospholipids). The reaction was stopped by addition of 0.1 ml of 2N HCl and 10% fatty acid-free BSA. Then the content was centrifuged and 140 μl of supernatant was carefully transferred to vial, scintillation cocktail was added, and the ^{14}C oleate was measured using scintillation counter. Enzyme activity is expressed as nanomoles of free fatty acid released per min/mg of protein at 37°C.	Vishwanath *et al.* (1996)

tumor necrosis factor (Feuerstein *et al.*, 1994), lipopolysaccharide (Huang & Kraus, 2016), and interferon-γ (Romero *et al.*, 2010). The $sPLA_2$ activity is found in numerous inflammatory fluids and plasma in the pathological situations. Detection of increased levels of $sPLA_2$ in plasma or biological fluids from patients with systemic or tissue-specific inflammatory disorders helped in understanding its pathophysiological role (Mehta *et al.*, 1990; Pruzanski *et al.*, 1992). Marked induction of the $sPLA_2$enzyme is observed in multiple pathological conditions, and it is considered as a major factor for the progression of various chronic diseases/disorders, including arthritis (Pruzanski *et al.*, 1985), diabetes (Ramanadham *et al.*, 2015), cardiovascular diseases (CVDs; Ravindran & Kurian, 2017), obesity (Hui, 2012), cancer (Peng *et al.*, 2020), eye disorders (Wei & Asbell, 2020), inflammatory bowel disease (Stokkers *et al.*, 1995), respiratory track inflammation (Rubin *et al.*, 2014), and autoimmune diseases (Cunningham *et al.*, 2006) (**Table 2**).

The discovery and characterization of $sPLA_2$ from the synovial fluids of the arthritis patients and its association with the pathophysiology of rheumatoid arthritis are the foundational studies to designate it as pro-inflammatory molecule (Vishwanath *et al.*, 1988). In arthritis, $sPLA_2$ is markedly upregulated, and high concentrations found in the synovial fluids may serve as its important biomarker. Several clinical studies have concluded that there is a proportional relationship between the serum $sPLA_2$ concentration and disease severity. In several acute inflammatory conditions such as pancreatitis (Mayer *et al.*, 1998), peritonitis (Uhl *et al.*, 1995), and sepsis (Tan & Goh, 2017), elevated serum $sPLA_2$ level was observed. Numerous studies highlight the potential for the use of $sPLA_2$ as biomarker for sepsis in adults (Nik Mansor *et al.*, 2018). Both $sPLA_2$ and arachidonic acid levels were found to be increased in bronchoalveolar lavage (BAL) fluid in patients with asthma and acute respiratory distress syndrome, and the level was correlated with the severity of the disease (Kim *et al.*, 1995). Plasma levels and activity of $sPLA_2$ have been assessed as biomarkers of CVD risk in hospital-based studies, and a multivariate

Table 2 Diseases associated with $sPLA_2$ enzyme.

S. No.	Diseases	$sPLA_2$	References
1.	**Inflammatory diseases** i. Arthritis ii. Septic shock iii. Pancreatitis iv. Burns v. Crush syndrome vi. Adult respiratory distress syndrome	Synovial fluid Serum Serum Serum Serum BAL fluid/serum	Kim *et al.* (1995); Masuda *et al.* (2005); Nevalainen (1988); Vadas *et al.* (1992); Yamada *et al.* (1998)
2.	**Allergic diseases** i. Allergic rhinitis ii. Bronchial asthma	Nasal fluid/serum BAL fluid/serum	Hallstrand *et al.* (2011)
3.	**Autoimmune diseases** i. Ulcerative colitis ii. Rheumatoid arthritis iii. Juvenile rheumatoid arthritis iv. Crohn's disease	Intestinal mucosa/ serum Synovial fluid/serum Serum Intestinal mucosa/ serum	Kim *et al.* (1995); Minami *et al.* (1993, 1994); Pruzanski *et al.* (1994)
4.	**Other diseases** i. Colon cancer ii. Prostate cancer iii. Typhoid fever iv. Atherosclerosis v. Myocardial infraction vi. Diabetes	Serum Serum Serum Serum Serum Serum	Kennedy *et al.* (1998); Keuter *et al.* (1995); Krakoff *et al.* (2003); Krijnen *et al.* (2006); Patel *et al.* (2008); Rosenson and Hurt-Camejo (2012)

analysis reveals that high $sPLA_2$ activity levels can be considered as an independent predictor of early atherosclerosis in metabolic syndrome subjects. High levels of $sPLA_2$ in the circulation have an independent risk factor for the presence of coronary artery disease (CAD) and predict future coronary events in patients with CAD (Mallat *et al.*, 2010). Apparently these studies substantiate the role of $sPLA_2$ in the progression of inflammatory conditions.

6. Hydrophobic $sPLA_2$ Inhibitors with Antioxidant Activity as Anti-inflammatory Molecules

As presented in the **Fig. 3**, regulation of inflammatory processes involving $sPLA_2$ makes this enzyme potential pharmacological target, and $sPLA_2$ inhibitors may be used in treating inflammatory diseases (Nanda *et al.*, 2007; Quach *et al.*, 2014). Various structurally different molecules have been studied for their inhibition of $sPLA_2$s. Before crystal structures of $sPLA_2$s were widely available,

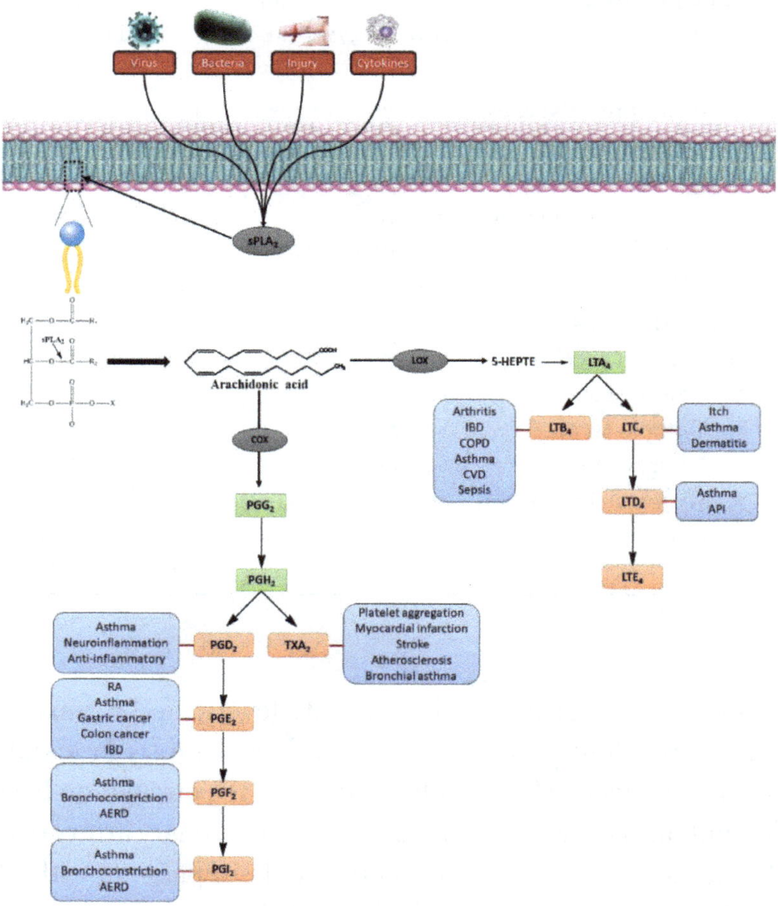

Fig. 3 Arachidonic acid pathway.

the first studied inhibitors were substrate analogs, manoalide from marine sponge and plant natural products (Lombardo & Dennis, 1985). The first potent and specific inhibitor of sPLA$_2$ was studied by Bristol-Myers Squibb in 1992 (Springer, 2001). It successfully reached Phase II clinical trials for treatment of psoriasis by topical application, but the studies were discontinued after confirmation that it could not reach the inner layer of the skin (Kokotou *et al.*, 2017). Various amide and sulfonamide inhibitors developed over the years proved to be valuable tools for mechanistic studies (Magrioti & Kokotos, 2010). Indole inhibitors, a comprehensively studied class of sPLA$_2$ inhibitors, have attracted the attention of several researchers as drug candidates (Dillard *et al.*, 1996).

Lilly Research Laboratory developed the highly potent sPLA$_2$ inhibitor molecule (LY315920) by chemical modification of a lead compound via molecular modeling techniques (Mihelich & Schevitz, 1999). This inhibitor, studied as a treatment for severe sepsis selective for sPLA$_2$, reached Phase II clinical trial, but the trials were discontinued when results did not meet expectations. A prodrug developed by Lilly was also used to study the possible role of sPLA$_2$ enzyme inhibitors in asthma. At the same time, a structurally similar, to Lilly's molecule, new inhibitor, namely Me-Indoxam was introduced by Shionogi. A few years later, when the full set of human sPLA$_2$s was known, indole-type inhibitors were developed that could somewhat distinguish the action of various sPLA$_2$s in cellular events.

Currently, the previously mentioned LY315920, also called Varespladib or A-001 with a hydrophobic index of XLogP3-AA = 2.8, together with Varespladib methyl or A-002 with a hydrophobic index of XLogP3-AA = 3.1 were clinically tested by Anthera Pharmaceuticals to treat CVDs (Leite *et al.*, 2009; Rosenson *et al.*, 2009). One of the most common interesting observed features of some of these compounds is their hydrophobicity. Detailed understanding of the molecular interactions of these test compounds with sPLA$_2$ enzymes enables us to underline the concept of hydrophobicity, that is, inhibitors which are cell-permeable and interact with hydrophobic substrate, may show greater effects clinically. In the quest for $sPLA_2$ inhibitors, our laboratory works extensively to identify and characterize the molecules which are both potent and hydrophobic. Some of the $sPLA_2$ inhibitors developed in our laboratory which falls in the category of "hydrophobicity and potency" are discussed.

Aristolochic acid (AA) is a plant-derived alkaloid isolated majorly from *Aristolochia* species and also from other species such as *Bragantia* and *Asarum*. AA has been used in traditional medicine to treat arthritis, gout, rheumatism, festering wounds, sepsis, and obstetrics. As demonstrated by Vishwanath *et al.*, AA has potent $sPLA_2$inhibitory activity, and later they reported the anti-inflammatory activity of AA (Vishwanath *et al.*, 1987). But unfortunately it was not developed into a potential anti-inflammatory drug because of severe side effects such as cancer, nephropathy, diarrhea, and paralysis this molecule may cause (Arlt *et al.*, 2002; Cosyns, 2003; Nortier & Vanherweghem, 2007). However, biochemical manufacturing companies including Sigma-Aldrich market it as a potent standard $sPLA_2$ inhibitor. The hydrophobic index of XLogP3-AA = 3.6, indicates the hydrophobic nature of aristolochic acid.

Further, to demonstrate the concept of hydrophobicity of $sPLA_2$ inhibitors, our laboratory begins screening and characterizing different endogenous antioxidants. The rationale for screening endogenous antioxidants is because of their involvement in regulation of inflammatory process. Enzymatic breakdown of arachidonic acid by COX and LXO releases free radicals, which may activate $sPLA_2$ enzyme directly, or they are involved in the peroxidation of various organelle membrane lipids, which sequentially activates $sPLA_2$ enzyme (Mori *et al.*, 2007). The activated $sPLA_2$ in turn repeats the cycle of downstream reactions more relentlessly, thereby producing a sea of inflammatory mediators, which may actually worsen the situation and results in chronic inflammatory reactions. Scavenging of these free radicals along with the inhibition of$sPLA_2$ is advantageous in the treatment of inflammatory

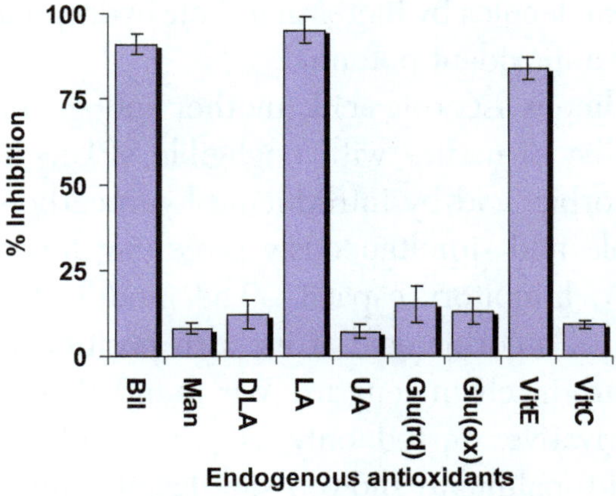

Fig. 4 Effect of hydrophilic and hydrophobic endogenous antioxidants on *in vitro* $sPLA_2$ activity. Bil, bilirubin; Man, mannitol; DLA, dihydrolipoic acid; LA, lipoic acid; UA, uric acid; Glu(rd), glutathione reduced; Glu(ox), glutathione oxidized; Vit E, vitamin E; Vit C, vitamin C.

diseases. Therefore, a single molecule which inhibits the enzymatic action of $sPLA_2$ along with potent free radical scavenger will be considered as therapeutically important anti-inflammatory drug. Among screened antioxidants we found that molecules which are hydrophobic in nature show strong $sPLA_2$ inhibition (**Fig. 4**).

α-Lipoic acid, an endogenous antioxidant molecule with hydrophobic as well as hydrophilic properties, is known to involve in regulation of number of physiological conditions and their pathologies. It inhibits pro-inflammatory $sPLA_2$ enzyme strongly with an IC_{50} of 0.75 μM by direct interaction with an enzyme as demonstrated by Jameel *et al.* (2006). Similarly, bilirubin, an endogenous antioxidant and a hydrophobic molecule made up of linear tetrapyrrole ring connected by a long chain of carbon is also shown to inhibit the catalytic activity of $sPLA_2$ enzyme with an IC_{50} of 10.00 μM. It is also shown to interact directly with $sPLA_2$ enzyme for its inhibition (Jameel *et al.*, 2005). On identification of these endogenous molecules as $sPLA_2$ inhibitors, we convinced with our hypothesis regarding the significance of hydrophobicity. However, to substantiate this further, we chemically modified few endogenous molecules by increasing their hydrophobicity without altering their antioxidant potential.

First in line is ascorbic acid, another endogenous antioxidant but hydrophilic in nature with negligible $sPLA_2$ inhibition. We modified ascorbic acid by introducing hydrocarbon tail to make it lipid-soluble and simultaneously screening for its pro-inflammatory $sPLA_2$ inhibitory capacity. The modification is done by esterification of ascorbic acid at its sixth position with fatty acid of various carbon chain lengths. We found that among all the obtained derivatives tested only ascorbic acid-6-myristate and ascorbic acid-6-palmitate showed significant inhibition of $sPLA_2$ and retained antioxidant property of parent compound (Mohamed *et al.*, 2010). However, ascorbic acid alone and its other derivatives having less than 13-carbon chain lengths fail to show significant $sPLA_2$ enzyme inhibition even at higher concentration, indicating that minimal degree of hydrophobicity is essential for inhibition.

In another study, the unconjugated bilirubin was chemically modified at its propionic acid site in order to increase the hydrophobicity; as a result six different molecules were synthesized. Each newly synthesized molecule tested for $sPLA_2$ inhibition, among them the dimethyl ester of bilirubin (BD1) shows $sPLA_2$ inhibitory activity and is nearly three times potent inhibitor than the parent molecule without losing its antioxidant property (Joshi, Umashankara, *et al.*, 2016). These studies demonstrated that increased hydrophobic interaction of molecule with $sPLA_2$ enzyme might have increased efficacy. Apart from demonstrating the $sPLA_2$ inhibition potential of these molecules, we also carried out interaction studies. Biophysical interaction studies such as circular dichroism and fluorescence studies and also *in silico* molecular docking studies give us clear evidence for the direct interaction of the inhibitors with $sPLA_2$ enzyme. Details regarding hydrophobic score (XLogP3-AA value), IC_{50} value, and molecular docking studies of these molecules with $sPLA_2$ are given in **Table 3**. After critically evaluating the studied molecules, researchers from our laboratory have confirmed that the antioxidant molecules with

Table 3 Hydrophobic score, IC_{50} value, and results of molecular docking studies of $sPLA_2$ inhibitors.

S. No.	Compound	Docking Result	Score (*S*)	Energy (*E*)	XLogP3-AA Value	IC_{50} Value (μM)	Reference
1.	α-Lipoic acid 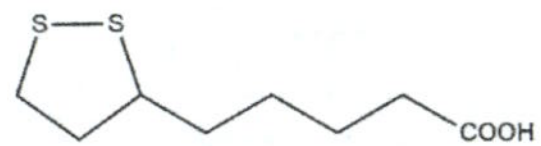		**−9.25**	**−40.68**	1.7	0.75–3.0	Jameel *et al.* (2006)
2.	Ascorbic acid-6-palmitate 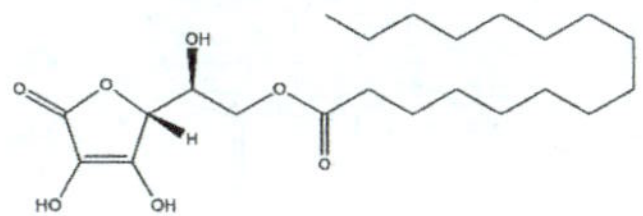	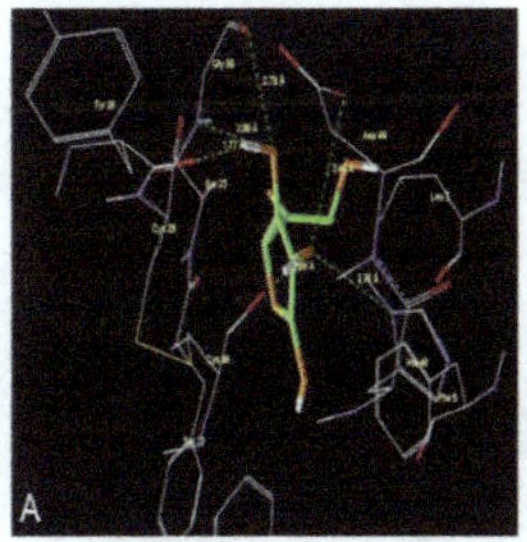	**−4.67**	**−29.44**	6.3	48.85	Mohamed *et al.* (2010)
3.	Unconjugated bilirubin 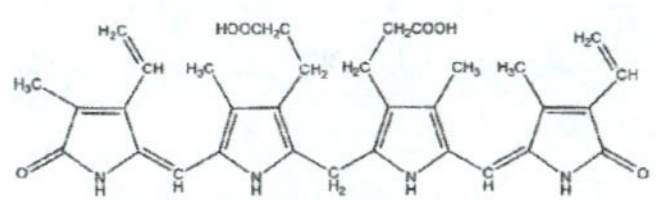	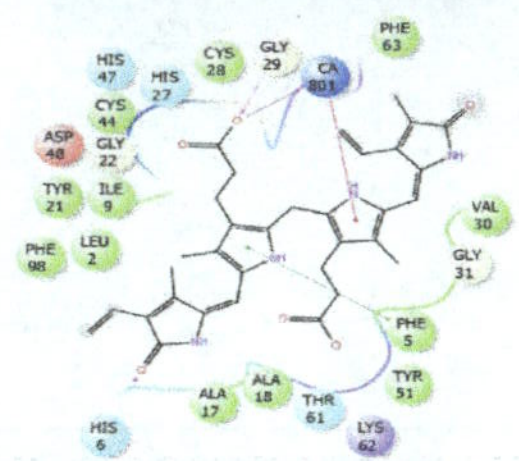	**−10.68**	**−61.95**	2.9	10.00	Jameel *et al.* (2005); Joshi, Umashankara, *et al.* (2016)

(*Continued*)

S. No.	Compound	Docking Result	Score (*S*)	Energy (*E*)	XLogP3-AA Value	IC_{50} Value (μM)	Reference
4.	Dimethyl ester of bilirubin 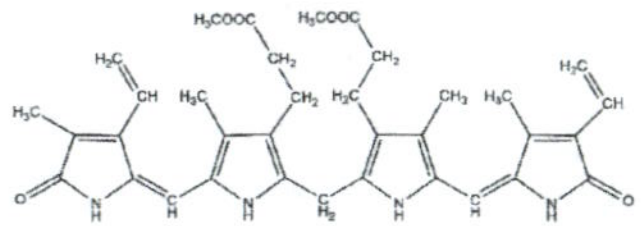	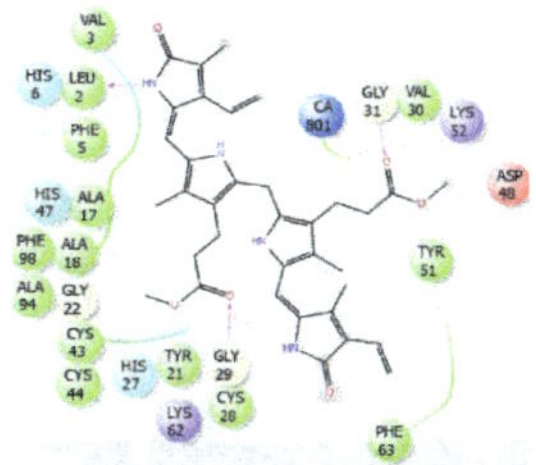	**−10.18**	**−58.63**	3.6	3.0–4.0	Joshi, Umashankara, *et al*. (2016)
5.	Aristolochic acid 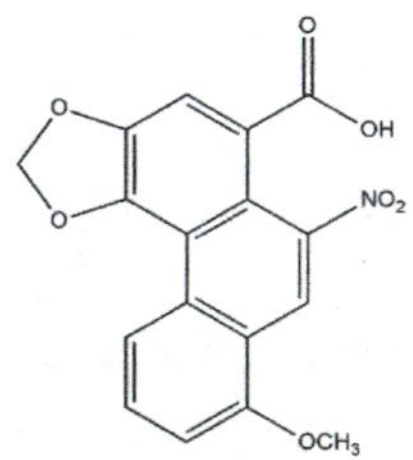	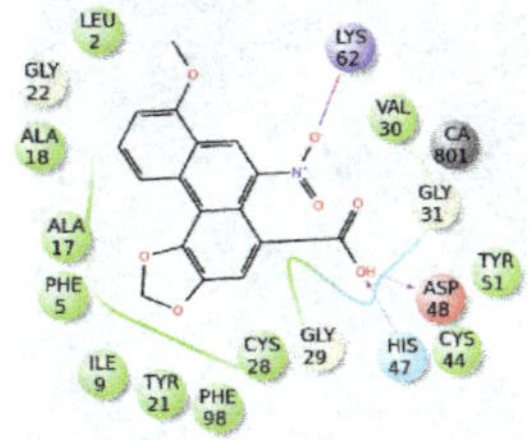	**−8.10**	**−46.03**	3.6	40.00	Vishwanath *et al*. (1987)
6.	Celastrol 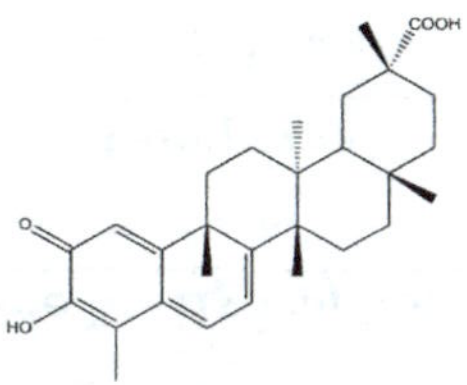	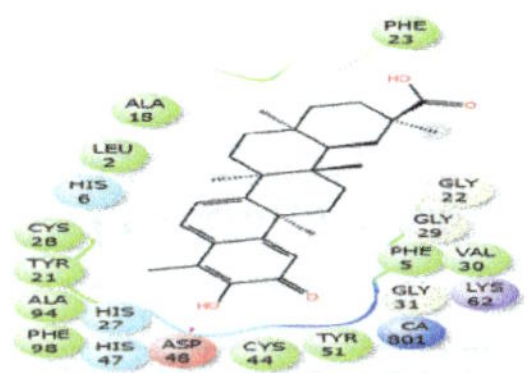	**−10.31**	**−51.28**	5.9	6.00	Joshi, Venkatesha, *et al*. (2016)

$sPLA_2$ inhibitory activity are lipid-soluble, whereas water-soluble antioxidants do not show any significant inhibition. From all the studies discussed above, it is quite evident that some degree of hydrophobicity is essential for the antioxidants to interact with $sPLA_2$ enzyme for its inhibition and anti-inflammatory activity.

Acknowledgments

M.D. Milan Gowda would like to thank University Grants Commission (UGC) Major Research Project [F. No. 43-41/2014 (SR)] for fellowship. K. Jayachandra [Letter No. 09/119(0207)2019-EMR-I] would like to thank UGC, New Delhi, for fellowship. Dr B.S. Vishwanath would like to thank UGC-BSR faculty [No. F.18-1/2011 (BSR)] for fellowship, and Department of Biotechnology (DBT) and Biotechnology Industry Research Assistance Council (BIRAC) (Proposal Ref. No. BT/AIR0492/PACE-15/18), New Delhi, for financial assistance. The authors thank Dr Riaz Mohamed and Dr Vikram Joshi for providing *in silico* studies pictures. Authors also thank Department of Studies in Biochemistry, University of Mysore (UOM), and Vijnana Bhavan, UOM.

References

Arlt, V. M., Stiborova, M., & Schmeiser, H. H. (2002). Aristolochic acid as a probable human cancer hazard in herbal remedies: A review, *17*(4), 265–277.

Aufenanger, J., Zimmer, W., & Kattermann, R. (1993). Characteristics and clinical application of a radiometric *Escherichia coli*-based phospholipase A2 assay modified for serum analysis, *39*(4), 605–613.

Bhat, M. K., & Gowda, T. V. (1989). Purification and characterization of a myotoxic phospholipase A2 from Indian cobra (Naja naja naja) venom, *27*(8), 861–873.

Chiurchiù, V., Leuti, A., & Maccarrone, M. (2018). Bioactive lipids and chronic inflammation: Managing the fire within, *9*, 38.

Chiurchiu, V., & Maccarrone, M. (2016). Bioactive lipids as modulators of immunity, inflammation and emotions, *29*, 54–62.

Cosyns, J.-P. (2003). Aristolochic acid and 'Chinese herbs nephropathy', *26*(1), 33–48.

Cunningham, T. J., Yao, L., Oetinger, M., Cort, L., Blankenhorn, E. P., & Greenstein, J. I. (2006). Secreted phospholipase A2 activity in experimental autoimmune encephalomyelitis and multiple sclerosis, *3*(1), 1–8.

Davies, P., Bailey, P. J., Goldenberg, M. M., & Ford-Hutchinson, A. W. (1984). The role of arachidonic acid oxygenation products in pain and inflammation, *2*(1), 335–357.

Dennis, E. A. (1994). Diversity of group types, regulation, and function of phospholipase A2, *269*(18), 13057–13060.

Dillard, R. D., Bach, N. J., Draheim, S. E., Berry, D. R., Carlson, D. G., Chirgadze, N. Y., Clawson, D. K., Hartley, L. W., Johnson, L. M., & Jones, N. D. (1996). Indole inhibitors of human nonpancreatic secretory phospholipase A2. 1. Indole-3-acetamides, *39*(26), 5119–5136.

Dinarello, C. A., & Wolff, S. M. (1993). The role of interleukin-1 in disease, *328*(2), 106–113.

Feuerstein, G., Liu, T., & Barone, F. C. (1994). Cytokines, inflammation, and brain injury: Role of tumor necrosis factor-alpha, *6*(4), 341–360.

Fonteh, A. N., Bass, D. A., Marshall, L. A., Seeds, M., Samet, J. M., & Chilton, F. H. (1994). Evidence that secretory phospholipase A2 plays a role in arachidonic acid release and eicosanoid biosynthesis by mast cells, *152*(11), 5438–5446.

Hallstrand, T. S., Lai, Y., Ni, Z., Oslund, R. C., Henderson Jr, W. R., Gelb, M. H., & Wenzel, S. E. (2011). Relationship between levels of secreted phospholipase A2 groups IIA and X in the airways and asthma severity, *41*(6), 801–810.

Hoffmann, G., Schmidt, D., Bastian, B., & Guder, W. (1986). Photometric determination of phospholipase A.

Huang, Z., & Kraus, V. B. (2016). Does lipopolysaccharide-mediated inflammation have a role in OA?, *12*(2), 123.

Hui, D. Y. (2012). Phospholipase A2 enzymes in metabolic and cardiovascular diseases, *23*(3), 235.

Jameel, N. M., Frey, B. M., Frey, F. J., Gowda, T. V., & Vishwanath, B. S. (2005). Inhibition of secretory phospholipase A2 enzyme by bilirubin: A new role as endogenous anti-inflammatory molecule, *276*(1), 219–225.

Jameel, N. M., Shekhar, M. A., & Vishwanath, B. S. (2006). α-Lipoic acid: An inhibitor of secretory phospholipase A2 with anti-inflammatory activity, *80*(2), 146–153.

Jimenez, M., Cabanes, J., Gandía-Herrero, F., Escribano, J., García-Carmona, F., & Perez-Gilabert, M. (2003). A continuous spectrophotometric assay for phospholipase A2 activity, *319*(1), 131–137.

Joshi, V., Umashankara, M., Ramakrishnan, C., Urs, A. N. N., Suvilesh, K. N., Velmurugan, D., Rangappa, K. S., & Vishwanath, B. S. (2016a). Dimethyl ester of bilirubin exhibits anti-inflammatory activity through inhibition of secretory phospholipase A2, lipoxygenase and cyclooxygenase, *598*, 28–39.

Joshi, V., Venkatesha, S. H., Ramakrishnan, C., Urs, A. N. N., Hiremath, V., Moudgil, K. D., Velmurugan, D., & Vishwanath, B. S. (2016b). Celastrol modulates inflammation through inhibition of the catalytic activity of mediators of arachidonic acid pathway: Secretory phospholipase A2 group IIA, 5-lipoxygenase and cyclooxygenase-2, *113*, 265–275.

Kennedy, B. P., Soravia, C., Moffat, J., Xia, L., Hiruki, T., Collins, S., Gallinger, S., & Bapat, B. (1998). Overexpression of the nonpancreatic secretory group II PLA2 messenger RNA and protein in colorectal adenomas from familial adenomatous polyposis patients, *58*(3), 500–503.

Keuter, M., Dharmana, E., Kullberg, B.-J., Schalkwijk, C., Gasem, M. H., Seuren, L., Djokomoeljanto, R., Dolmans, W. M., Bosch, H.v.d., & van der Meer, J. W. M. (1995). Phospholipase A2 is a circulating mediator in typhoid fever, *172*(1), 305–308.

Kim, D., Fukuda, T., Thompson, B. T., Cockrill, B., Hales, C., & Bonventre, J. V. (1995). Bronchoalveolar lavage fluid phospholipase A2 activities are increased in human adult respiratory distress syndrome, *269*(1), L109–L118.

Kim, R. R., Chen, Z., Mann, T. J., Bastard, K., Scott, K., & Church, W. B. (2020). Structural and functional aspects of targeting the secreted human group IIA phospholipase A2, *25*(19), 4459.

Kokotou, M. G., Limnios, D., Nikolaou, A., Psarra, A., & Kokotos, G. (2017). Inhibitors of phospholipase A2 and their therapeutic potential: An update on patents (2012–2016), *27*(2), 217–225.

Kotas, M. E., & Medzhitov, R. (2015). Homeostasis, inflammation, and disease susceptibility, *160*(5), 816–827.

Krakoff, J., Funahashi, T., Stehouwer, C. D., Schalkwijk, C. G., Tanaka, S., Matsuzawa, Y., Kobes, S., Tataranni, P. A., Hanson, R. L., & Knowler, W. C. (2003). Inflammatory markers, adiponectin, and risk of type 2 diabetes in the Pima Indian, *26*(6), 1745–1751.

Krijnen, P. A., Meischl, C., Nijmeijer, R., Visser, C. A., Hack, C. E., & Niessen, H. W. M. (2006). Inhibition of sPLA2-IIA, C-reactive protein or complement: New therapy for patients with acute myocardial infarction?, *6*(2), 111–121.

Kuehl, F. A., & Egan, R. W. (1980). Prostaglandins, arachidonic acid, and inflammation, *210*(4473), 978–984.

Lee, W.-H., Toyama, M. H., Soares, A. M., Giglio, J. e. R., Marangoni, S., & Polikarpov, I. (1999). Crystallization and preliminary X-ray diffraction studies of piratoxin III, a D-49 phospholipase A2 from the venom of *Bothrops pirajai*, *55*(6), 1229–1230.

Leite, J. O., Vaishnav, U., Puglisi, M., Fraser, H., Trias, J., & Fernandez, M. L. (2009). A-002 (Varespladib), a phospholipase A2 inhibitor, reduces atherosclerosis in guinea pigs, *9*(1), 1–9.

Lombardo, D., & Dennis, E. A. (1985). Cobra venom phospholipase A2 inhibition by manoalide. A novel type of phospholipase inhibitor, *260*(12), 7234–7240.

Magee, W., & Thompson, R. (1960). The estimation of phospholipase A activity in aqueous systems, *77*(3), 526–534.

Magrioti, V., & Kokotos, G. (2010). Phospholipase A2 inhibitors as potential therapeutic agents for the treatment of inflammatory diseases, *20*(1), 1–18.

Mallat, Z., Lambeau, G., & Tedgui, A. (2010). Lipoprotein-associated and secreted phospholipases A_2 in cardiovascular disease: Roles as biological effectors and biomarkers. *Circulation*, *122*(21), 2183–2200.

Masuda, S., Murakami, M., Komiyama, K., Ishihara, M., Ishikawa, Y., Ishii, T., & Kudo, I. (2005). Various secretory phospholipase A2 enzymes are expressed in rheumatoid arthritis and augment prostaglandin production in cultured synovial cells, *272*(3), 655–672.

Mayer, J., Rau, B., Grewe, M., Schoenberg, M. H., Nevalainen, T. J., & Beger, H. G. (1998). Secretory phospholipase A2 in patients with infected pancreatic necroses in acute pancreatitis, *17*(3), 272–277.

Medzhitov, R. (2008). Origin and physiological roles of inflammation, *454*(7203), 428–435.

Mehta, D., Gupta, S., Gaur, S. N., Gangal, S. V., & Agrawal, K. P. (1990). Increased leukocyte phospholipase A2 activity and plasma lysophosphatidylcholine levels in asthma and rhinitis and their relationship to airway sensitivity to histamine, *142*(1), 157–161.

Mihelich, E. D., & Schevitz, R. W. (1999). Structure-based design of a new class of anti-inflammatory drugs: Secretory phospholipase A2 inhibitors, SPI, *1441*(2–3), 223–228.

Minami, T., Tojo, H., Shinomura, Y., Komatsubara, T., Matsuzawa, Y., & Okamoto, M. (1993). Elevation of phospholipase A2 protein in sera of patients with Crohn's disease and ulcerative colitis, *88*(7).

Minami, T., Tojo, H., Shinomura, Y., Matsuzawa, Y., & Okamoto, M. (1994). Increased group II phospholipase A2 in colonic mucosa of patients with Crohn's disease and ulcerative colitis, *35*(11), 1593–1598.

Mohamed, R., Dharmappa, K., Tarannum, S., Jameel, N., Kannum, S., Ashrafulla, H., Rai, L., Jmd' Souza, C., Shekhar, M., & Vishwanath, B. S. (2010). Chemical modification of ascorbic acid and evaluation of its lipophilic derivatives as inhibitors of secretory phospholipase A2 with anti-inflammatory activity, *345*(1), 69–76.

Mori, T., Ito, S., Namiki, M., Suzuki, T., Kobayashi, S., Matsubayashi, K., & Sawaguchi, T. (2007). Involvement of free radicals followed by the activation of phospholipase A2 in the mechanism that underlies the combined effects of methamphetamine and morphine on subacute toxicity or lethality in mice: Comparison of the therapeutic potential of fullerene, mepacrine, and cooling, *236*(3), 149–157.

Nair, B., Nair, C., & Elliott, W. (1976). Temperature stability of phospholipase A activity — II variations in optimum temperature of phospholipases A2 from various snake venoms, *14*(1), 43–47.

Nanda, B., Nataraju, A., Rajesh, R., Rangappa, K., Shekar, M., & Vishwanath, B. S. (2007). PLA2 mediated arachidonate free radicals: PLA2 inhibition and neutralization of free radicals by anti-oxidants — A new role as anti-inflammatory molecule, *7*(8), 765–777.

Naugler, W. E., & Karin, M. (2008). The wolf in sheep's clothing: The role of interleukin-6 in immunity, inflammation and cancer, *14*(3), 109–119.

Nevalainen, T. J. (1988). Phospholipase A2 in acute pancreatitis, *23*(8), 897-904.

Nik Mansor, N. N., Leong, T. T., Safitri, E., Futra, D., Ahmad, N. S., Nasuruddin, D. N., Itnin, A., Zaini, I. Z., Arifin, K. T., & Heng, L. Y. (2018). An amperometric biosensor for the determination of bacterial sepsis biomarker, secretory phospholipase group 2-IIA using a tri-enzyme system, *18*(3), 686.

Nikolaou, A., Kokotou, M. G., Vasilakaki, S., & Kokotos, G. (2019). Small-molecule inhibitors as potential therapeutics and as tools to understand the role of phospholipases A2, *1864*(6), 941–956.

Nortier, J. L., & Vanherweghem, J.-L. (2007). For patients taking herbal therapy — Lessons from aristolochic acid nephropathy, *22*(6), 1512–1517.

Patel, M. I., Kurek, C., & Dong, Q. J. T. (2008). The arachidonic acid pathway and its role in prostate cancer development and progression, *179*(5), 1668–1675.

Peng, Z., Chang, Y., Fan, J., Ji, W., & Su, C. (2020). Phospholipase A2 superfamily in cancer.

Pérez-Jeldres, T., Tyler, C. J., Boyer, J. D., Karuppuchamy, T., Yarur, A., Giles, D. A., Yeasmin, S., Lundborg, L., Sandborn, W. J., & Patel, D. R. (2019). Targeting cytokine signaling and lymphocyte traffic via small molecules in inflammatory bowel disease: JAK inhibitors and S1PR agonists, *10*, 212.

Piomelli, D., & Greengard, P. (1991). Bidirectional control of phospholipase A2 activity by Ca^{2+}/calmodulin-dependent protein kinase II, cAMP-dependent protein kinase, and casein kinase II, *88*(15), 6770–6774.

Pruzanski, W., Albin-Cook, K., Laxer, R., MacMillan, J., Stefanski, E., Vadas, P., & Silverman, E. (1994). Phospholipase A2 in juvenile rheumatoid arthritis: Correlation to disease type and activity, *21*(10), 1951–1954.

Pruzanski, W., Scott, K., Smith, G., Rajkovic, I., Stefanski, E., & Vadas, P. (1992). Enzymatic activity and immunoreactivity of extracellular phospholipase A2 in inflammatory synovial fluids, *16*(5), 451–457.

Pruzanski, W., Vadas, P., Stefanski, E., & Urowitz, M. J. (1985). Phospholipase A2 activity in sera and synovial fluids in rheumatoid arthritis and osteoarthritis. Its possible role as a proinflammatory enzyme, *12*(2), 211–216.

Quach, N. D., Arnold, R. D., & Cummings, B. S. (2014). Secretory phospholipase A2 enzymes as pharmacological targets for treatment of disease, *90*(4), 338–348.

Ramanadham, S., Ali, T., Ashley, J. W., Bone, R. N., Hancock, W. D., & Lei, X. (2015). Calcium-independent phospholipases A2 and their roles in biological processes and diseases, *56*(9), 1643–1668.

Ravindran, S., & Kurian, G. A. (2017). The role of secretory phospholipases as therapeutic targets for the treatment of myocardial ischemia reperfusion injury, *92*, 7–16.

Romero, C. R., Herzig, D. S., Etogo, A., Nunez, J., Mahmoudizad, R., Fang, G., Murphey, E., Toliver⊠Kinsky, T., & Sherwood, E. R. (2010). The role of interferon⊠γ in the pathogenesis of acute intra⊠abdominal sepsis, *88*(4), 725–735.

Rosenson, R. S., Hislop, C., McConnell, D., Elliott, M., Stasiv, Y., Wang, N., Waters, D. D., & PLASMA Investigators (2009). Effects of 1-H-indole-3-glyoxamide (A-002) on concentration of secretory phospholipase A2 (PLASMA study): A phase II double-blind, randomised, placebo-controlled trial, *373*(9664), 649–658.

Rosenson, R. S., & Hurt-Camejo, E. (2012). Phospholipase A2 enzymes and the risk of atherosclerosis, *33*(23), 2899–2909.

Rubin, B. K., Priftis, K. N., Schmidt, H. J., & Henke, M. O. (2014). Secretory hyperresponsiveness and pulmonary mucus hypersecretion, *146*(2), 496–507.

Scott, D. L., & Sigler, P. B. (1994). Structure and catalytic mechanism of secretory phospholipases A2, *45*, 53–88.

Springer, D. M. (2001). An update on inhibitors of human 14 kDa type II s PLA2 in development, *7*(3), 181–198.

Stokkers, P., Camoglio, L., & Van Deventer, S. J. (1995). Tumor necrosis factor (TNF) in inflammatory bowel disease: Gene polymorphisms, animal models, and potential for anti-TNF therapy, *47*(1–2), 97–103.

Tan, T. L., & Goh, Y. Y. (2017). The role of group IIA secretory phospholipase A2 (sPLA2-IIA) as a biomarker for the diagnosis of sepsis and bacterial infection in adults — A systematic review, *12*(7), e0180554.

Tessmer, M. H., Anderson, D. M., Buchaklian, A., Frank, D. W., & Feix, J. B. (2017). Cooperative substrate-cofactor interactions and membrane localization of the bacterial phospholipase A2 (PLA2) enzyme, ExoU, *292*(8), 3411–3419.

Uhl, W., Beger, H., Hoffmann, G., Hanisch, E., Schild, A., Waydhas, C., Entholzner, E., Müller, K., Kellermann, W., & Vogeser, M. (1995). A multicenter study of phospholipase A2 in patients in intensive care units, *180*(3), 323–331.

Vadas, P., Scott, K., Smith, G., Rajkovic, I., Stefanski, E., Schouten, B., Singh, R., & Pruzanski, W. (1992). Serum phospholipase A2 enzyme activity and immunoreactivity in a prospective analysis of patients with septic shock, *50*(11), 807–811.

Verheij, H., Slotboom, A., & De Haas, G. H. (1981). Structure and function of phospholiphase A2. *Reviews of Physiology, Biochemistry and Pharmacology*, 91, 91–203

Vishwanath, B., Fawzy, A., & Franson, R. (1988). Edema-inducing activity of phospholipase A2 purified from human synovial fluid and inhibition by aristolochic acid, *12*(6), 549–561.

Vishwanath, B. S., Eichenberger, W., Frey, F. J., & Frey, B. M. (1996). Interaction of plant lipids with 14 kDa phospholipase A2 enzymes, *320*(1), 93–99.

Vishwanath, B. S., Kini, R. M., & Gowda, T. V. (1987). Characterization of three edema-inducing phospholipase A2 enzymes from habu (*Trimeresurus flavoviridis*) venom and their interaction with the alkaloid aristolochic acid, *25*(5), 501–515.

Wei, Y., & Asbell, P. (2020). sPLA2-IIa participates in ocular surface inflammation in humans with dry eye disease, *201*, 108209.

Yamada, Y., Endo, S., Kamei, Y., Minato, T., Yokoyama, M., Taniguchi, S., Nakae, H., Inada, K., & Ogawa, M. (1998). Plasma levels of type II phospholipase A2 and nitrite/nitrate in patients with burns, *24*(6), 513–517.

https://doi.org/10.1142/9789811254796_0003

3 Exploring the Shock and Kill Strategy to Eradicate Latent HIV-1 Infection

Mohd. Aqueel Khan, Rajaram Abhirami, and Sanjeev Kumar Singh*

Computer Aided Drug Designing & Molecular Modelling Lab, Department of Bioinformatics, Alagappa University, Karaikudi 630004, Tamil Nadu, India

Abstract

Human immunodeficiency virus type 1 (HIV-1) infections have been prevailing worldwide since the last three decades. Yet, no permanent cure is available. Currently, combinations of antiretroviral therapy (cART) are available for treatment that successfully helps in the management of disease and reducing the global burden of death. However, cART fails in eradicating the virus because HIV-1 latency comprises a silent, replication-competent viral DNA present in between the host genome known as provirus. The provirus is mainly dominant in the resting memory $CD4^+$ T cells, macrophages, and other cells. Scientists have been exploring various strategies to address the problem of viral latency. So far, Shock and Kill strategy shows promising result in reactivating the virus using latency reversal agents that produce viral progeny cleared by either host immune systems or viral cytopathic effect. This chapter mainly focuses on understanding

*Corresponding author: e-mail: skysanjeev@gmail.com

the Shock and Kill approach to resume the transactivator of transcription-mediated viral transcription.

1. Introduction

Acquired immunodeficiency syndrome (AIDS) is a sexually transmitted disease caused by human immunodeficiency virus (HIV). According to UNAIDS Factsheet, in 2020, there were 38 million active cases and 32.7 million deaths worldwide. HIV belongs to the viral family Retroviridae and class *Lentivirus*; it is further divided into two subtypes, namely HIV-1 and HIV-2 (Blood, 2016). HIV-1 has higher prevalence around the world than HIV-2 (Buonaguro *et al.*, 2007). Sub-Saharan Africa is the major hotspot of two-third HIV-1-infected cases (Kharsany & Karim, 2016). HIV-1 cases are mostly seen in the developing countries and also in the Eastern Europe and Central Asia (Shao & Williamson, 2012). A combination of antiretroviral therapy (cART) has been successfully used in the management of a disease, which targets various stages of viral life cycle and thereby diminishes the morbidity and mortality associated with AIDS (Arts & Hazuda, 2012; Khan *et al.*, 2020; Panwar *et al.*, 2019). However, cART failed due to HIV-1 latency, because it represents a major barrier in completely eradicating the virus. HIV-1 latency consists of a transcriptionally silent, replication-competent viral DNA present in between the host genome, termed provirus. The provirus is mainly present in the resting memory $CD4^+$ T cells, macrophages, and other cells (monocytes, microglial cells, etc.) (Honeycutt *et al.*, 2017; Kwon *et al.*, 2020). The small pool of cells, harboring the transcriptionally silent provirus, is termed as HIV-1 latent reservoirs (Cohn *et al.*, 2020). These reservoirs hide in the anatomical sites and tissue sanctuaries, which makes cART difficult to reach them, and thus virus escapes from the cART and host defense mechanism (Castro-Gonzalez *et al.*, 2018; Chun *et al.*, 2015; Dahabieh *et al.*, 2015; Siliciano & Greene, 2011). The estimated size of the latent reservoir is 10–100 copies per million of infected cells (Crooks *et al.*, 2015). Once the patient interrupts the treatment in between, virus again emerges from the reservoirs within 2–3 weeks (Davey *et al.*, 1999). Still, no inhibitor is available for blocking the ongoing viral transcription in these infected cells. The mechanism of latency is very complex. Several studies have tried to explain this mechanism but not understood completely (Nikolai & Feng, 2017; Razooky *et al.*, 2015). HIV contains two transcriptionally important regulatory proteins, namely transactivator of transcription (TAT) and regulator of virion expression protein (Rev).

TAT is a key controller of viral transcription that binds to the transactivation response element (TAR) RNA element, a stem-loop structure initially produced at the 5 end of HIV-1 promoter region. Later, TAT elongates the TAR RNA by hijacking the host positive transcription elongation factor b (P-TEFb) which releases the paused RNA Pol II. Currently, "Shock and Kill" strategy is utmost promising in reactivating the latent infected cells using latency-reversing agents (LRAs), which further leads to clearance of latent cells via host-mediated immune or viral cytopathic effect (Deeks, 2012; Kim *et al.*, 2018). During the clinical trials, several LRAs (disulfiram, panobinostat, romidepsin, vorinostat) have shown the promising results in activating the viral gene expression but failed in clearing the latent infected cells (Archin *et al.*, 2017; Darcis *et al.*, 2017; Elliott *et al.*, 2015; Rasmussen *et al.*, 2014). Hence, there is an urgent need of novel potent LRAs that can reactivate the latent cells and also reduce size of viral reservoirs.

2. Molecular Basis of Understanding the Shock and Kill Approach

HIV-1 infects the active $CD4^+$ T cells and enters inside the host cells where it releases the genomic RNA and converts into double-stranded complimentary DNA (cDNA) (Chandra *et al.*,

2021). Next, cDNA moves toward the nucleus and gets attached in between the host DNA, which further leads the viral genes and proteins to virions assembly (Yadav & Singh, 2003, 2005). During this step, sometimes latency occurs instead of regular viral production, which produces the minimal or null HIV-1 transcripts. A recent study has shown the establishment of latency in the resting memory $CD4^+$ T cells and also directly via activated primary $CD4^+$ T cells (Chavez *et al.*, 2015). The viral latency is enforced in the resting memory $CD4^+$ T cells due to the presence of epigenetic modifiers, transcriptional interference, sequestration of host transactional factors, and lack of TAT protein (Turner & Margolis, 2017; Yukl *et al.*, 2009). The epigenetic modifiers comprise histone deacetylases (HDACs), histone lysine methyltransferases present at the viral 5′ LTR promoter leads to condense of chromatin regions and restricts the RNA Pol II to initiate viral transcription. A recent work has shown that H3K27me, H3K9, and other epigenetic factors are important for the viral latency maintenance and establishment (Nguyen *et al.*, 2017). The latent $CD4^+$ T cells comprises several important host factors such as P-TEFb, nuclear factor of activated T-cells, and NF-κB, which remains isolated in the cytoplasm and lacks the essential post-translational modifications for the stimulation. The active HIV-1 transcription requires both host transcription factors and viral TAT proteins, which usually remains suppressed during the latency. Initially, viral DNA is transcribed by the RNA pol II that produces approximately 59-nucleotide-long TAR RNA, and further stops due to the presence of DRB sensitivity-inducing factor (DSIF) and negative elongation factor (NELF). To overcome this barrier, HIV-1 produces the TAT protein that hijacks the host P-TEFb complex to release the paused transcription elongation process (Mousseau *et al.*, 2016; Peterlin & Price, 2006). Scientists believed that the Shock and Kill strategy will play an important role in the functional curing of HIV-1 infection.

3. Shock and Kill Strategy

The reemergence of latently infected cells, after a treatment gap, causes the major barrier in eradicating the HIV-1. The Shock and Kill approach involves first reactivating certain cells with LRAs (shock) and then killing those reactivated cells (kill), either through the immune system or the virus-induced cytopathic effect or cART as shown in **Fig. 1** (Kim *et al.*, 2018). The first attempts to cause latency reversal included activating T cells with interleukin-2 (IL-2), which shows the low infectious units per million cells but no difference in viral DNA levels (Fun *et al.*, 2017). IL-2 in conjunction with anti-CD3 antibodies176 shows significant side effects, resultant generation of early antibodies against the anti-CD3 antibodies, thereby restricting the stimulatory effect. The mainstream latency-reversing compounds function by releasing the sequestered cellular transcription factors or altering the epigenetic regulation through Bromodomain and extra-terminal (BET) inhibitors, DNA methyltransferase inhibitors, and protein kinase C (PKC) agonists, and so on. The use of HDAC inhibitors such as vorinostat, panobinostat, and romidepsin to remodel the chromatin has been the most studied pathway for HIV-1 reactivation. Several theories are proposed for understanding the failure in clearing the reactivated cells, including the anti-apoptotic action of some viral proteins like TAT, Nef, and Vpr or deficiency of the CTL response mediated by HDAC inhibitors (Timilsina & Gaur, 2016). Most reports

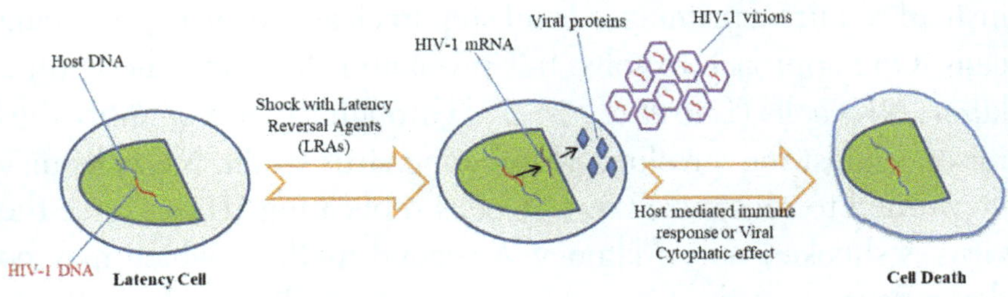

Fig. 1 Schematic representation of Shock and Kill approach.

indicate LRAs alone are not sufficient in killing the reactivated cells (Pardons *et al.*, 2019). Thus, in order to enhance the "kill" process, several approaches have been proposed, including the use of antibodies, chimeric antigen receptor T cells, therapeutic vaccination, and pro-apoptotic compounds [second mitochondria-derived activator of caspases (SMAC) mimetic, Bcl-2 antagonists, PI3K/Akt inhibitors, and RIG-I inducers). However, there is still a long way for "Shock and Kill" approach to be considered as a viable HIV-1 cure technique. Furthermore, deeper understanding of HIV-1 integration sites role in latency reversal is essential in finding a suitable LRA cocktail to induce HIV-1 reactivation regardless of the position of provirus in the genome.

Several compounds are used to give "Shock," including cytokines (Chun *et al.*, 1998), bromodomain inhibitors (Boehm *et al.*, 2013), disulfiram (Doyon *et al.*, 2013), PKC agonists (Williams *et al.*, 2004), histone methyltransferase inhibitors (HMTIs) (Bouchat *et al.*, 2012), and HDAC inhibitors, and so on (Archin *et al.*, 2009). Since there are many molecular pathways involved in latency modulation, a hybrid solution is essential to achieve the level of reactivation required for the immune system to recognize the infected cell. Indeed, synergy for HIV reactivation was observed in some of the LRAs studied in combination strategies. For the "Kill" approach, it was initially believed that the immune system could clear the actively infected cell after exposure to a "Shock" compound. Unfortunately, this proved difficult as the immune system may be unable to perform this function alone, and instead require a priming second step to clear the virus-producing cells. One approach to solve this problem is to utilize the natural killer (NK) cells (Luo *et al.*, 2017). Through the use of antibodies raised against the envelope of infecting virus strain, NK cells may be primed to recognize $CD4^+$ T cells replicating HIV-1, once the virus is shocked out of latency. A second method, which may be dependent upon the host immune system, utilizes a dual-affinity retargeting proteins to target the actively replicating viral progeny.

The above-mentioned two methods, paired with a LRA, show the potential to clear latent HIV-1 reservoir. The success of the "Shock and Kill" approach may depend upon the multiple rounds of treatment with activating or killing compounds in order to destroy the latently infected cells.

4. HIV-1 TAT Protein

4.1. Structural Features and Functions

HIV-1 TAT is minor regulatory protein (86–101 amino acids) (Clark *et al.*, 2017; Williams *et al.*, 2020). Among all the HIV-1 proteins, TAT is an important target of latency, essential for viral transcription. The viral TAT protein is coded via two exons of length 1–72 and 73–102 amino acids, respectively. The first exon (1–72 amino acids) is mainly dominant and consists of five regions: N-terminus, cysteine, hydrophobic, basic, and glutamine, whereas second exon consists of C-domain as shown in **Fig. 2**. The TAT activation domain (1–48 amino acids) binds mainly with P-TEFb (CycT1 subunit), to mediate transactivation at 5′ LTR promoter. The cysteine-rich domain comprises mainly cysteine residue at various positions (22, 25, 27, 30, 31, and 34) in the TAT, which helps in making the disulfide bonds (intermolecular). The cysteine-rich domain along with the core helps in the binding of various cofactors such as HATs, CBP/p300, and Sp1 (Marzio *et al.*, 1998). TAT basic domain (49–57 amino acids) binds with TAR element that contains signal for the nuclear localization

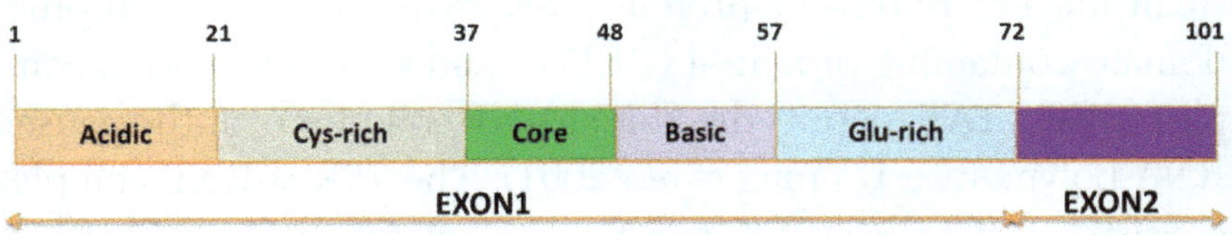

Fig. 2 Representations of viral TAT domains.

(nucleus) of infected cell (Kurnaeva *et al.*, 2019). The TAT domains are functionally overlying each other and contain only the limited number of conserved residues in the full length of protein (Li *et al.*, 2012).

The Apo TAT protein shows the highest flexibility in the solution structure, and it depends on solvent polarity (Shojania & O'Neil, 2006). Moreover, TAT is a highly disordered protein, intensely bound with TAR element, P-TEFb complex, respectively (Zhang *et al.*, 2000). The experimental resolved TAT structure (2.1 Å) shows interaction and conformational changes with P-TEFb (CycT1/CDK9) complex (Tahirov *et al.*, 2010). In this study, they have crystallized the TAT transactivation domain (1–48 amino acids) along with the P-TEFb. The viral TAT structure consists of a coil, two helices, tail, and zinc ions. Earlier studies have also shown that TAT majorly interacts with the CycT1 (cysteine 261) through a zinc-mediated bridge (Garber *et al.*, 1998). TAT mainly involves in both the latency formation and revival (Razooky *et al.*, 2015). TAT initiates the transcription of HIV-1 mRNA, resulting in the production of various viral proteins. Therefore, HIV-1 needs the TAT for lifecycle, nuclear translocation, viral RNA binding, transactivation of LTR promoter, and so on.

4.2. TAT-mediated HIV-1 transcription

Initially, RNA polymerase II starts the viral transcription and pauses after producing the TAR RNA. Next, TAT hijacks the P-TEFb complex to activate the paused transcription elongation process. In search of active P-TEFb, TAT intermingles with the small nuclear ribonucleoprotein (7SK snRNP) complex, bromodomain-containing protein-4 (BRD4), and super-elongation complex (SEC). TAT recruits the 7SK snRNP complex over the paused RNA polymerase II (Yang *et al.*, 2001). The 7SK snRNP complex consists of P-TEFb, 7SK snRNA, La-related protein (LaRP7), methylphosphate capping enzyme (MePCE), and hexamethylene bisacetamide-inducible protein 1/2 (HEXIM1/2). P-TEFb is suppressed by the HEXIM1 present inside the 7SK snRNP complex (Kwak & Lis, 2013; Lin *et al.*, 2002). TAT binds with the cyclin T1 via activation domain and relocates the HEXIM1, resulting in the release of active P-TEFb (Rice, 2017). TAT induces conformational changes in P-TEFb leading to activation of the CDK9 and later directly transfers the active P-TEFb to the nascent TAR RNA element (stem-loop), and finally recruits the SEC. Next, P-TEFb catalytic kinase domain phosphorylates the CTD of RNA polymerase II, DSIF, and NELF-E subunit, resulting in the discharge of halt RNA polymerase II complex (Czudnochowski *et al.*, 2012; Kim *et al.*, 2002). In general, other than TAT several other proteins also interact with P-TEFb to discharge the halt RNA polymerase II complex such as BRD4, Mediator, NF-κB, and c-Myc. In the latency-infected cell, both the TAT and CycT1 represent the low level. TAT also facilitates the histone acetyltransferase (HAT) over chromatin to acetylate histone (H3, H4). During the early transcription elongation, HAT acetylates the TAT (lysine 50 residues) to dissociate from the TAR RNA. Later, TAT recruits the SWI/SNF complex for remodeling the nucleosomes for the active transcription (Mahmoudi *et al.*, 2006). The primary $CD4^+$ cells model shows that increased level of active P-TEFb is needed for reactivation of viral transcription (Tyagi *et al.*, 2010). Recently, several scientific groups have investigated the "Shock and Kill" approach to eradicate the latent cells and reservoirs (Divsalar *et al.*, 2020; Lichterfeld, 2020; Margolis *et al.*, 2016; Walker-Sperling *et al.*, 2016).

5. LRAs

LRAs are small molecules used for the reactivation of latency cells. Currently, several LRAs are available but unable to decrease the number of viral reservoirs. Several assays (qPCR, qVOA, TILDA, RNA FISH/flow method) are used to determine the effect of LRAs on the size of viral reservoirs by measuring the level of viral RNA or DNA (Grau-Expósito *et al.*, 2017; Laird *et al.*, 2016; Procopio *et al.*, 2015). LRAs can be classified into six different categories shown in **Table 1**.

- Histone post-translational modification modulators
- Non-histone chromatin modulators
- NF-κB stimulators
- TLR agonists
- Extracellular stimulators
- Miscellaneous

5.1. Histone Post-translational Modification Modulators

The histone modulators influence the provirus reactivation by modulating simple protein tail modifications at the nucleosomes of the incorporated HIV-1. The histone protein methyltransferase and HDAC inhibitors are the common LRAs. However, novel compounds targeting the uncommon protein modifications have been recently identified, such as *vorinostat*, *romidepsin*, *DZNep*, *Na-Cro*, and *MG-149*.

5.2. Non-histone Chromatin Modulators

The non-histone modulators have the ability to influence the existence and action of alternate chromatin components like transcription factors, besides NF-κB, DNA methylation, and numerous functional proteins. *JQ1*, *OTX-015*, *BAF inhibitors*, *5-aza-2′-deoxycytidine*, *AV6*, and *HODHBt* are some of the most well-known examples of this class.

5.3. NF-κB Stimulators

These stimulators are PKC agonists that activate the NF-κB leading to nuclear localization and resultant reactivation of viral transcription. This class consists of potent LRAs, and also causes

Table 1 Latency reversal agents and their mechanism of action.

Type	Compounds	Function	Reference
Cytokines	IL-2, IL-6,TNF-α	Cytokines influence the viral expression by stimulating the infected $CD4^+$ T cells.	Chun *et al*. (1998)
Bromodomain inhibitors	JQ1	Inhibits the binding of BRD4 with the P-TEFb complex.	Li *et al*. (2013)
	I-BET		Boehm *et al*. (2013)
	I-BET151		
	MS417		
	OTX015		Lu *et al*. (2016)
P-TEFb-releasing agents	HMBA	Releases P-TEFb from the 7SK snRNP complex using PI3K/Akt pathway.	Contreras *et al*. (2007)
	Disulfiram		Doyon *et al*. (2013)
PKC agonists	Prostratin	PKCs phosphorylate IBs, which then degrade to produce NF-B, an HIV replication enzyme.	Williams *et al*. (2004)
	Bryostatin-1		Dias *et al*. (2015)
	Ingenol		Jiang *et al*. (2014)
	Phorbol-13-stearate		Márquez *et al*. (2008)
HMTIs	Chaetocin	Inhibits the Suv39H1 (H3K9 trimethylation), G9a (H3K9 dimethylation) function through competitive or uncompetitive binding with *S*-adenosylmethionine.	Bernhard *et al*. (2011)
	BIX-01294		Bouchat *et al*. (2012)
Histone deacetylase (HDAC) inhibitors	SAHA	Inhibits the removal of an acetyl group from histones by HDACs. This keeps chromatin relaxed and conducive to transcription.	Archin *et al*. (2009)
	Panobinostat		Palmer & Crowe (2014)
	Romidepsin		Wei *et al*. (2014)
	Entinostat		Wightman *et al*. (2013)
	Givinostat		Banga *et al*. (2015)
	Belinostat		Rasmussen *et al*. (2013)
	Valproic acid		Routy *et al*. (2012)

an inflammatory response in the body. The examples of this class are *PMA*, *prostratin derivatives*, *ingenols*, and *SMAC mimetics*.

5.4. TLR Agonists

TLR agonists function by reactivating the provirus transcription via triggering the TLR-based innate immune response that further helps in recognizing the immune system to kill infected cells. The examples of this class are *CL413*, *GS-986*, *GS-9840*, *3M-002*, and *MGN*.

5.5. Extracellular Stimulators

This category encompasses the compounds that interact with extracellular receptors and trigger the molecular pathways (intracellular) resulting in the reactivation of latent HIV-1 cells. It can differ significantly depending on the upstream positioning. *TNF*, *PHA*, *cytokines*, *antibodies*, and *rGal9* are some notable examples.

5.6. Miscellaneous

This group consists of all uncommon compounds which modulate the specific cellular pathways but their mode of action is unknown. *Disulfiram*, *BMS-936559*, and *Ixazomib* are three notable examples of this group.

6. Concluding Remarks

The understanding of latent reservoirs establishment and their maintenance is crucial for eradicating the HIV-1 infection. During the infection some part of active $CD4^+$ T cells converts into latency cells. These latency cells remain dormant without producing any genes or proteins or virions till the patient taking treatment. Once patient interrupts the treatment, virus again remerges from these latent cells or reservoirs and produce infectious virions. Hence, “Shock and Kill” seems a promising approach to reactivate the latent cells using LRAs and later killed by either host immune system or viral cytopathic effects or cART. Therefore, future studies should be emphasized on finding new promising LRAs to reactivate the latent cells without causing global T cells activation.

Acknowledgment

The authors thankfully acknowledge the AURF and MHRD-Rashtriya Uchchatar Shiksha Abhiyan (RUSA) Phase 2.0 [Grant no. F. 24-51/ 2014-U, Policy (TN Multi-Gen), Dept. of Edn., Govt. of India, Dated 09.10.2018].

References

Archin, N. M., Espeseth, A., Parker, D., Cheema, M., Hazuda, D., & Margolis, D. M. (2009). Expression of latent HIV induced by the potent HDAC inhibitor suberoylanilide hydroxamic acid. *AIDS Research and Human Retroviruses*, *25*(2), 207–212.

Archin, N. M., Kirchherr, J. L., Sung, J. A., Clutton, G., Sholtis, K., Xu, Y., & Margolis, D. M. (2017). Interval dosing with the HDAC inhibitor vorinostat effectively reverses HIV latency. *Journal of Clinical Investigation*, *127*(8), 3126–3135.

Arts, E. J., & Hazuda, D. J. (2012). HIV-1 antiretroviral drug therapy. *Cold Spring Harbor Perspectives in Medicine*, *2*(4), a007161.

Banga, R., Procopio, F. A., Cavassini, M., & Perreau, M. (2016). In vitro reactivation of replication-competent and infectious HIV-1 by histone deacetylase inhibitors. *Journal of Virology*, *90*(4), 1858–1871.

Blood, G. A. C. (2016). Human immunodeficiency virus (HIV). *Transfusion Medicine and Hemotherapy*, *43*(3), 203.

Boehm, D., Calvanese, V., Dar, R. D., Xing, S., Schroeder, S., Martins, L., & Ott, M. (2013). BET bromodomain-targeting compounds reactivate HIV from latency via a TAT-independent mechanism. *Cell Cycle*, *12*(3), 452–462.

Bouchat, S., Gatot, J. S., Kabeya, K., Cardona, C., Colin, L., Herbein, G., & Van Lint, C. (2012). Histone methyltransferase inhibitors induce HIV-1 recovery in resting CD4+ T cells from HIV-1-infected HAART-treated patients. *Aids*, *26*(12), 1473–1482.

Bernhard, W., Barreto, K., Saunders, A., Dahabieh, M. S., Johnson, P., & Sadowski, I. (2011). The Suv39H1 methyltransferase inhibitor chaetocin causes induction of integrated HIV-1 without producing a T cell response. *FEBS Letters*, *585*(22), 3549–3554.

Buonaguro, L., Tornesello, M. L., & Buonaguro, F. M. (2007). Human immunodeficiency virus type 1 subtype distribution in the worldwide epidemic: Pathogenetic and therapeutic implications. *Journal of Virology*, *81*(19), 10209–10219.

Castro-Gonzalez, S., Colomer-Lluch, M., & Serra-Moreno, R. (2018). Barriers for HIV cure: The latent reservoir. *AIDS Research and Human Retroviruses*, *34*(9), 739–759.

Chandra, I., Prabhu, S.V., Nayak, C., & Singh, S.K. (2021). E-pharmacophore based screening to identify potential HIV-1 gp120 and CD4 interaction blockers for wild and mutant types. *SAR and QSAR in Environmental Research*, *32*(5), 353–377.

Chavez, L., Calvanese, V., & Verdin, E. (2015). HIV latency is established directly and early in both resting and activated primary CD4 T cells. *PLoS Pathogens*, *11*(6), e1004955.

Chun, T. W., Engel, D., Mizell, S. B., Ehler, L. A., & Fauci, A. S. (1998). Induction of HIV-1 replication in latently infected CD4+ T cells using a combination of cytokines. *The Journal of Experimental Medicine*, *188*(1), 83–91.

Chun, T. W., Moir, S., & Fauci, A. S. (2015). HIV reservoirs as obstacles and opportunities for an HIV cure. *Nature Immunology*, *16*(6), 584–589.

Contreras, X., Barboric, M., Lenasi, T., & Peterlin, B. M. (2007). HMBA releases P-TEFb from HEXIM1 and 7SK snRNA via PI3K/Akt and activates HIV transcription. *PLoS Pathogens*, *3*(10), e146.

Clark, E., Nava, B., & Caputi, M. (2017). TAT is a multifunctional viral protein that modulates cellular gene expression and functions. *Oncotarget*, *8*, 27569–27581.

Crooks, A. M., Bateson, R., Cope, A. B., Dahl, N. P., Griggs, M. K., Kuruc, J. D., & Archin, N. M. (2015). Precise quantitation of the latent HIV-1 reservoir: Implications for eradication strategies. *The Journal of Infectious Diseases*, *212*(9), 1361–1365.

Czudnochowski, N., Bösken, C. A., & Geyer, M. (2012). Serine-7 but not serine-5 phosphorylation primes RNA polymerase II CTD for P-TEFb recognition. *Nature Communications*, *3*(1), 1–12.

Dahabieh, M. S., Battivelli, E., & Verdin, E. (2015). Understanding HIV latency: The road to an HIV cure. *Annual Review of Medicine*, *66*, 407–421.

Darcis, G., Bouchat, S., Kula, A., Van Driessche, B., Delacourt, N., Vanhulle, C., & Van Lint, C. (2017). Reactivation capacity by latency-reversing agents ex vivo correlates with the size of the HIV-1 reservoir. *AIDS*, *31*(2), 181–189.

Davey, R. T., Bhat, N., Yoder, C., Chun, T. W., Metcalf, J. A., Dewar, R., & Lane, H. C. (1999). HIV-1 and T cell dynamics after interruption of highly active antiretroviral therapy (HAART) in patients with a history of sustained viral suppression. *Proceedings of the National Academy of Sciences*, *96*(26), 15109–15114.

Deeks, S. G. (2012). Shock and kill. *Nature*, *487*(7408), 439–440.

Díaz, L., Martínez-Bonet, M., Sánchez, J., Fernández-Pineda, A., Jiménez, J. L., Muñoz, E., & Muñoz-Fernández, M. Á. (2015). Bryostatin activates HIV-1 latent expression in human astrocytes through a PKC and NF-κB-dependent mechanism. *Scientific Reports*, *5*(1), 1–12.

Divsalar, D. N., Simoben, C. V., Schonhofer, C., Richard, K., Sippl, W., Ntie-Kang, F., & Tietjen, I. (2020). Novel histone deacetylase inhibitors and HIV-1 latency-reversing agents identified by large-scale virtual screening. *Frontiers in Pharmacology*, *11*, 905.

Doyon, G., Zerbato, J., Mellors, J. W., & Sluis-Cremer, N. (2013). Disulfiram reactivates latent HIV-1 expression through depletion of the phosphatase and tensin homolog. *AIDS*, *27*(2), F7–F11.

Elliott, J. H., McMahon, J. H., Chang, C. C., Lee, S. A., Hartogensis, W., Bumpus, N., & Lewin, S. R. (2015). Short-term administration of disulfiram for reversal of latent HIV infection: A phase 2 dose-escalation study. *The Lancet HIV*, *2*(12), e520–e529.

Fun, A., Mok, H. P., Wills, M. R., & Lever, A. M. (2017). A highly reproducible quantitative viral outgrowth assay for the measurement of the replication-competent latent HIV-1 reservoir. *Scientific Reports*, *7*, 43231.

Garber, M. E., Wei, P., KewalRamani, V. N., Mayall, T. P., Herrmann, C. H., Rice, A. P., & Jones, K. A. (1998). The interaction between HIV-1 TAT and human cyclin T1 requires zinc and a critical cysteine residue that is not conserved in the murine CycT1 protein. *Genes & Development*, *12*(22), 3512–3527.

Grau-Expósito, J., Serra-Peinado, C., Miguel, L., Navarro, J., Curran, A., Burgos, J., Ocaña, I., Ribera, E., Torrella, A., Planas, B., Badía, R., Castellví, J., Falcó, V., Crespo, M., & Buzon, M. J. (2017). A novel single-cell FISH-flow assay identifies effector memory CD4+ T cells as a major niche for HIV-1 transcription in HIV-infected patients. *mBio*, *8*(4), e00876-17.

Honeycutt, J. B., Thayer, W. O., Baker, C. E., Ribeiro, R. M., Lada, S. M., Cao, Y., & Garcia, J. V. (2017). HIV persistence in tissue macrophages of humanized myeloid-only mice during antiretroviral therapy. *Nature Medicine*, *23*(5), 638–643.

Jiang, G., Mendes, E. A., Kaiser, P., Sankaran-Walters, S., Tang, Y., Weber, M. G., & Dandekar, S. (2014). Reactivation of HIV latency by a newly modified Ingenol derivative via protein kinase Cδ–NF-κB signaling. *AIDS (London, England)*, *28*(11), 1555.

Khan, M. A., Gupta, K. K., & Singh, S. K. (2020). A review on pharmacokinetics properties of antiretroviral drugs to treat HIV-1 infections. *Current Computer-aided Drug Design*, *17*, 1–15.

Kharsany, A. B., & Karim, Q. A. (2016). HIV infection and AIDS in sub-Saharan Africa: Current status, challenges and opportunities. *The Open AIDS Journal*, *10*, 34.

Kwon, K. J., Timmons, A. E., Sengupta, S., Simonetti, F. R., Zhang, H., Hoh, R., & Siliciano, R. F. (2020). Different human resting memory CD4+ T cell subsets show similar low inducibility of latent HIV-1 proviruses. *Science Translational Medicine*, *12*(528).

Kim, Y., Anderson, J. L., & Lewin, S. R. (2018). Getting the "Kill" into "Shock and Kill": strategies to eliminate latent HIV. *Cell Host & Microbe*, *23*(1), 14–26.

Kim, Y. K., Bourgeois, C. F., Isel, C., Churcher, M. J., & Karn, J. (2002). Phosphorylation of the RNA polymerase II carboxyl-terminal domain by CDK9 is directly responsible for human immunodeficiency virus type 1 TAT-activated transcriptional elongation. *Molecular and Cellular Biology*, *22*(13): 4622–4637.

Kurnaeva, M. A., Sheval, E. V., Musinova, Y. R., & Vassetzky, Y. S. (2019). TAT basic domain: A "Swiss army knife" of HIV-1 TAT? *Reviews in Medical Virology*, *29*(2), e2031.

Kwak, H., & Lis, J. T. (2013). Control of transcriptional elongation. *Annual Review of Genetics*, *47*, 483–508.

Laird, G. M., Rosenbloom, D. I., Lai, J., Siliciano, R. F., & Siliciano, J. D. (2016). Measuring the frequency of latent HIV-1 in resting $CD4^+$ T cells using a limiting dilution coculture assay. *Methods in Molecular Biology (Clifton, N.J.)*, *1354*, 239–253.

Li, L., Dahiya, S., Kortagere, S., Aiamkitsumrit, B., Cunningham, D., Pirrone, V., Nonnemacher, M. R., & Wigdahl, B. (2012). Impact of TAT genetic variation on HIV-1 disease. *Advances in Virology*, *2012*, 123605.

Li, Z., Guo, J., Wu, Y., & Zhou, Q. (2013). The BET bromodomain inhibitor JQ1 activates HIV latency through antagonizing Brd4 inhibition of TAT-transactivation. *Nucleic Acids Research*, *41*(1), 277–287.

Lichterfeld, M. (2020). Reactivation of latent HIV moves shock-and-kill treatments forward. *Nature*, *578*(7793), 42–43.

Lin, X., Taube, R., Fujinaga, K., & Peterlin, B. M. (2002). P-TEFb containing cyclin K and Cdk9 can activate transcription via RNA. *The Journal of Biological Chemistry*, *277*(19), 16873–16878.

Lu, P., Qu, X., Shen, Y., Jiang, Z., Wang, P., Zeng, H., & Zhu, H. (2016). The BET inhibitor OTX015 reactivates latent HIV-1 through P-TEFb. *Scientific Reports*, *6*(1), 1–13.

Luo, Z., Li, Z., Martin, L., Hu, Z., Wu, H., Wan, Z., & Jiang, W. (2017). Increased natural killer cell activation in HIV-infected immunologic non-responders correlates with CD4+ T cell recovery after antiretroviral therapy and viral suppression. *PLoS One*, *12*(1), e0167640.

Mahmoudi, T., Parra, M., Vries, R. G., Kauder, S. E., Verrijzer, C. P., Ott, M., & Verdin, E. (2006). The SWI/SNF chromatin-remodeling complex is a cofactor for TAT transactivation of the HIV promoter. *Journal of Biological Chemistry*, *281*(29), 19960–19968.

Margolis, D. M., Garcia, J. V., Hazuda, D. J., & Haynes, B. F. (2016). Latency reversal and viral clearance to cure HIV-1. *Science*, *353*(6297).

Márquez, N., Calzado, M. A., Sánchez-Duffhues, G., Pérez, M., Minassi, A., Pagani, A., & Muñoz, E. (2008). Differential effects of phorbol-13-monoesters on human immunodeficiency virus reactivation. *Biochemical Pharmacology*, *75*(6), 1370–1380.

Marzio, G., Tyagi, M., Gutierrez, M. I., & Giacca, M. (1998). HIV-1 TAT transactivator recruits p300 and CREB-binding protein histone acetyltransferases to the viral promoter. *Proceedings of the National Academy of Sciences*, *95*(23), 13519–13524.

Mousseau, G., & Valente, S. T. (2016). Didehydro-cortistatin A: A new player in HIV-therapy? *Expert Review of Anti-infective Therapy*, *14*(2), 145–148.

Nguyen, K., Das, B., Dobrowolski, C., & Karn, J. (2017). Multiple histone lysine methyltransferases are required for the establishment and maintenance of HIV-1 latency. *MBio*, *8*(1), e00133-17.

Nikolai, B. C., & Feng, Q. (2017). HIV latency gets a new Histone mark. *Cell Host & Microbe*, *21*(5), 549–550.

Pardons, M., Fromentin, R., Pagliuzza, A., Routy, J. P., & Chomont, N. (2019). Latency-reversing agents induce differential responses in distinct memory CD4 T cell subsets in individuals on antiretroviral therapy. *Cell Reports*, *29*(9), 2783–2795.

Peterlin, B. M., & Price, D. H. (2006). Controlling the elongation phase of transcription with P-TEFb. *Molecular Cell*, *23*(3), 297–305.

Palmer, C. S., & Crowe, S. M. (2014). Panobinostat clinical trial highlights the challenges towards an HIV cure. *The Lancet HIV*, *1*(3), e103.

Panwar, U., Chandra, I., Selvaraj, C., & Singh, S. K. (2019). Current computational approaches for the development of anti-HIV inhibitors: An overview. *Current Pharmaceutical Design*, *25*, 3390–3405.

Panwar, U., & Singh, S. K. (2021). In silico virtual screening of potent inhibitor to hamper the interaction between HIV-1 integrase and LEDGF/p75 interaction using E-pharmacophore modeling, molecular docking, and dynamics simulations. *Computational Biology and Chemistry*, *93*, 107509.

Procopio, F. A., Fromentin, R., Kulpa, D. A., Brehm, J. H., Bebin, A. G., Strain, M. C., Richman, D. D., O'Doherty, U., Palmer, S., Hecht, F. M., Hoh, R., Barnard, R. J., Miller, M. D., Hazuda, D. J., Deeks, S. G., Sékaly, R. P., & Chomont, N. (2015).

A novel assay to measure the magnitude of the inducible viral reservoir in HIV-infected individuals. *EBioMedicine*, *2*(8), 874–883.

Rasmussen, T. A., Søgaard, O. S., Brinkmann, C., Wightman, F., Lewin, S. R., Melchjorsen, J., & Tolstrup, M. (2013). Comparison of HDAC inhibitors in clinical development: Effect on HIV production in latently infected cells and T-cell activation. *Human Vaccines & Immunotherapeutics*, 9(5), 993–1001.

Rasmussen, T. A., Tolstrup, M., Brinkmann, C. R., Olesen, R., Erikstrup, C., Solomon, A., & Søgaard, O. S. (2014). Panobinostat, a histone deacetylase inhibitor, for latent-virus reactivation in HIV-infected patients on suppressive antiretroviral therapy: A phase 1/2, single group, clinical trial. *The Lancet HIV*, *1*(1), e13–e21.

Razooky, B. S., Pai, A., Aull, K., Rouzine, I. M., & Weinberger, L. S. (2015). A hardwired HIV latency program. *Cell*, *160*(5), 990–1001.

Rice, A. P. (2017). The HIV-1 TAT protein: Mechanism of action and target for HIV-1 cure strategies. *Current Pharmaceutical Design*, *23*(28), 4098–4102.

Routy, J. P., Tremblay, C. L., Angel, J. B., Trottier, B., Rouleau, D., Baril, J. G., & Boulassel, M. R. (2012). Valproic acid in association with highly active antiretroviral therapy for reducing systemic HIV-1 reservoirs: Results from a multicentre randomized clinical study. *HIV Medicine*, *13*(5), 291–296.

Shao, Y., & Williamson, C. (2012). The HIV-1 epidemic: Low-to middle-income countries. *Cold Spring Harbor Perspectives in Medicine*, *2*(3), a007187.

Shojania, S., & O'Neil, J. D. (2006). HIV-1 TAT is a natively unfolded protein: The solution conformation and dynamics of reduced HIV-1 TAT-(1–72) by NMR spectroscopy. *Journal of Biological Chemistry*, *281*(13), 8347–8356.

Siliciano, R. F., & Greene, W. C. (2011). HIV latency. *Cold Spring Harbor Perspectives in Medicine*, *1*(1), a007096.

Tahirov, T. H., Babayeva, N. D., Varzavand, K., Cooper, J. J., Sedore, S. C., & Price, D. H. (2010). Crystal structure of HIV-1 TAT complexed with human P-TEFb. *Nature*, *465*(7299), 747–751.

Timilsina, U., & Gaur, R. (2016). Modulation of apoptosis and viral latency — An axis to be well understood for successful cure of human immunodeficiency virus. *The Journal of General Virology*, *97*(4), 813–824.

Turner, A. M. W., & Margolis, D. M. (2017). Focus: Infectious diseases: Chromatin regulation and the histone code in HIV LATENCY. *The Yale Journal of Biology and Medicine*, *90*(2), 229.

Tyagi, M., Pearson, R. J., & Karn, J. (2010). Establishment of HIV latency in primary CD4+ cells is due to epigenetic transcriptional silencing and P-TEFb restriction. *Journal of Virology*, *84*(13), 6425–6437.

Walker-Sperling, V. E., Pohlmeyer, C. W., Tarwater, P. M., & Blankson, J. N. (2016). The effect of latency reversal agents on primary CD8+ T cells: Implications for Shock and Kill strategies for human immunodeficiency virus eradication. *EBioMedicine*, *8*, 217–229.

Williams, M. E., Zulu, S. S., Stein, D. J., Joska, J. A., & Naudé, P. J. W. (2020). Signatures of HIV-1 subtype B and C TAT proteins and their effects in the neuropathogenesis of HIV-associated neurocognitive impairments. *Neurobiology of Disease*, *136*, 104701.

Williams, S. A., Chen, L. F., Kwon, H., Fenard, D., Bisgrove, D., Verdin, E., & Greene, W. C. (2004). Prostratin antagonizes HIV latency by activating NF-κB. *Journal of Biological Chemistry*, *279*(40), 42008–42017.

Wei, D. G., Chiang, V., Fyne, E., Balakrishnan, M., Barnes, T., Graupe, M., & Cihlar, T. (2014). Histone deacetylase inhibitor romidepsin induces HIV expression in CD4 T cells from patients on suppressive antiretroviral therapy at concentrations achieved by clinical dosing. *PLoS Pathogens*, *10*(4), e1004071.

Wightman, F., Lu, H. K., Solomon, A. E., Saleh, S., Harman, A. N., Cunningham, A. L., & Lewin, S. R. (2013). EntinosTAT is a histone deacetylase inhibitor selective for class 1 histone deacetylases and activates HIV production from latently infected primary T cells. *AIDS (London, England)*, *27*(18), 2853.

Yadav, A., & Singh, S. K. (2003). Pharmacophoric features of nucleosidic HIV-1RT inhibitors. *Bioorganic & Medicinal Chemistry*, *11*(8), 1801–1807.

Yadav, A., & Singh, S. K. (2005). Common binding mode for structurally and chemically diverse non-nucleosidic HIV-1RT inhibitors. *Journal of Molecular Structure: THEOCHEM*, *723*(1–3), 205–209.

Yang, Z., Zhu, Q., Luo, K., & Zhou, Q. (2001). The 7SK small nuclear RNA inhibits the CDK9/cyclin T1 kinase to control transcription. *Nature*, *414*(6861), 317–322.

Yukl, S., Pillai, S., Li, P., Chang, K., Pasutti, W., Ahlgren, C., Havlir, D., Strain, M., Günthard, H., Richman, D., Rice, A. P., Daar, E., Little, S., & Wong, J. K. (2009). Latently-infected CD4+ T cells are enriched for HIV-1 TAT variants with impaired transactivation activity. *Virology*, *387*(1), 98–108.

Zhang, J., Tamilarasu, N., Hwang, S., Garber, M. E., Huq, I., Jones, K. A., & Rana, T. M. (2000). HIV-1 TAR RNA enhances the interaction between TAT and cyclin T1. *Journal of Biological Chemistry*, *275*(44), 34314–34319.

https://doi.org/10.1142/9789811254796_0004

4 Therapeutic Target Identification and Evaluation using Machine Learning

Sreetama Das[†,‡], Kavyashree Manjunath[§], Ansuman Biswas[¶] and Kanagaraj Sekar[*,||]

[†]*Robert Bosch Engineering and Business Solutions, Bangalore, India*
[‡]*GSK, India*
[§]*Centre for Chemical Biology and Therapeutics, Institute for Stem Cell Science and Regenerative Medicine, Bangalore, India*
[¶]*Simons Centre for the Study of Living Machines, National Centre for Biological Sciences, Bangalore, India*
[||]*Computational Data Sciences, Indian Institute of Science, Bangalore, India*

Abstract

The challenges and failures in the drug discovery process in different stages not only delay the discovery but also increase the average expenses in this. Finding the suitable druggable target is not easy as on an average a drug may bind with at least nine protein targets. Technological developments lead to explosion of data and human intervention is not possible to analyse and choose the best. High speed computers along with fast analyses using Artificial intelligence and Machine learning are the only alternatives to overcome this complicated problem. This chapter mainly deals with the utilisation of machine learning models in

*Corresponding author: e-mail: sekar@iisc.ac.in

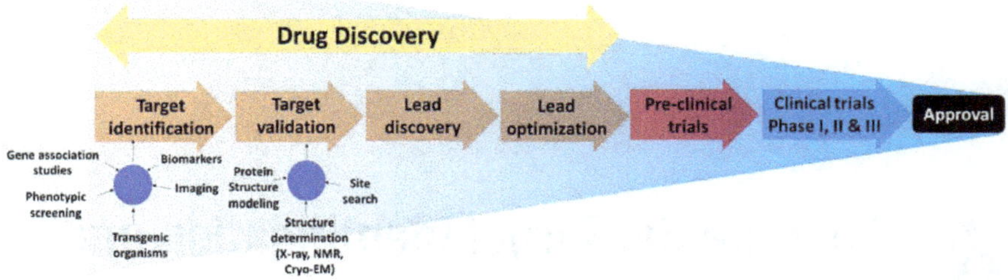

Fig. 1 Stages of drug development.

drug design and development pipeline , especially in the identification of targets and evaluation

1. Introduction

Drug discovery pipelines have typically been affected by lengthy development times and high costs, with average expenses of approximately 2.6 billion US dollars and taking up to 12 years to reach patients (Chan *et al.*, 2019). This can be attributed to the challenges and failures arising in different stages of the drug development process (**Fig. 1**) (Maia *et al.*, 2020; Waring *et al.*, 2015), namely, in appropriate target identification, lead generation and optimization, and finally clinical trials (Hingorani *et al.*, 2019). The first key step in drug development involves the identification of the therapeutic target molecule, typically a protein but could also be nucleic acids (Holt *et al.*, 2011; Yu *et al.*, 2020). The target should satisfy several properties like a proven role in causing disease, be druggable (i.e., can be modulated by a drug), amenable to high-throughput screening, and be modulated without adverse effects (Gashaw *et al.*, 2011). Partial availability of knowledge about disease biology at the molecular level, and the infeasibility of experimentally evaluating the entire druggable proteome make target selection such a daunting task. The emergence of omics technologies has led to an explosion of data on gene expression profiles, gene regulatory networks, protein–protein interaction, and so on. Effectively analyzing these data to identify biologically relevant patterns is key to identifying good drug targets. Post the identification of the therapeutic target, the drug design process can follow either the structure-based or ligand-based methods (Sliwoski *et al.*, 2014). In structure-based drug design, prior knowledge of the three-dimensional (3D) structure of the target protein is required. Chemical libraries of ligand molecules are screened, based on shape and charge complementarity of the target molecule and the ligand, to identify "hits" — potential molecules which can bind to the target. These hits are further screened to identify "leads" which can inhibit the function of the target upon binding. On the other hand, ligand-based drug design strategy is preferred in the absence of structural data. Prior knowledge of known binders to a target molecule is utilized to design new leads using pharmacophore modeling or quantitative structure–activity relationship (Sliwoski *et al.*, 2014; Yang, 2010). The lead identification stage is followed by several iterations of optimization of the molecules, and validation through *in vitro* and *in vivo* studies, to generate compounds with favorable physicochemical and pharmacokinetic properties. The candidate molecules from this stage undergo animal testing for toxicity and other adverse effects, and only the best candidates proceed to clinical trials for further tests of safety and efficacy in humans. Evidently, the drug discovery process is complex and several of the lead molecules fail at different stages of the pipeline, thereby making it a costly affair.

Rapid developments in computing power, memory storage, and algorithms have facilitated the storage, retrieval, and computational analyses of the vast amounts of data generated from high-throughput experiments and those deposited into open-access scientific databases. Such *in silico* analyses provide cost savings in the drug development pipeline through a reduction in the number of expensive experiments conducted, and have been employed for modeling the 3D structures of target molecules (Moult *et al.*, 2018), sampling the target protein conformational space to account for structural flexibility and identify allosteric binding sites or cryptic pockets (Davis & Baker, 2009; Hernández-

Rodríguez *et al.*, 2016), performing multiscale simulations on large spatiotemporal scales (Amaro & Mulholland, 2018), virtual screening of compound databases, and *de novo* drug design (Maia *et al.*, 2020; Sliwoski *et al.*, 2014). An attractive alternative to drug discovery is the use of drug repurposing (Pushpakom *et al.*, 2019), wherein new therapeutic uses are identified for approved or investigational drugs. Here too, *in silico* approaches play a key role in identifying the candidate molecule for the chosen disease. Well-known examples include Minoxidil (an antihypertensive vasodilator repurposed to treat hair loss; Abels & Soeberdt, 2019), aspirin (nonsteroidal anti-inflammatory drug repurposed for treating cardiovascular and cerebrovascular diseases; Montinari *et al.*, 2019), sildenafil (antihypertensive repositioned to treat erectile dysfunction; Ashburn & Thor, 2004), and so on. Such an approach reduces the time and cost of drug development and the risk of failure during clinical trials due to prior safety assessments.

The huge volumes, variety, and complexity of the data undergoing analysis in the drug development pipeline make it a particularly suitable avenue for the application of machine learning techniques. Machine learning involves training a computer algorithm to learn patterns from data in an automated manner, without the specification of explicit rules by humans. Recent advancements in graphics processing unit technology and the explosion of "Big Data" have led to a renewed interest in machine learning and, in particular, its subfield deep learning (Hinton *et al.*, 2012; Hirschberg & Manning, 2015; LeCun *et al.*, 2015; Russakovsky *et al.*, 2015). This has profoundly impacted several domains of healthcare like genomics (Angermueller *et al.*, 2016; Hampel *et al.*, 2012; Jones *et al.*, 2017), medical imaging-based diagnostics (Abedin *et al.*, 2019; Dong *et al.*, 2017; Ertosun & Rubin, 2015; Esteva *et al.*, 2017; Gulshan *et al.*, 2016; Litjens *et al.*, 2016, 2017; Liu *et al.*, 2017; Ortiz *et al.*, 2016; Paluru *et al.*, 2021; Pereira *et al.*, 2016; Pinaya *et al.*, 2016; Van Grinsven *et al.*, 2016; Varshni *et al.*, 2019; Yahalomi *et al.*, 2019), point-of-care diagnostics, wearables, and implantables (An *et al.*, 2021; Benjamens *et al.*, 2020; Witt *et al.*, 2019; Yang, 2014), assistive technologies (Poggi & Mattoccia, 2016), medical informatics (Artemov *et al.*, 2016; Ithapu *et al.*, 2015; Jagannatha & Yu, 2016; Katzman *et al.*, 2018; Miotto *et al.*, 2016; Wickramasinghe, 2017), and public health research (Zhao *et al.*, 2015; Zou *et al.*, 2016). While the pharmaceutical industry has been a relatively late adopter of machine learning (ML), the aforementioned advances have provided an impetus to its use in different stages of the drug development pipeline.

This chapter discusses the advances made by machine learning, including state-of-the-art techniques, in therapeutic protein target identification and the early stages of structure-based drug design (target structure modeling and binding pocket identification). We also discuss the challenges of applying machine learning in drug design and possible future directions. Given the breadth of the field, there are separate reviews describing the application of machine learning for the target identification phase (Kandoi *et al.*, 2015), protein structure prediction (Gao *et al.*, 2020; Kandathil *et al.*, 2019; Kuhlman & Bradley, 2019; Torrisi *et al.*, 2020; Zhang, 2020), ligand binding site prediction (Zhao *et al.*, 2020) or structure-based drug design (Batool *et al.*, 2019; Lipinski *et al.*, 2019; Maia *et al.*, 2020), but none on the use of machine learning for protein structure modeling from experimental data. The present chapter addresses this lacuna and also provides a holistic view of techniques used to enhance the understanding of the target molecule, with a view to introducing the readers to the gamut of recent developments in this field.

2. Brief Background to Machine Learning and Deep Learning

Given the rapid developments in the field of machine learning and the diverse terms used to describe them in common parlance [artificial intelligence (AI), machine learning, and deep learning, to name a few], we start with descriptions of the context behind the usage of these different terms. AI focuses on devising machines with "human-like intelligence" for problem solving. While general AI is hard to implement, there are far more examples of "narrow

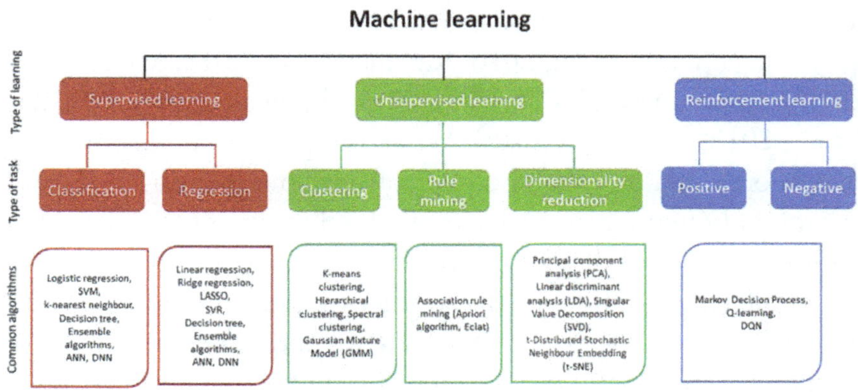

Fig. 2 Different types of machine learning models.

AI," or "weak AI," which simulate human-like intelligence for solving well-defined tasks. Much of this is powered by the field of machine learning (ML) and involves the use of algorithms which can "learn" from data and then detect patterns or predict future instances, without being explicitly programmed via rules to do so. The predictive performance of ML algorithms improves with the quality and quantity of data available. Such a technique is useful when the underlying relationship among the predictor variables (i.e., the independent variables or input features) and the response variable (the dependent variable or target variable to be determined) is not known and cannot be easily expressed as a mathematical function.

There are three main types of ML techniques — supervised, unsupervised, and reinforcement learning (**Fig. 2**). In supervised learning, the input data have paired sets of values of the independent and dependent variables (also referred to as "features" and "response," respectively), and the model can be trained to predict future instances of the dependent variable which can be either a category (classification) or a continuous variable (regression). On the other hand, unsupervised learning is used to discover patterns and spatially order the data points based on their similarities or differences, when the values of the response variable are not available in the input data (commonly referred to as unlabeled data). In practice, data labeling is an expensive task and the amount of unlabeled data often exceeds the labeled data available. Hence, a semi-supervised learning approach is used, which is a combination of unsupervised learning to group the data and supervised learning to infer the labels of the unlabeled data. Finally, in reinforcement learning, a system of rewards and penalties is employed to train the ML model, through trial and error, to make a sequence of decisions to achieve its goal in an uncertain and potentially complex environment. The outcome is the development of decision-making capability under specified constraints (task-associated rewards and penalties); no response variable is predicted unlike in supervised learning. Several well-known algorithms exist to perform each of these learning tasks. An overview of these ML techniques is provided in **Fig. 2**, and readers are referred to existing literature for a detailed exposition (Yang *et al.*, 2019).

A particularly interesting ML algorithm is the artificial neural network (ANN), which is structured as layers of interconnected nodes and is inspired by how the brain functions using its network of neurons. ANNs can be used to model complex underlying relationships in the data by increasing the number of nodes per layer and the number of layers in the network. This has given rise to the field of deep learning (DL) (Esteva *et al.*, 2019), where multiple layers of nodes are stacked next to each other to create a "deep" neural network (DNN). Such an architecture acts as an automated feature extractor by learning high-level patterns from the data in a hierarchical manner, whereas traditional ML utilizes task-appropriate features as input and thereby requires human intervention. DL algorithms can also accept heterogeneous data types as input, making them particularly suitable for healthcare applications. Another interesting aspect is that the performance of deep learning algorithms continues to improve as the dataset size is increased, in contrast to traditional ML approaches. However, DL algorithms generally require more compute power for data processing and training, compared to classical ML. As a result, recent advancements in computational hardware have driven the development of a wide variety of DNN algorithms (Ravì *et al.*, 2016) that have been applied for complex tasks like image recognition (analyzing images for object classification and pixel-wise image segmentation) and natural language processing (NLP, analyzing text data).

The choice of ML algorithm is driven by the problem to be addressed, as well as the type and amount of data available. A typical machine learning pipeline involves the following steps. First, the data are randomly partitioned into the "train," "validation," and "test" sets. When data are scarce, a technique called *k*-fold cross-validation may also be applied on the training set instead of setting aside a separate validation dataset. Subsequently, the training data samples are scaled and the same transformations are applied to the samples in the validation and the test sets. The ML algorithm is then trained on the train set and its performance is evaluated on the validation set. Several iterations of this step are performed to "tune" the model, that is, to find the optimal values of the model parameters. A well-tuned model should generalize well to unseen data. Underfitting is said to occur when the model is too simple and performs poorly on both the train and the validation datasets (high error), while an overfitted model is too complex and performs very well on training data (low error) but poorly on the validation data (high error). Overfitting can be taken care of by implementing regularization techniques which penalize the use of excess parameters as model complexity increases. Once the model performance is deemed satisfactory based on its performance during validation, it is evaluated on the independent test set using metrics like root mean square error (for regression problem) or accuracy, precision, recall, and F1-score (for classification). Several open-source software libraries like Scikit-Learn, Keras, TensorFlow, and so on, are now available to implement various steps in an ML pipeline.

3. ML in Drug Target Identification

A typical drug development pipeline involves drug discovery, preclinical and clinical studies, followed by approval (Patrick, 2013). The core of the development process lies in the initial stage of target identification, target validation, lead discovery and its optimization, which plays a critical role in the success of the project and is also the second-most time taking process (~4.5 years) after the clinical trial phase (Paul *et al.*, 2010). The first step, namely, target identification requires knowledge of the role of the target in the disease phenotype. A typical "target" could be any of the biological molecules like enzyme, ion channel receptors, DNA/RNA, metabolites, and so on which are relevant to the disease or pathological condition in question and can interact with drug molecules to modulate or cure the disease state (Imming *et al.*, 2006; Knowles & Gromo, 2003).

Prior to the target identification for a specific disease, it is imperative to diagnose the disease accurately. Statistical analyses of high-throughput clinical data (patients data) provide insights into the changes (upregulation or downregulation) in expression profiles of specific genes, which can be used as biomarkers for detecting disease (skin disease, different cancers, Alzheimer's disease, etc.) (Ashkani & Naidoo, 2016; Fortino *et al.*, 2020; Jin *et al.*, 2021; Su *et al.*, 2020). For example, extracellular glycan expression is altered in cancerous cells due to changes in the gene expression levels of different glycosyltransferase (GTase) enzymes, which are responsible for the biosynthesis of glycans. Machine learning models have been applied on the microarray data of 210 such GTase genes from 1893 cancer samples, to classify cancer types (Ashkani & Naidoo, 2016). A new machine learning-based tool, ECmarker, has also been developed to predict the biomarkers from gene expression data for specific disease phenotypes (Jin *et al.*, 2021).

Approaches like forward genetics, reverse genetics, and chemical-genetic (forward and reverse) screening have also been employed to investigate the specific genes related to a disease (Stockwell, 2000). In the forward genetic approach, a model organism is subjected to randomized mutations, and the phenotypic changes owing to such mutations are studied. Among the observed phenotypes, the ones which are similar to the phenotypes of the diseased state would help to determine the possible mutations which have caused the disease. On the other hand, in reverse genetics, a single gene is mutated to understand its role on the phenotype. In the forward chemical-genetic approach, a library of small molecules is screened for a specific phenotype of interest in a model organism. The compounds eliciting the desired phenotypic change are added to DNA microarrays to identify the gene of interest from changes in expression levels. Finally, in the reverse chemical-genetic approach, a known target is screened using ligands to find the resulting phenotype (Stockwell, 2000).

Both the forward approaches (genetic and chemical) are high-throughput experimental methods, wherein the cells are screened for phenotypic changes arising from the effect of either the gene mutation or the compound, respectively. Imaging techniques like fluorescence microscopy are often used for phenotypic screening, wherein different physical properties of the cell organelles (shape, intensity, texture, staining intensity) and cell viability features are extracted (Caicedo *et al.*, 2017; Grys *et al.*, 2017; Zanella *et al.*, 2010). The scale of such studies has necessitated the use of automated imaging and image-processing methods (Caicedo *et al.*, 2016). Several image analysis tools (e.g., "ilastik," "CellClassifier," etc.) have been developed where machine learning techniques like random forest, deep convolutional neural network (CNN), and support vector machine are utilized to classify the cells based on the phenotypic features (Rämö *et al.*, 2009; Sommer *et al.*, 2011). Post the identification of the target gene from the disease phenotype, efforts are concentrated toward obtaining its sequence and 3D structure to facilitate structure-based drug discovery.

The wealth of information available in different databases (e.g., protein–protein interactions, gene expression data, protein structure coordinates, results from biochemical experiments) as well as in scientific literature makes them potent sources for knowledge mining using computational techniques. The BeFree (Bravo *et al.*, 2015) text mining system, developed to identify relationships between biomedical entities using NLP, has been used to create the DisGeNET (Piñero *et al.*, 2020) database containing a collection of genes and their variants associated with human disease.

Such databases can be used for identifying novel drug targets. Other studies include the use of a decision tree-based classifier (ML algorithm) on a dataset containing the transcription profile, subcellular location, and gene interaction network topological features to predict druggable and morbid genes□ (Costa *et al.*, 2010), and a support vector machine-based classifier to identify genome-wide anticancer drug targets, using mRNA expression data, DNA copy number, and gene activity ranking profile scores□ (Jeon *et al.*, 2014). A recent study has even demonstrated the use of a deep learning model, with features derived from different chemical, genomic, phenotypic, and cellular networks, to identify drug targets (Zeng *et al.*, 2020).

4. ML in Protein Structure Modeling

Post the selection of a target protein, it is important to identify druggable pockets on its surface, which requires its 3D structure. The 3D coordinates of the target molecule can be obtained from either theoretical models or experimental methods like X-ray crystallography, nuclear magnetic resonance, and cryo-electron microscopy (cryoEM). Experimental structure determination is a time-consuming process and has its own challenges (Slabinski *et al.*, 2007), which has spurred the development of computational structure prediction methods. However, prior to determining the 3D structure of a protein, valuable insights can be obtained from its sequence, for example, its secondary structure information, solvent accessibility of residues, backbone dihedral angle, contact map, possible disordered regions, and so on, which are termed as protein structure annotation (PSA) (Torrisi *et al.*, 2020). The PSA attributes can be divided in two categories, namely, one-dimensional (1D) annotations (secondary structure, solvent accessibility) and 2D annotations (contact map, torsional angles, etc.). Both classical ML algorithms (k-Nearest Neighbor, support vector machine, linear regression) (Kuang *et al.*, 2004; Levin, 1997; Li & Pan, 2001) and deep learning-based methods have been employed to predict 1D annotations with high accuracy (Wang, Ma, *et al.*, 2016; Wang, Peng, *et al.*, 2016). Several 2D PSA predictors like β-sheet pairing (Cheng & Baldi, 2005), disulfide bonds (Ceroni *et al.*, 2006), contact maps (Tegge *et al.*, 2009), and multiclass contact maps (Kukic *et al.*, 2014; Wang *et al.*, 2017) have also been developed using DL algorithms like recursive neural networks and deep residual neural networks algorithms.

Protein structure prediction methods are classified into two major categories, namely, "template-based" structure prediction methods like homology modeling and threading, using already available homologous structures (Qu *et al.*, 2009), and "*ab initio*" methods that require a deeper understanding of the principles of protein folding and often involve the use of accurate potential functions (Bonneau & Baker, 2001). Both strategies utilize 1D and 2D PSA for structure predictions. For example, contact maps were utilized as constraints in 3D structure reconstruction (Vassura *et al.*, 2008). Earlier studies have also used different parameters like conservation and correlated mutations, extracted from multiple sequence alignments, to infer contact maps from sequence data (Göbel *et al.*, 1994). Support vector machines, neural networks (Cheng & Baldi, 2007; Fariselli *et al.*, 2001), and, off late, deep learning have aided the process of contact map prediction. The predicted contact maps, secondary structure information, and other PSA are utilized to predict the 3D structure, which is further refined with a reconstruction algorithm by optimizing the energy function and using simulated annealing (Kukic *et al.*, 2014) to generate a relatively accurate 3D model. *Ab initio* modeling has seen a significant advancement in recent years with the DL-based algorithm AlphaFold that used deep learning to predict pairwise residue distance map (as opposed to a contact map) and optimized the resulting potential function to yield a model of protein 3D structure (AlQuraishi, 2019; Senior *et al.*, 2020), and its latest variant AlphaFold2 which achieved accuracies comparable to experimental structures for several test proteins (Jumper *et al.*, 2020).

Despite the recent developments in computational protein fold prediction from sequence, protein structures continue to be also derived experimentally since they provide insights into conformational variability in and around the ligand binding site, its electrostatic properties, functionally important dynamical features, allosteric sites, and other relevant information. Comparative analysis of the structures of homologous proteins also helps in understanding subtle variations in the target residues between pathogenic and non-pathogenic variants. Together, this knowledge helps to narrow down on the target residues for inhibitor design with high specificity. For example, the thymidylate kinase (TMK) enzyme from pox virus has 42% sequence identity with its human homolog. But crystal structures of the human and pox virus TMK enzymes demonstrated crucial differences in dimeric assembly, a feature which was utilized to design inhibitors specific to the viral TMK (Caillat *et al.*, 2008).

Protein structure determination through X-ray crystallography faces a bottleneck in obtaining diffraction quality crystals. Crystallization is an expensive and time-consuming process with an overall low success rate of 2%–10% (Terwilliger *et al.*, 2009). The physical basis of enhancing the crystallizability of a protein is still under study. One of the factors impacting the crystallizability of a protein is protein surface entropy; reducing the surface entropy through site directed mutagenesis can enhance protein crystallizability (Derewenda & Vekilov, 2006). Several studies have attempted to predict the crystallizability of a protein sequence using machine learning (Mizianty & Kurgan, 2011; Wang *et al.*, 2014; Wang, Feng, *et al.*, 2016), wherein several physicochemical features were extracted from the protein sequences and utilized as inputs to train the ML models. A recent study (Elbasir *et al.*, 2019) demonstrated the use of DeepCrystal, a tool based on CNNs, in classifying crystallizable versus non-crystallizable protein sequences. It works with the sequence directly and does not require various physicochemical properties from protein sequences to be provided as feature inputs, and has been demonstrated to outperform other methods.

The search for a suitable crystallization condition that can yield diffraction quality crystals involves several unknown parameters like temperature, pH, buffer, additives, sample concentrations, and types of the solvents. Different combinations of these factors result in hundreds of crystallization conditions, which are to be added to the ultrapure protein solution during every crystallization trial. Moreover, the time required for a chemical cocktail to yield crystals is unknown beforehand. Hence, for every protein, one has to monitor hundreds of crystallization droplets over months through a microscope and investigate if any of them result in a positive outcome. An automated approach to identify protein crystals from negative outcomes (salt crystals, no crystal growth, precipitate) would be helpful in this regard. The Machine Recognition of Crystallization Outcomes (MARCO) database [MAchine Recognition of Crystallization Outcomes (MARCO), 2017] is a source of almost half a million annotated images of crystallization drops and has been utilized for automating the process of protein crystal detection among hundreds of droplets with various outcomes other than protein crystals. A four way classification algorithm, using a deep CNN model and trained on the MARCOS database, has been able to identify the droplets with protein crystals from outliers successfully, with more than 94% of the droplet images from the test dataset being correctly labeled (Bruno *et al.*, 2018). A recent development in this domain is the tool Polo (Holleman *et al.*, 2021), which not only provides CNN-based classification of the droplet images, but also provides the option of comparing the crystallization cocktails by assigning scores to the images.

Post the successful growth of protein crystals, they are irradiated with X-ray beams and the diffraction images are collected for subsequent analysis. Occasionally, the crystallization trials yield microcrystals which are subjected to serial crystallography using X-ray free-electron laser to model the protein structure. Serial crystallography requires the collection of thousands of diffraction images (Bücker *et al.*, 2020) in order to obtain reasonable completeness of the data. The quality of diffraction may differ from one crystal to another, as well as across different orientations of the same crystal. Manually screening these large numbers of images to assess the quality of diffraction is a challenging task. In order to develop an automated image screening method, a new serial crystallography dataset called DiffraNet consisting of approximately 25,000 real and synthetic (generated through simulation) images was generated (Souza *et al.*, 2019) and the performances of multiple ML models (random forest, SVM, and CNN) to classify the images among five classes (blank, no-crystal, weak, good, and strong diffraction patterns) were evaluated on this dataset. The models were trained solely on the synthetic images and tested on both the real and synthetic images. The CNN model (deep learning-based model) performed the best, with classification accuracies of 94.5% and 98.5% on real and synthetic images, respectively.

In the protein structure determination pipeline, the image processing step is succeeded by the calculation of structure factors (SFs) from the intensity values extracted from diffraction images. The electron density map, which is used to interpret the protein's 3D structure, is subsequently computed from the SFs. SF has a phase component which cannot be deduced directly from the intensities computed from diffraction data; the determination of "missing" phases is a classic problem in the field of crystallography (Rupp, 2009). Multiple techniques have been developed to derive phase information. With the available phases and SFs, the electron density map is calculated and the protein chain model is optimized manually, to fit into this density map, with a subsequent refinement step to evaluate how well the model can explain the experimental diffraction data. Many of the steps in the structure determination pipeline are performed manually and require an experienced crystallographer, especially in case of challenging datasets. As a result, machine learning has found utility to improve several steps of this pipeline. For example, a recent study demonstrated the application of Bayesian machine learning in improving the single-wavelength X-ray anomalous diffraction-based phase determination method (Garcia-Bonete & Katona, 2019). ML models have also been applied to automate the density map interpretation (DiMaio *et al.*, 2008) while building the protein model through map tracing. A tool named TEXTAL has been developed (DiMaio *et al.*, 2008; Gopal *et al.*, 2005) which trains a neural network model to identify the location of the backbone and side chain atoms of a protein molecule in a density map, built from a relatively low resolution data (2.2–3.0 □). Finally, deep learning has been used to improve the protein structure refinement process during experimental model building (Hiranuma *et al.*, 2021).

Apart from X-ray crystallography, cryo-EM is another experimental technique to determine protein 3D structure, especially where the molecules are recalcitrant to crystallization. State-of-the-art cryo-EM can even produce high-resolution maps (Nakane *et al.*, 2020). Protein structure determination through cryo-EM requires extensive data analysis and interpretation. Deep learning has been used to assist in several of these steps, for example, in picking a single protein particle from 2D micrograph (Al-Azzawi *et al.*, 2020), predicting the backbone structure (Si *et al.*, 2020), and interpreting protein dynamics (Matsumoto *et al.*, 2021).

5. ML in Protein Binding Site Discovery

After elucidating the 3D structure, identification of the druggable binding pocket on the protein surface is an important step in structure-based drug design. Traditional site discovery methods mostly relied on geometry, evolutionary information, or energy-based features for the identification of ligand binding sites on protein structures (Jiménez *et al.*, 2017). Recent studies have utilized deep learning-based models to identify pockets from either protein structures (Jiménez *et al.*, 2017; Kozlovskii & Popov, 2020; Pu *et al.*, 2019), or sequence (Cui *et al.*, 2019), or identify similar binding pockets in different target proteins (Simonovsky & Meyers, 2020). Apart from pocket identification, a novel deep learning-based tool called Deep Docking was able to carry out accurate docking of billions of small molecules onto multiple target proteins at rapid pace (Gentile *et al.*, 2020). This enables the screening of huge small molecule libraries against target proteins in a short period of time.

6. Challenges

A key challenge in developing supervised ML models is the availability of sufficient, good-quality labeled data (Bender & Cortes-Ciriano, 2021), which is often expensive to obtain. While semi-supervised learning is a possible solution, the implicit assumption is that the unlabeled data follow the same distribution as the labeled data, which may not always be true (Yang *et al.*, 2019). Alternate approaches involve the use of simulated data, augmented data from simple image transformations (rotation, flipping, brightness changes, etc. applied to images) or generated using DL models such as generative adversarial network (Ching *et al.*, 2018), or using text-mining to generate annotations (Dong *et al.*, 2017). However, not all such augmentations will be feasible for different types of biological data. Often, annotated data are available with individual organizations but cannot be shared because of privacy concerns or IP sharing issues. Application of federated learning (Chen *et al.*, 2020; Rieke *et al.*, 2020) in such cases can help develop better models which benefit from the entire data without having to share the data explicitly among the different organizations.

A second challenge is the use of features appropriate to the problem, which largely drives the success of ML approaches. Feature engineering is time-consuming and often driven by the experience of the human researcher working on the problem. Moreover, heavily engineered features, or features derived by neural networks from raw data, are not easily interpretable. While such ML models may yield highly accurate results, the logic behind the prediction is not always evident, leading to hesitancy in their adoption. Hence, the development of explainable or interpretable machine learning techniques is an area of active research (Jiménez-Luna *et al.*, 2020).

A third challenge is the repeatability of results of an ML algorithm on the same dataset, especially with neural networks, because of variations in initial weights, model hyperparameter values, randomization, sequence of training examples, implementation environment, hardware differences, and so on. This has necessitated the development and implementation of tools to track model training metadata (Hartley & Olsson, 2020).

7. Conclusion and Future Direction

The present chapter has described how a plethora of methods utilizing machine learning models have eased early steps of the drug design and development pipeline, especially target identification and evaluation. These efforts not only bring down the cost of drug design, but also save valuable time. While the concepts of machine learning have been in existence for decades, recent technical advancements coupled with the rapid expansion of available biological data have facilitated the application of ML methods to solve some of the long-standing problems in the drug development pipeline. There exists a tremendous potential for the application of these methods to discover drugs against neglected tropical diseases and rare diseases (Winkler, 2021), different cancers (Kadurin *et al.*, 2017), or find new antibiotics (Stokes *et al.*, 2020), thereby strengthening our arsenal against deadly diseases.

References

Abedin, J., Antony, J., McGuinness, K., Moran, K., O'Connor, N. E., Rebholz-Schuhmann, D., & Newell, J. (2019). Predicting knee osteoarthritis severity: Comparative modeling based on patient's data and plain X-ray images. *Scientific Reports*, 9(1), 1–11.

Abels, C., & Soeberdt, M. (2019). Can we teach old drugs new tricks? — Repurposing of neuropharmacological drugs for inflammatory skin diseases. *Experimental Dermatology*, *28*(9), 1002–1009.

Al-Azzawi, A., Ouadou, A., Max, H., Duan, Y., Tanner, J. J., & Cheng, J. (2020). DeepCryoPicker: Fully automated deep neural network for single protein particle picking in cryo-EM. *BMC Bioinformatics*, *21*(1), 1–38.

AlQuraishi, M. (2019). AlphaFold at CASP13. *Bioinformatics*, *35*(22), 4862–4865.

Amaro, R. E., & Mulholland, A. J. (2018). Multiscale methods in drug design bridge chemical and biological complexity in the search for cures. *Nature Reviews Chemistry*, *2*(4), 1–12.

An, R., Huang, Y., Man, Y., Valentine, R. W., Kucukal, E., Goreke, U., Sekyonda, Z., Piccone, C., Owusu-Ansah, A., Ahuja, S., & Little, J. A. (2021). Emerging point-of-care technologies for anemia detection. *Lab on a Chip*, *21*, 1843–1865.

Angermueller, C., Pärnamaa, T., Parts, L., & Stegle, O. (2016). Deep learning for computational biology. *Molecular Systems Biology*, *12*(7), 878.

Artemov, A. V., Putin, E., Vanhaelen, Q., Aliper, A., Ozerov, I. V., & Zhavoronkov, A. (2016). Integrated deep learned transcriptomic and structure-based predictor of clinical trials outcomes. *BioRxiv*, 095653.

Ashburn, T. T., & Thor, K. B. (2004). Drug repositioning: Identifying and developing new uses for existing drugs. *Nature Reviews Drug Discovery*, *3*(8), 673–683.

Ashkani, J., & Naidoo, K. J. (2016). Glycosyltransferase gene expression profiles classify cancer types and propose prognostic subtypes. *Scientific Reports*, *6*(1), 1–8.

Batool, M., Ahmad, B., & Choi, S. (2019). A structure-based drug discovery paradigm. *International Journal of Molecular Sciences*, *20*(11), 2783.

Bender, A., & Cortes-Ciriano, I. (2021). Artificial intelligence in drug discovery: What is realistic, what are illusions? Part 1: Ways to make an impact, and why we are not there yet. *Drug Discovery Today*, *26*, 511–524.

Benjamens, S., Dhunnoo, P., & Meskó, B. (2020). The state of artificial intelligence-based FDA-approved medical devices and algorithms: An online database. *npj Digital Medicine*, *3*(1), 1–8.

Bonneau, R., & Baker, D. (2001). Ab initio protein structure prediction: Progress and prospects. *Annual Review of Biophysics and Biomolecular Structure*, *30*(1), 173–189.

Bravo, À., Piñero, J., Queralt-Rosinach, N., Rautschka, M., & Furlong, L. I. (2015). Extraction of relations between genes and diseases from text and large-scale data analysis: Implications for translational research. *BMC Bioinformatics*, *16*(1), 1–17.

Bruno, A. E., Charbonneau, P., Newman, J., Snell, E. H., So, D. R., Vanhoucke, V., Watkins, C. J., Williams, S., & Wilson, J. (2018). Classification of crystallization outcomes using deep convolutional neural networks. *PLoS One*, *13*(6), e0198883.

Bücker, R., Hogan-Lamarre, P., Mehrabi, P., Schulz, E. C., Bultema, L. A., Gevorkov, Y., Brehm, W., Yefanov, O., Oberthür, D., Kassier, G. H., & Miller, R. D. (2020).

Serial protein crystallography in an electron microscope. *Nature Communications*, *11*(1), 1–8.

Caicedo, J. C., Cooper, S., Heigwer, F., Warchal, S., Qiu, P., Molnar, C., Vasilevich, A. S., Barry, J. D., Bansal, H. S., Kraus, O., & Wawer, M. (2017). Data-analysis strategies for image-based cell profiling. *Nature Methods*, *14*(9), 849–863.

Caicedo, J. C., Singh, S., & Carpenter, A. E. (2016). Applications in image-based profiling of perturbations. *Current Opinion in Biotechnology*, *39*, 134–142.

Caillat, C., Topalis, D., Agrofoglio, L. A., Pochet, S., Balzarini, J., Deville-Bonne, D., & Meyer, P. (2008). Crystal structure of poxvirus thymidylate kinase: An unexpected dimerization has implications for antiviral therapy. *Proceedings of the National Academy of Sciences*, *105*(44), 16900–16905.

Ceroni, A., Passerini, A., Vullo, A., & Frasconi, P. (2006). DISULFIND: A disulfide bonding state and cysteine connectivity prediction server. *Nucleic Acids Research*, *34*(suppl_2), W177–W181.

Chan, H. C. S., Shan, H., Dahoun, T., Vogel, H., & Yuan, S. (2019). Advancing drug discovery via artificial intelligence. *Trends in Pharmacological Sciences*. doi:10.1016/j.tips.2019.06.004

Chen, S., Xue, D., Chuai, G., Yang, Q., & Liu, Q. (2020). FL-QSAR: A federated learning based QSAR prototype for collaborative drug discovery. *Bioinformatics, 36*(22–23), 5492–5498.

Cheng, J., & Baldi, P. (2005). Three-stage prediction of protein β-sheets by neural networks, alignments and graph algorithms. *Bioinformatics*, *21*(suppl_1), i75–i84.

Cheng, J., & Baldi, P. (2007). Improved residue contact prediction using support vector machines and a large feature set. *BMC Bioinformatics*, *8*(1), 1–9.

Ching, T., Himmelstein, D. S., Beaulieu-Jones, B. K., Kalinin, A. A., Do, B. T., Way, G. P., … & Greene, C. S. (2018). Opportunities and obstacles for deep learning in biology and medicine. *Journal of the Royal Society Interface*, *15*(141), 20170387.

Costa, P. R., Acencio, M. L., & Lemke, N. (2010, December). A machine learning approach for genome-wide prediction of morbid and druggable human genes based on systems-level data. *BMC Genomics*, *11*(5), 1–15.

Cui, Y., Dong, Q., Hong, D., & Wang, X. (2019). Predicting protein-ligand binding residues with deep convolutional neural networks. *BMC Bioinformatics*, *20*(1), 1–12.

Davis, I. W., & Baker, D. (2009). RosettaLigand docking with full ligand and receptor flexibility. *Journal of Molecular Biology*, *385*(2), 381–392.

Derewenda, Z. S., & Vekilov, P. G. (2006). Entropy and surface engineering in protein crystallization. *Acta Crystallographica Section D: Biological Crystallography*, *62*(1), 116–124.

DiMaio, F., Soni, A., & Shavlik, J. (2008). Machine learning in structural biology: Interpreting 3D protein images. In *Introduction to machine learning and bioinformatics* (pp. 237–276). Chapman & Hall/CRC Press.

Dong, Y., Pan, Y., Zhang, J., & Xu, W. (2017, July). Learning to read chest X-ray images from 16000+ examples using CNN. In *2017 IEEE/ACM international conference on connected health: Applications, systems and engineering technologies (CHASE)* (pp. 51–57). IEEE.

Elbasir, A., Moovarkumudalvan, B., Kunji, K., Kolatkar, P. R., Mall, R., & Bensmail, H. (2019). DeepCrystal: A deep learning framework for sequence-based protein crystallization prediction. *Bioinformatics*, *35*(13), 2216–2225.

Ertosun, M. G., & Rubin, D. L. (2015). Automated grading of gliomas using deep learning in digital pathology images: A modular approach with ensemble of convolutional neural networks. In *AMIA annual symposium proceedings* (Vol. 2015, p. 1899). American Medical Informatics Association.

Esteva, A., Kuprel, B., Novoa, R. A., Ko, J., Swetter, S. M., Blau, H. M., & Thrun, S. (2017). Dermatologist-level classification of skin cancer with deep neural networks. *Nature*, *542*(7639), 115–118.

Esteva, A., Robicquet, A., Ramsundar, B., Kuleshov, V., DePristo, M., Chou, K., Cui, C., Corrado, G., Thrun, S., & Dean, J. (2019). A guide to deep learning in healthcare. *Nature Medicine*, *25*(1), 24–29.

Fariselli, P., Olmea, O., Valencia, A., & Casadio, R. (2001). Prediction of contact maps with neural networks and correlated mutations. *Protein Engineering*, *14*(11), 835–843.

Fortino, V., Wisgrill, L., Werner, P., Suomela, S., Linder, N., Jalonen, E., Suomalainen, A., Marwah, V., Kero, M., Pesonen, M., & Lundin, J. (2020). Machine-learning-driven biomarker discovery for the discrimination between allergic and irritant contact dermatitis. *Proceedings of the National Academy of Sciences*, *117*(52), 33474–33485.

Gao, W., Mahajan, S. P., Sulam, J., & Gray, J. J. (2020). Deep learning in protein structural modeling and design. *Patterns*, 100142.

Garcia-Bonete, M. J., & Katona, G. (2019). Bayesian machine learning improves single-wavelength anomalous diffraction phasing. *Acta Crystallographica Section A: Foundations and Advances*, *75*(6), 851–860.

Gashaw, I., Ellinghaus, P., Sommer, A., & Asadullah, K. (2011). What makes a good drug target? *Drug Discovery Today*, *16*(23–24), 1037–1043.

Gentile, F., Agrawal, V., Hsing, M., Ton, A. T., Ban, F., Norinder, U., Gleave, M. E., & Cherkasov, A. (2020). Deep docking: A deep learning platform for augmentation of structure based drug discovery. *ACS Central Science*, *6*(6), 939–949.

Kandoi, G., Acencio, M. L., & Lemke, N. (2015). Prediction of druggable proteins using machine learning and systems biology: A mini-review. *Frontiers in Physiology*, *6*, 366.

Katzman, J. L., Shaham, U., Cloninger, A., Bates, J., Jiang, T., & Kluger, Y. (2018). DeepSurv: Personalized treatment recommender system using a Cox proportional hazards deep neural network. *BMC Medical Research Methodology*, *18*(1), 1–12.

Knowles, J., & Gromo, G. (2003). Target selection in drug discovery. *Nature Reviews Drug Discovery*, *2*(1), 63–69.

Kozlovskii, I., & Popov, P. (2020). Spatiotemporal identification of druggable binding sites using deep learning. *Communications Biology*, *3*(1), 1–12.

Kuang, R., Leslie, C. S., & Yang, A. S. (2004). Protein backbone angle prediction with machine learning approaches. *Bioinformatics*, *20*(10), 1612–1621.

Kuhlman, B., & Bradley, P. (2019). Advances in protein structure prediction and design. *Nature Reviews Molecular Cell Biology*, *20*(11), 681–697.

Kukic, P., Mirabello, C., Tradigo, G., Walsh, I., Veltri, P., & Pollastri, G. (2014). Toward an accurate prediction of inter-residue distances in proteins using 2D recursive neural networks. *BMC Bioinformatics*, *15*(1), 1–15.

LeCun, Y., Bengio, Y., & Hinton, G. (2015). Deep learning. *Nature*, *521*(7553), 436–444.

Levin, J. M. (1997). Exploring the limits of nearest neighbour secondary structure prediction. *Protein Engineering*, *10*(7), 771–776.

Li, X., & Pan, X. M. (2001). New method for accurate prediction of solvent accessibility from protein sequence. *Proteins: Structure, function, and bioinformatics*, *42*(1), 1–5.

Lipinski, C. F., Maltarollo, V. G., Oliveira, P. R., da Silva, A. B., & Honorio, K. M. (2019). Advances and perspectives in applying deep learning for drug design and discovery. *Frontiers in Robotics and AI*, *6*, 108.

Litjens, G., Kooi, T., Bejnordi, B. E., Setio, A. A. A., Ciompi, F., Ghafoorian, M., Van Der Laak, J. A., Van Ginneken, B., & Sánchez, C. I. (2017). A survey on deep learning in medical image analysis. *Medical Image Analysis*, *42*, 60–88.

Litjens, G., Sánchez, C. I., Timofeeva, N., Hermsen, M., Nagtegaal, I., Kovacs, I., Hulsbergen-Van De Kaa, C., Bult, P., Van Ginneken, B., & Van Der Laak, J. (2016). Deep learning as a tool for increased accuracy and efficiency of histopathological diagnosis. *Scientific Reports*, *6*(1), 1–11.

Liu, C., Cao, Y., Alcantara, M., Liu, B., Brunette, M., Peinado, J., & Curioso, W. (2017, September). TX-CNN: Detecting tuberculosis in chest X-ray images using convolutional neural network. In *2017 IEEE International Conference on Image Processing (ICIP)* (pp. 2314–2318). IEEE.

Machine Recognition of Crystallization Outcomes (MARCO) (2017). https://marco.ccr.buffalo.edu/

Maia, E. H. B., Assis, L. C., de Oliveira, T. A., da Silva, A. M., & Taranto, A. G. (2020). Structure-based virtual screening: From classical to artificial intelligence. *Frontiers in Chemistry*, *8*.

Matsumoto, S., Ishida, S., Araki, M., Kato, T., Terayama, K., & Okuno, Y. (2021). Extraction of protein dynamics information from cryo-EM maps using deep learning. *Nature Machine Intelligence*, *3*(2), 153–160.

Miotto, R., Li, L., Kidd, B. A., & Dudley, J. T. (2016). Deep patient: An unsupervised representation to predict the future of patients from the electronic health records. *Scientific Reports*, *6*(1), 1–10.

Mizianty, M. J., & Kurgan, L. (2011). Sequence-based prediction of protein crystallization, purification and production propensity. *Bioinformatics*, *27*(13), i24–i33.

Montinari, M. R., Minelli, S., & De Caterina, R. (2019). The first 3500 years of aspirin history from its roots – A concise summary. *Vascular Pharmacology*, *113*, 1–8.

Moult, J., Fidelis, K., Kryshtafovych, A., Schwede, T., & Tramontano, A. (2018). Critical assessment of methods of protein structure prediction (CASP) — Round XII. *Proteins: Structure, Function, and Bioinformatics*, *86*, 7–15.

Nakane, T., Kotecha, A., Sente, A., McMullan, G., Masiulis, S., Brown, P. M., … & Scheres, S. H. (2020). Single-particle cryo-EM at atomic resolution. *Nature*, *587*(7832), 152–156.

Ortiz, A., Munilla, J., Gorriz, J. M., & Ramirez, J. (2016). Ensembles of deep learning architectures for the early diagnosis of the Alzheimer's disease. *International Journal of Neural Systems*, *26*(7), 1650025.

Paluru, N., Dayal, A., Jenssen, H. B., Sakinis, T., Cenkeramaddi, L. R., Prakash, J., & Yalavarthy, P. K. (2021). Anam-Net: Anamorphic depth embedding-based lightweight CNN for segmentation of anomalies in COVID-19 chest CT images. *IEEE Transactions on Neural Networks and Learning Systems*, *32*(3), 932–946.

Patrick, G. L. (2013). *An introduction to medicinal chemistry*. Oxford University Press.

Paul, S. M., Mytelka, D. S., Dunwiddie, C. T., Persinger, C. C., Munos, B. H., Lindborg, S. R., & Schacht, A. L. (2010). How to improve R&D productivity: The pharmaceutical industry's grand challenge. *Nature Reviews Drug Discovery*, *9*(3), 203–214.

Pereira, S., Pinto, A., Alves, V., & Silva, C. A. (2016). Brain tumor segmentation using convolutional neural networks in MRI images. *IEEE Transactions on Medical Imaging*, *35*(5), 1240–1251.

Pinaya, W. H., Gadelha, A., Doyle, O. M., Noto, C., Zugman, A., Cordeiro, Q., Jackowski, A. P., Bressan, R. A., & Sato, J. R. (2016). Using deep belief network modelling to characterize differences in brain morphometry in schizophrenia. *Scientific Reports*, *6*(1), 1–9.

Piñero, J., Ramírez-Anguita, J. M., Saüch-Pitarch, J., Ronzano, F., Centeno, E., Sanz, F., & Furlong, L. I. (2020). The DisGeNET knowledge platform for disease genomics: 2019 update. *Nucleic Acids Research*, *48*(D1), D845–D855.

Poggi, M., & Mattoccia, S. (2016, June). A wearable mobility aid for the visually impaired based on embedded 3D vision and deep learning. In *2016 IEEE Symposium on Computers and Communication (ISCC)* (pp. 208–213). IEEE.

Pu, L., Govindaraj, R. G., Lemoine, J. M., Wu, H. C., & Brylinski, M. (2019). Deep-Drug3D: Classification of ligand-binding pockets in proteins with a convolutional neural network. *PLoS Computational Biology*, *15*(2), e1006718.

Pushpakom, S., Iorio, F., Eyers, P. A., Escott, K. J., Hopper, S., Wells, A., … & Pirmohamed, M. (2019). Drug repurposing: Progress, challenges and recommendations. *Nature Reviews Drug Discovery*, *18*(1), 41–58.

Qu, X., Swanson, R., Day, R., & Tsai, J. (2009). A guide to template based structure prediction. *Current Protein and Peptide Science*, *10*(3), 270–285.

Rämö, P., Sacher, R., Snijder, B., Begemann, B., & Pelkmans, L. (2009). CellClassifier: Supervised learning of cellular phenotypes. *Bioinformatics*, *25*(22), 3028–3030.

Ravì, D., Wong, C., Deligianni, F., Berthelot, M., Andreu-Perez, J., Lo, B., & Yang, G. Z. (2016). Deep learning for health informatics. *IEEE Journal of Biomedical and Health Informatics*, *21*(1), 4–21.

Rieke, N., Hancox, J., Li, W., Milletari, F., Roth, H. R., Albarqouni, S., … & Cardoso, M. J. (2020). The future of digital health with federated learning. *npj Digital Medicine*, *3*(1), 1–7.

Rupp, B. (2009). *Biomolecular Crystallography: Principles, Practice, and Application to Structural Biology*. Garland Science.

Russakovsky, O., Deng, J., Su, H., Krause, J., Satheesh, S., Ma, S., … & Fei-Fei, L. (2015). ImageNet large scale visual recognition challenge. *International Journal of Computer Vision*, *115*(3), 211–252.

Senior, A. W., Evans, R., Jumper, J., Kirkpatrick, J., Sifre, L., Green, T., Qin, C., Žídek, A., Nelson, A. W., Bridgland, A., & Penedones, H. (2020). Improved protein structure prediction using potentials from deep learning. *Nature*, *577*(7792), 706–710.

Si, D., Moritz, S. A., Pfab, J., Hou, J., Cao, R., Wang, L., Wu, T., & Cheng, J. (2020). Deep learning to predict protein backbone structure from high-resolution cryo-EM density maps. *Scientific Reports*, *10*(1), 1–22.

Simonovsky, M., & Meyers, J. (2020). DeeplyTough: Learning structural comparison of protein binding sites. *Journal of Chemical Information and Modeling*, *60*(4), 2356–2366.

Slabinski, L., Jaroszewski, L., Rodrigues, A. P., Rychlewski, L., Wilson, I. A., Lesley, S. A., & Godzik, A. (2007). The challenge of protein structure determination — Lessons from structural genomics. *Protein Science*, *16*(11), 2472–2482.

Sliwoski, G., Kothiwale, S., Meiler, J., & Lowe, E. W. (2014). Computational methods in drug discovery. *Pharmacological Reviews*, *66*(1), 334–395.

Sommer, C., Straehle, C., Koethe, U., & Hamprecht, F. A. (2011, March). Ilastik: Interactive learning and segmentation toolkit. In *2011 IEEE International Symposium on Biomedical Imaging: From Nano to Macro* (pp. 230–233). IEEE.

Souza, A., Oliveira, L. B., Hollatz, S., Feldman, M., Olukotun, K., Holton, J. M., Cohen, A. E., & Nardi, L. (2019). Deepfreak: Learning crystallography diffraction patterns with automated machine learning. *arXiv preprint arXiv:1904.11834*.

Stockwell, B. R. (2000). Chemical genetics: Ligand-based discovery of gene function. *Nature Reviews Genetics*, *1*(2), 116–125.

Stokes, J. M., Yang, K., Swanson, K., Jin, W., Cubillos-Ruiz, A., Donghia, N. M., … & Collins, J. J. (2020). A deep learning approach to antibiotic discovery. *Cell*, *180*(4), 688–702.

Su, C., Tong, J., & Wang, F. (2020). Mining genetic and transcriptomic data using machine learning approaches in Parkinson's disease. *npj Parkinson's Disease*, *6*(1), 1–10.

Tegge, A. N., Wang, Z., Eickholt, J., & Cheng, J. (2009). NNcon: Improved protein contact map prediction using 2D-recursive neural networks. *Nucleic Acids Research*, *37*(suppl_2), W515–W518.

Terwilliger, T. C., Stuart, D., & Yokoyama, S. (2009). Lessons from structural genomics. *Annual Review of Biophysics*, *38*, 371–383.

Torrisi, M., Pollastri, G., & Le, Q. (2020). Deep learning methods in protein structure prediction. *Computational and Structural Biotechnology Journal*, *18*, 1301–1310.

Van Grinsven, M. J., van Ginneken, B., Hoyng, C. B., Theelen, T., & Sánchez, C. I. (2016). Fast convolutional neural network training using selective data sampling: Application to hemorrhage detection in color fundus images. *IEEE Transactions on Medical Imaging*, *35*(5), 1273–1284.

Varshni, D., Thakral, K., Agarwal, L., Nijhawan, R., & Mittal, A. (2019, February). Pneumonia detection using CNN based feature extraction. In *2019 IEEE International Conference on Electrical, Computer and Communication Technologies (ICECCT)* (pp. 1–7). IEEE.

Vassura, M., Margara, L., Di Lena, P., Medri, F., Fariselli, P., & Casadio, R. (2008). Reconstruction of 3D structures from protein contact maps. *IEEE/ACM Transactions on Computational Biology and Bioinformatics*, *5*(3), 357–367.

Wang, H., Feng, L., Zhang, Z., Webb, G. I., Lin, D., & Song, J. (2016). Crysalis: An integrated server for computational analysis and design of protein crystallization. *Scientific Reports*, *6*(1), 1–14.

Wang, H., Wang, M., Tan, H., Li, Y., Zhang, Z., & Song, J. (2014). PredPPCrys: Accurate prediction of sequence cloning, protein production, purification and crystallization propensity from protein sequences using multi-step heterogeneous feature fusion and selection. *PLoS One*, *9*(8), e105902.

Wang, S., Ma, J., & Xu, J. (2016). AUCpreD: Proteome-level protein disorder prediction by AUC-maximized deep convolutional neural fields. *Bioinformatics*, *32*(17), i672–i679.

Wang, S., Peng, J., Ma, J., & Xu, J. (2016). Protein secondary structure prediction using deep convolutional neural fields. *Scientific Reports*, *6*(1), 1–11.

Wang, S., Sun, S., Li, Z., Zhang, R., & Xu, J. (2017). Accurate de novo prediction of protein contact map by ultra-deep learning model. *PLoS Computational Biology*, *13*(1), e1005324.

Waring, M. J., Arrowsmith, J., Leach, A. R., Leeson, P. D., Mandrell, S., Owen, R. M., Pairaudeau, G., Pennie, W. D., Pickett, S. D., Wang, J., & Wallace, O. (2015). An analysis of the attrition of drug candidates from four major pharmaceutical companies. *Nature Reviews Drug Discovery*, *14*(7), 475–486.

Wickramasinghe, N. (2017). Deepr: A convolutional net for medical records.

Winkler, D. A. (2021). Use of artificial intelligence and machine learning for discovery of drugs for neglected tropical diseases. *Frontiers in Chemistry*, *9*, 39.

Witt, D. R., Kellogg, R. A., Snyder, M. P., & Dunn, J. (2019). Windows into human health through wearables data analytics. *Current Opinion in Biomedical Engineering*, *9*, 28–46.

Yahalomi, E., Chernofsky, M., & Werman, M. (2019, July). Detection of distal radius fractures trained by a small set of X-ray images and faster R-CNN. In *Intelligent computing: Proceedings of the computing conference* (pp. 971–981). Cham: Springer.

Yang, G. (2014). *Body sensor networks* (2nd ed., G. Z. Yang, Ed.). London: Springer.

Yang, S. Y. (2010). Pharmacophore modeling and applications in drug discovery: Challenges and recent advances. *Drug Discovery Today*, *15*(11–12), 444–450.

Yang, X., Wang, Y., Byrne, R., Schneider, G., & Yang, S. (2019). Concepts of artificial intelligence for computer-assisted drug discovery. *Chemical Reviews*, *119*(18), 10520–10594.

Yu, A. M., Choi, Y. H., & Tu, M. J. (2020). RNA Drugs and RNA targets for small molecules: Principles, progress, and challenges. *Pharmacological Reviews*, *72*(4), 862–898.

Zanella, F., Lorens, J. B., & Link, W. (2010). High content screening: Seeing is believing. *Trends in Biotechnology*, *28*(5), 237–245.

Zeng, X., Zhu, S., Lu, W., Liu, Z., Huang, J., Zhou, Y., Fang, J., Huang, Y., Guo, H., Li, L., & Trapp, B. D. (2020). Target identification among known drugs by deep learning from heterogeneous networks. *Chemical Science*, *11*(7), 1775–1797.

Zhang, Y. (2020). Toward the solution of the protein⊠structure prediction problem. *The FASEB Journal*, *34*(S1), 1.

Zhao, J., Cao, Y., & Zhang, L. (2020). Exploring the computational methods for protein-ligand binding site prediction. *Computational and Structural Biotechnology Journal*, *18*, 417–426.

Zhao, L., Chen, J., Chen, F., Wang, W., Lu, C. T., & Ramakrishnan, N. (2015, November). Simnest: Social media nested epidemic simulation via online semi-supervised deep learning. In *2015 IEEE International Conference on Data Mining* (pp. 639–648). IEEE.

Zou, B., Lampos, V., Gorton, R., & Cox, I. J. (2016, April). On infectious intestinal disease surveillance using social media content. In *Proceedings of the 6th International Conference on Digital Health Conference* (pp. 157–161).

https://doi.org/10.1142/9789811254796_0005

5 Proteases as Therapeutic Targets: A Structural Biology Perspective

Yeu Khai Choong[†], Mahalashmi Srinivasan[†], and Chacko Jobichen[*,‡]

[†]*Department of Biological Sciences, National University of Singapore, Singapore 117557*
[‡]*Centre for Advanced Microscopy, Australian National University, Canberra, Australian Capital Territory, Australia*

Abstract

Proteases are enzymes produced by various living organisms and these enzymes help to cleave proteins into smaller fragments. They are widely involved in biological activities such as gene expression, immunological defense, migration, and cell death. Protease inhibitors play a role in suppressing this unwanted biological activity that could benefit the host. Proteases hydrolyze or cleave peptide bonds of protein substrate based on the arrangement of amino acid residues before and/or after the cleavage site. They specifically cleave protein substrates through the binding interaction of residues within the protease active site to the substrate cleavage site. This chapter shows the general classification of proteases and outlines the importance of protease-inhibitor interaction. The detailed knowledge about the interaction of proteases and inhibitors can be unravelled using the structural biology, especially by determining the structures of protease-inhibitor complexes. Examples of various protease structures

*Corresponding author: e-mail: Jobichen.Chacko@u.nus.edu

along with the bound inhibitors are detailed in this chapter. These structural details will help us to design and create suitable small molecule or drug, targeting the substrate binding site. Additionally, the existing inhibitors can be further modified to increase the binding affinity and to improve the inhibitory effects leading to the generation of potential drugs targeting proteases.

1. Introduction

Proteases are enzymes produced in various living organisms for breaking down proteins into smaller fragments. Proteolytic activity has been an important event in all living organisms, and it plays various roles including host defense and virulence.

Proteases are classified into six subgroups based on their specific mechanism of action (Rao *et al.*, 1998): (1) aspartic proteases, which contain a pair of aspartic acid residues at their active sites and cleave protein at low optimum pH (pH 3–4); (2) cysteine proteases, which contain a cysteine–histidine dyad at their catalytic sites; (3) glutamic proteases, which contain a glutamic acid residue within the active site; (4) metalloproteases, which represent proteases that require at least one metal ion for activity; (5) serine proteases, which contain serine residue at their active sites; and (6) threonine proteases, which contain a theronine residue within the active site (**Table 1**).

Serine proteases, which belong to enzyme class 3.4.21, is an endopeptidase (Rao *et al.*, 1998). Roles of serine proteases range from blood coagulation to inflammatory responses. However, overexpression of these proteases leads to pathogenesis and even cancer. Thus, deciphering the structure of such proteases aids in drug discovery and identification/synthesis of suitable inhibitors. Most of the serine proteases conserve serine, aspartic acid, and histidine residues, which forms the catalytic triad (Blow *et al.*, 1969; **Fig. 1**), aiding the easy transfer of protons in and out of the catalytic region. Though the structure and sequence alignments reveal maximum identity, certain structural differences in their binding pockets help us to identify their unique substrates; and to study a

Table 1 Various types of proteases and their specific inhibitors.

Type of Protease	Mechanism of Action	Native Proteases (PDB code)	Protease–inhibitor Complex (PDB code)
Aspartic proteases	• Presence of a pair of aspartic acid residue at the active site, which is required for catalytic activity. • Activity happens optimally at low pH.	• Pepsin A (3UTL) • HIV-1 retropepsin (3HVP) • DNA-damage-inducible protein 1 (4Z2Z)	• Pepsin-pepstatin (1PSO) • HIV-1 protease-ritonavir (1RL8)
Cysteine proteases	• Presence of cysteine–histidine dyad at the catalytic sites. • Reducing agents are needed for retention of catalytic activity. • Catalytic triad: Cys-His-Asp.	• Papain (9PAP) • Clostripain (3UWS) • Streptopain (2UZJ)	• Papain-E64 (1PE6) • Clostripain- Ac-VLTK-AOMK (4YEC) • Streptopain-SpeB 2477 (4RKX)
Glutamic proteases	• Presence of glutamic acid residue at the active site, which is required for catalytic activity.	• Scytalidopepsin B (1S2K)	• Scytalidopepsin B-TA1 (2IFW)
Metalloproteases	• Presence of bound divalent cation for activity.	• Thermolysin (2TLX) • Human angiotensin converting enzyme-related carboxypeptidase (ACE2) (1R42)	• Thermolysin-phosphoramidon (5TMN) • ACE2-MLN-4760 (1R4L)
Serine proteases	• Presence of serine residue at the active site, which is required for catalytic activity. • Catalytic triad: Ser-His-Asp.	• Chymotrypsin (8GCH) • Subtilisin (1SBC) • Thrombin (1ABI)	• Subtilisin-chymotrypsin inhibitor (2SNI) • Thrombin-rhodniin (1TBQ)
Theorine proteases	• Presence of threonine residue at the active site, which is required for catalytic activity. • Catalytic triad: Thr-Ser-Cys.	• γ-Glutamyltransferase 1 (GGT1) (4Z9O)	• GGT1-ACPB (6XPB)

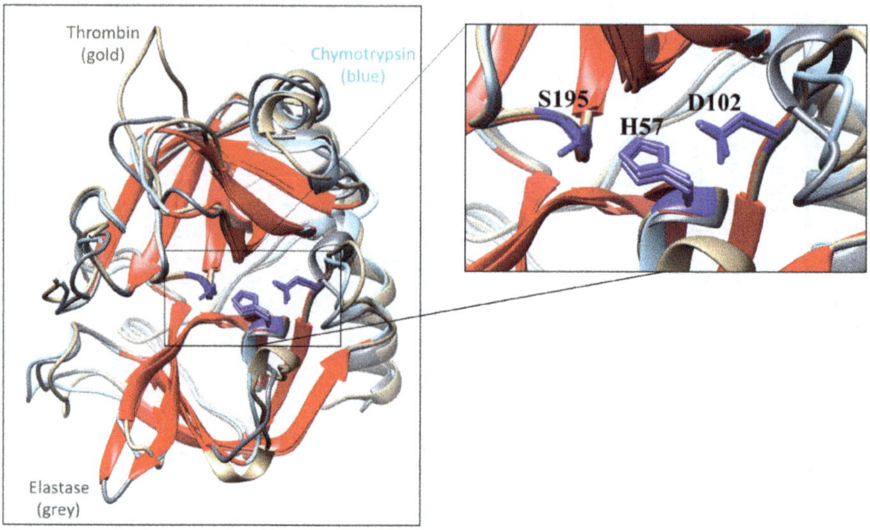

Fig. 1 Superimposition of α-thrombin (PDB 1ABI; gold), γ-chymotrypsin A (PDB 8GCH; blue), and elastase (PDB 1QNJ; gray) representing in cartoon. Red cartoon representation shows the six-stranded β-barrel at each domain. The zoomed-in view of catalytic triad (H57, D102, and S195) is shown in blue stick.

wide range of possible downstream activities. For example, serine proteinases of the chymotrypsin family contain two domains of similar structure, each consisting of a six-stranded β-barrel (Lesk & Fordham, 1996; **Fig. 1**). These two domains are believed to have arisen by gene duplication and divergence. The two domains pack together asymmetrically, with the residues of the catalytic triad lying between them. The catalytic triad in chymotrypsin family is formed by residues Asp102-His57-Ser195.

This chapter aims to provide the recent developments in the use of proteases and protease inhibitors as potential drug targets with a structure-based perspective.

1.1. Protease Substrate Specificity

Proteases hydrolyze or cleave peptide bonds of protein substrate based on the arrangement of amino acid residues before and/or

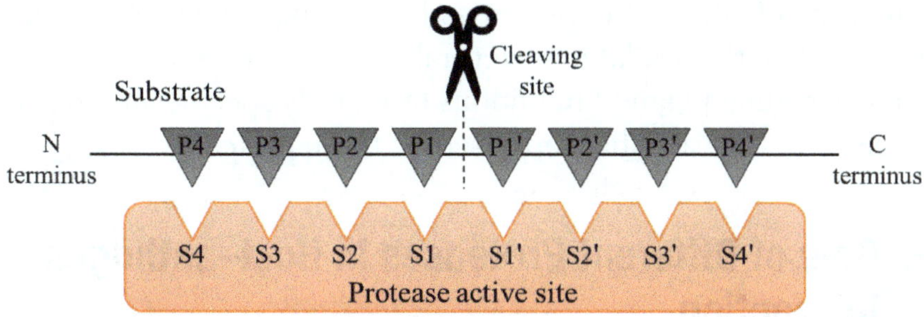

Fig. 2 Protease substrate specificity. Residues in substrate are numbered in P4–P4′, and the corresponding residues in protease active site are numbered in S4–S4′. The substrate cleavage occurs after P1 position.

after the cleavage site. They specifically cleave protein substrates (from N-, C-terminal, or in the middle of the substrate) through the binding interaction of residues within the protease active site to the substrate cleavage site. The protease active site residues are composed of contiguous pockets termed subsites (Harper & Berger, 1972). Each subsite pocket binds to a corresponding residue in the substrate sequence. According to this definition, amino acid residues in the substrate sequence are labeled as "-P4 - P3 - P2 - P1 - P1′ - P2′ - P3′ - P4′-," (the cleaving site is located between the P1 and P1′ positions), while the subsites in the active site are labeled as "-S4 - S3 - S2 - S1 - S1′ - S2′ - S3′ - S4′-" (**Fig. 2**).

Serine proteases are involved in numerous biological processes (Stroud, 1974), such as digesting food, blood coagulation, fighting infections, and helping sperm to enter eggs (Stroud, 1974). Blow *et al.* (1969) examined the structure of chymotrypsin using X-ray crystallography, and identified that His57 and Ser195 residues were close to each other in the structure, forming a hydrogen bond. Similarly, Asp102 residue was also close to His57, but it is located on the other side of the Ser195 (Blow *et al.*, 1969). This specific arrangement of His, Ser, and Asp has been found in many proteases, and it is known as the catalytic triad. The amino acid sequence can be very different from each other; however, by analyzing the arrangement of the catalytic triad (His-Ser-Asp), we can easily identify if the proteases belong to serine protease family. Based on the available structural information, researchers may carry out some planned mutations to identify specific amino acids involved in the catalytic steps used by these proteases.

2. Role of Different Proteases in Host–pathogen Interaction

Proteases are produced in living organism; they can be found in human, bacteria, plant, and virus. They are involved in many crucial biological processes. We will briefly discuss about various serine proteases found in living organisms, and how they are involved in host–pathogen interaction.

2.1. Human Proteases

Serine proteases in humans are expressed in endosomal vesicles of cells of the human immune system like the granzymes in lymphocytes, neutrophil proteases in granulocytes, and tryptase and chymase in mast cells. These proteases play important roles in the inflammatory response, tissue remodeling, pathogen clearance. and cell apoptosis (Heutinck *et al.*, 2010).

The zymogen form of the chymase (PDB: 1NN6) (Reiling *et al.*, 2003) exhibits a canonical trypsin fold that comprises two, six-stranded β-barrels, whereas the β-tryptase is a tetramer that has enzymatic activity which requires heparin binding to maintain functional and structural stability (Rohr *et al.*, 2006). Chymase protease is the major non-angiotensin converting enzyme (ACE), angiotensin II-generating enzyme in human tissues, and it is involved in various physiological processes (ranging from inflammation to hypertension) (Reiling *et al.*, 2003). By looking into the crystal structure, they have shown that the position of 180s (Pro185A-Asp194) and autolysis loop (Gly142-Thr154) of the zymogen are synergistic structural elements that appear to prevent premature proteolysis by chymase.

On the other hand, Rohr *et al.* (2006) showed that the β-tryptase has increased catalytic activity than the α-tryptase. The structure of the α-tryptase monomer resembles the other trypsin-like serine proteinases, which comprises two six-stranded β-barrels, two α-helices, and a short helical turn (Rohr *et al.*, 2006). They compared the α- and β-tryptase, and revealed that Asp216 is the key residue responsible for the inactivity of α-tryptase, as it locks the 214–220 segment of this enzyme in the closed conformation (Rohr *et al.*, 2006).

2.2. Plant Proteases

Similar to human, plants also have serine proteases. They are mainly found in the seeds. Several subtilisin-like serine proteases can be found in plant pollen. They have shown to improve membrane permeability by disrupting the transmembrane adhesion proteins (occludin, claudin-1, ZO-1, and E-cadherin), resulting IgE antibody production (Runswick *et al.*, 2007; Vinhas *et al.*, 2011). In another scenario, chitinase-producing plants could degrade chitin effectively. Chitin is a major structural component of fungal cell walls. However, some fungi possess the ability to secrete chitin-binding effector proteins, which could protect the cell walls from chitinase. Fungi, such as *Fusarium*, *Verticillium*, and *Botrytis cinerea*, are able to secret metalloproteases and serine proteases that are responsible in cleaving the chitinase, resulting in a lower antifungal activity (Jashni *et al.*, 2015).

Yano *et al.* (1998) reported that xylanase from *Trichoderma viride* (TvX) could induce an oxidative burst and cell death in cultured tobacco cells. In the following year, with this established system, they managed to inhibit only the oxidative burst of cells with N-acetyl-L-cysteine. Interestingly, they discovered an inhibitor of serine proteases that could inhibit the TvX-induced cell death, suggesting that serine proteases play an important role in signal transduction in its signaling pathway (Yano *et al.*, 1999).

2.3. Bacterial Proteases

Similarly, bacterial proteases play important roles in pathogenicity, cell viability, and stress response (Culp & Wright, 2017). For instance, *Clavibacter michiganensis* subsp. *michiganensis* causes wilt and canker in tomato plants. Though *pat-1* gene encodes a putative serine protease which belongs to the chymotrypsin subfamily S1A, which is partially responsible for the virulence of the bacteria, nucleotide sequence analysis revealed seven other pseudogenes (*chpA*, *ChpB*, *ChpC*, *ChpD*, *ChpE*, *ChpF*, *ChpG*) whose proteins are homologous to Pat-1. Sequence alignment of all these proteins revealed the presence of a conserved His, Ser, and Asp catalytic residues at their active sites. These pseudogenes possess internal frameshifts and in frame stop codon which leads to the synthesis of nonfunctional proteins, except for *ChpC*, *ChpE*, *ChpF*, and *ChpG*. Knockout of this putative *ChpC* gene led to the reduction in bacterial virulence and growth. Similarly, *Aeromonas sobria* which causes gastroenteritis encodes serine protease (ASP) which is part of the virulence mechanism. ASP is a kexin-like serine protease (Murakami *et al.*, 2012), that belongs to the subtilisin family characterized by the catalytic Asp, His, and Ser triad. The overall structure of ASP resembles Kex2, a Ca^{2+}-dependent serine protease from *Saccharomyces cerevisiae*. Though the N-terminal domain of ASP represents the catalytic subtilisin domain of Kex2 and the C-terminal domain is structurally similar to Kex2, ASP has an extra occluding region close to its active site (PDB: 3HJR) that may have a role in substrate specificity. A nicked form of ASP shows increased cleavage pattern of small peptide substrates than the native form (Kobayashi *et al.*, 2009).

2.4. Viral Proteases

Proteases are not only limited to bacteria. They are widely present in viruses, namely, alphaviruses, adenoviruses, picornaviruses, human immunodeficiency virus (HIV), Hepatitis C Virus (HCV), herpesviruses, and flaviviruses (Sharma & Gupta, 2017). While the first three viruses encode for mostly cysteine proteases and HIV encodes for aspartic proteases, the rest encode for serine proteases.

Non-structural protein NS3-4A is one of the HCV serine proteases, which has the catalytic subunit NS3 and an activating cofactor protein NS4A. NS3 plays a role in the maturation of the viral polyprotein (De Francesco & Steinkühler, 2000), NS4A is required for the proteolytic processing of the HCV polyprotein (Tanji *et al.*, 1995), and residues 21–34 are required to fully activate the NS3 protease (Lin *et al.*, 1995). Crystal structure of the NS3–NS4A protease reveals that the cofactor protein assumes an extended structure and forms a β-strand conformation which exclusively interacts with the N-terminal barrel of NS3 (De Francesco & Steinkühler, 2000). The N-terminal region of NS3 is probably disordered when not engaged in the interaction with NS4A, thus providing an explanation for the enhanced metabolic stability of the NS3–NS4A complex with respect to the uncomplexed enzyme (Tanji *et al.*, 1995).

Herpes simplex virus 1 (HSV-1) protease is essential for viral growth and auto processing, and interacts with the native substrate ICP35 to alter the capsid conformation, thereby enabling a proper DNA packaging (Matusick-Kumar *et al.*, 1994). Human cytomegalovirus (HCMV) protease undergoes an autocatalytic cleavage between the residues 143 and 209, where the cleavage at residue 143 produces a two-chain form of the protease that is still catalytically active (Holwerdas *et al.*, 1994; Loveland *et al.*, 2005). Both herpesvirus protease in HSV-1 and HCMV contain a central, mostly antiparallel, seven-stranded β-barrel, surrounded by eight helices. The active site of the protease contains a novel Ser132-His63-His157 catalytic triad (Sharma & Gupta, 2017).

Flavivirus protease is normally referred to as NS2B–NS3 protease, which cleaves the joints of NS2A–NS2B, NS2B–NS3, NS3–

NS4A, and NS4B–NS5 proteins, which is essential for maturation of these viral proteins (Pierson & Kielian, 2013).

In structures of Dengue virus, West Nile virus, and Zika virus NS2B–NS3 proteases, the folds of NS3 in various X-ray structures are almost identical as reviewed by Li and Kang (2020). The N-terminal domain of NS3 contains two β-barrels, and each barrel consists of six β-strands. The catalytic triad formed by His, Asp, and Ser residues is absolutely conserved among these proteases. The cofactor region of NS2B adopts two different conformations in some crystal structures. In the absence of NS3pro, the free cofactor region of NS2B is unstructured in solution. The N-terminal part of the cofactor region forms a stable complex with NS3 and exists as a β-strand which itself stabilizes NS3 protein. Nonetheless, in the presence of the C-terminal part of the cofactor, the protease activity gets enhanced (Li & Kang, 2020).

3. Importance of Protease Inhibitors

Proteases play several important roles in a variety of microbial and viral pathophysiological conditions, including acquired immune deficiency syndrome (AIDS), staphylococcal infections, candidiasis, and malaria, as well as in some cancers. Therefore, the identification and development of protease inhibitors as therapeutic agents against disease-causative proteases are very crucial (**Table 1**). In recent years, researchers have begun to look into protease inhibitors combating other conditions, such as fungal infections, viral infections, parasites, and even cancers. For example, protease inhibitors are commonly used along with other treatment to treat HIV. Protease inhibitors will not cure HIV, but help to stop HIV from reproducing by blocking the proteases' activity. This itself could help to lower the body's viral load, and slow down the progression of HIV from developing into AIDS. In severe acute respiratory syndrome coronavirus 2 (SARS-CoV-2), furin proteases and TMPRSS2 serine proteases target Spike glycoprotein by cleaving at S1/S2 site and S2/S2′ site, respectively, allowing the viral entry. Both proteases are important for Spike glycoprotein activation. Protease inhibitor targeting furin (e.g., MI-1851) and/or TMPRSS2 proteases (e.g., Camostat mesylate, aprotinin, MI-432, and nafamostat mesylate) suppress the activation and reducing the viral entry (Sivaraman *et al.*, 2021). On the other hand, Immunoglobulin A1 proteases (IgA1 proteases) are serine proteases from pathogenic bacteria, which enable colonization of human mucosal surfaces by cleaving the secreted IgA antibodies, resulting in the disruption of immunity responses. Inactivation of proteolytic event of IgA1 proteases could reduce bacterial colonization and infections. Only two inhibitors, substrate analog inhibitors (Burton *et al.*, 1988) and small synthetic peptide inhibitors (Bachovchin *et al.*, 1990) of *Neisseria gonorrhoeae* IgA1 proteases, have been reported in the last decade. To date, there are no further advances in development of IgA1 protease inhibitors.

Unfortunately, resistance may develop against protease inhibitor, especially when the inhibitor is used at suboptimal concentrations. The initial resistance mutations against the protease inhibitors could be different between them; however, the mutations are more likely to be located near the substrate binding site of the proteases (van Maarseveen & Boucher, 2006). Mutation of certain amino acid residues of the proteases will change the structure of the substrate-binding site, hence interfering the binding of protease inhibitor to the proteases, resulting in resistance to protease inhibitors.

4. Protease–protease Inhibitor Interactions

There are a lot of protease–protease inhibitor (small molecule/drug/ligand) structures deposited in Protein Data Bank (PDB). Here, we will show four different pairs of protease–protease inhibitor complex, and how these protease inhibitors inhibit their respective proteases.

4.1. Cell Envelop Proteinases (ScpC-AEBSF)

Streptococcus pyogenes (Group A *Streptococcus*) is a bacterium that causes diseases like pharyngitis, impetigo, and necrotizing

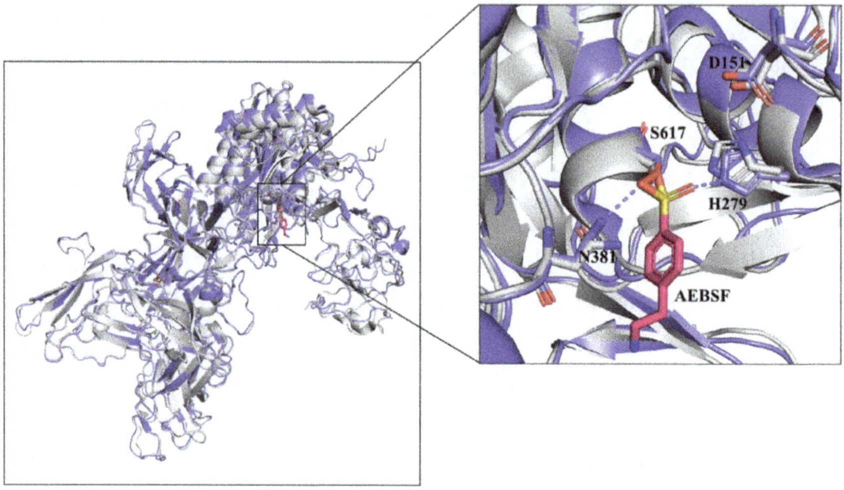

Fig. 3 Superimposition of ScpC proteases (PDB 5XYR; gray) and ScpC-AEBSF complex (PDB 5XYA; blue). The AEBSF is covalently linked to the ScpC at the active site of S617. The stick representation shows the substrate-binding sites and catalytic site residue. H279 residue is shifted away from D151 when interacting with AEBSF.

fasciitis. ScpC (SpyCEP) is a 180-kDa surface-exposed, subtilisin-like serine protease that helps *S. pyogenes* to evade the innate immune response by cleaving and inactivating C-X-C chemokines. ScpC cleaves the last 14 C-terminal amino acids of interleukin 8 (IL-8 or CXCL8) and impairs essential IL-8 signaling processes. Recently we determined the structure of this multidomain protease ScpC, consisting of nine structural domains, of which the first five domains are required for catalytic activity (PDB: 5XYA) (Jobichen *et al.*, 2018). The C-terminal domains of this protease are similar to collagen-binding and pilin proteins, suggesting an additional role for ScpC in pathogenesis. The overall structure of ScpC catalytic domain (Cat domain) is similar to subtilisin-like proteases but it showed specific structural differences to dictate its specificity toward C-X-C chemokines. This study also showed that ScpC does not undergo structural rearrangement upon maturation. The structure of ScpC–AEBSF inhibitor complex (**Fig. 3**) revealed that the bound inhibitor breaks the hydrogen bond between active site residues, thereby inhibiting the catalysis.

ScpC undergoes an autocatalytic cleavage between Gln244 and Ser245, resulting in two polypeptide chains that assemble together forming the active protease. Previously, it was reported that the region harboring the autocatalytic cleavage site, stretching from Gln213 to Asp272, is completely disordered. Our recent studies have shown that a deletion mutant (ScpCΔ60) of this region forms a single polypeptide chain (PDB: 7EDD) (Jobichen *et al.*, 2021), and ScpCΔ60 is an active protease capable of cleaving its substrate IL-8 in a manner comparable to that of the wild type.

4.2. Human Neutrophil Elastase — Ecotin

Human neutrophil elastase (hNE), a natural human serine protease, plays an important role during inflammatory host defense mechanism; however, their upregulated expression leads to cancer. Ecotin (ET) strongly inhibits S1A family serine proteases, which includes the hNE. We determined the structure of hNE-ET complex (PDB 7CBK), and the complex appears as a heterotetramer in the asymmetric unit, consisting a dimer of ET with two independent molecules of hNE binding to each molecule of ET (Jobichen *et al.*, 2020). ET has two binding sites with hNE, allowing them to achieve high-affinity binding (Ki = 0.012 nM): (1) the primary binding site of ET (Ser79–Ala86) interacts with the subsite of hNE, and (2) the secondary binding site involves the interaction between the region of the 60s loop (Leu64–Tyr69) of ET and several residues in hNE (**Fig. 4**). The primary and secondary binding sites are 24.2 Å apart. In addition, the secondary binding site forms a larger buried surface, and hence leads to the inhibition of the protease (Jobichen *et al.*, 2020). This study provides an insight to researchers or medical personnel to develop specific probes or inhibitors targeting hNE, which could help in therapeutic drug development in the future.

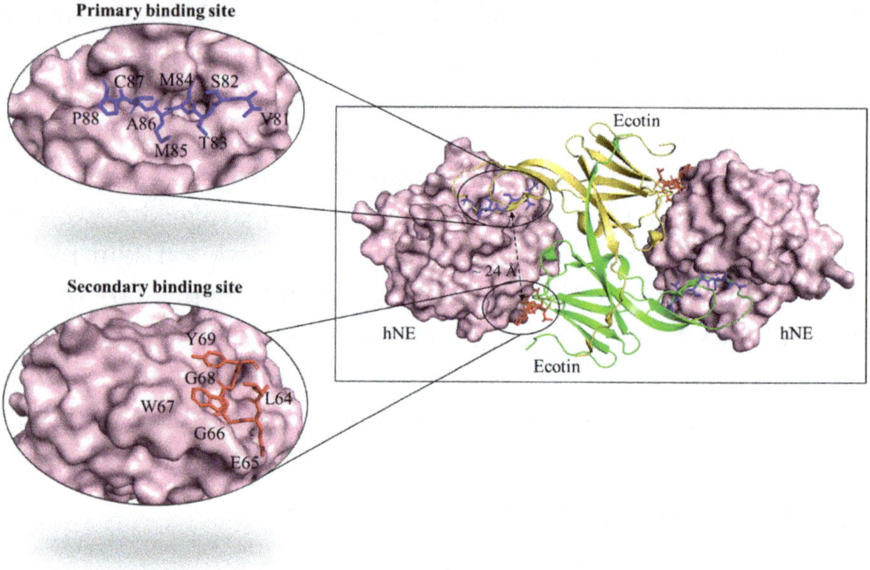

Fig. 4 Complex structure of human neutrophil elastase (surface representation) and ecotin (cartoon representation). Interacting residues of primary binding sites and secondary binding sites are represented in blue and red sticks, respectively. The distance between the primary and secondary site is about 24 Å apart.

4.3. Thrombin–CrSPI

The Kazal family is one of the 18 families of serine protease inhibitors. It is mainly categorized into classical and nonclassical inhibitors. The positions of the Cys residues involved in disulfide bond formation are different among the classical and nonclassical Kazal-type inhibitors (Tschesche *et al.*, 1987). The inhibitors contain a surface exposed reactive site loop (RSL). Domain 1 of CrSPI-1 is a close homolog to the domain 1 of rhodniin (a known thrombin inhibitor), sharing 42% of sequence identity. However, the CrSPI-1-D1 does not inhibit thrombin (Giri *et al.*, 2010). The rhodniin–thrombin complex structure revealed that the N-terminal domain of rhodniin interacts with the active-site cleft of thrombin (PDB: 1TBQ). Based on this rhodniin–thrombin complex, Pankaj *et al.* constructed a model for CrSPI-1-D1–thrombin complex. In

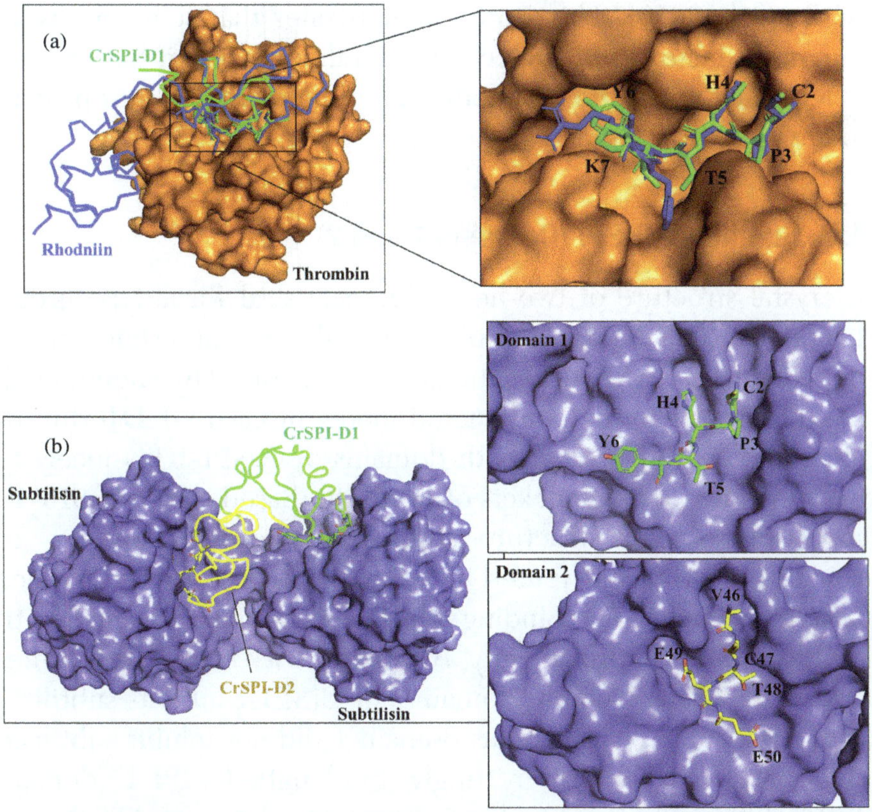

Fig. 5 Reactive site loop (RSL) of CrSPI in domains 1 and 2 in protease–inhibitor complex. (a) Model of CrSPI-D1 in complex with thrombin is shown by superimposing CrSPI-D1 to rhodniin–thrombin complex. Thrombin is represented in orange surface, while rhodniin inhibitor is represented in blue ribbon/stick. CrSPI-D1 superimposed to this complex, is represented in green ribbon/stick, and labeled in zoomed view. (b) CrSPI–subtilisin complex (subtilisin in surface representation and CrSPI in ribbon/stick representation) shows the interacting site of CrSPI at both domains. Interacting residues of domains 1 and 2 of CrSPI are shown in green and yellow stick in zoomed view, respectively.

this model, the RSL of CrSPI-1-D1 nicely fits in the active site of the thrombin (**Fig. 5a**). This allows the group to introduce mutations in the RSL region of CrSPI-1-D1, enabling the inhibitor to target thrombin. The modified CrSPI-1-D1 (Thr4Ala, Tyr5Lys, Lys6His, and Pro7Arg) inhibits thrombin with IC50 of 26.3 nM

(Giri *et al.*, 2010). This study demonstrates that sequence is an important factor for the specificity of inhibitor, and it has created a significant application to modify a multidomain inhibitor protein to target several proteases.

4.4. Subtilisin–CrSPI (Domains 1 and 2)

A crystal structure of two-headed nonclassical Kazal-type group 1 inhibitor (CrSPI-1) in complex with subtilisin, at a stoichiometric ratio of 1:2 (CrSPI-1 to subtilisin) was reported by Shenoy *et al.* (2011). Similar to the constructed model of CrSPI-1-D1–thrombin complex, the RSL of both domains of CrSPI-1 fits nicely to the substrate binding pockets of subtilisin. Based on the CrSPI-1–subtilisin complex structure (**Fig. 5b**), the RSL residues of domains 1 and 2 contributed to 445 and 530 Å^2 of buried surface area, respectively. The binding interfaces of domains 1 and 2 with subtilisin were approximately 76% and 90%, respectively (Shenoy *et al.*, 2011). Notably, domain 2 of CrSPI-1 inhibits subtilisin with a Ki of 2.5 nM, whereas domain 1 did not inhibit subtilisin (Jiang *et al.*, 2009). Interestingly, full-length CrSPI-1 (domain 1+2) inhibits subtilisin at a lower Ki value of 1.43 nM. ITC experiments on full-length CrSPI-1 further revealed the presence of two non-identical binding sites, one domain binds to one subtilisin molecule (Shenoy *et al.*, 2011). This result suggests that domain 2 of CrSPI-1 binds to subtilisin molecule first (at a higher affinity), followed by the binding of domain 1 to another molecule of subtilisin (at a lower affinity; Shenoy *et al.*, 2011).

5. Summary

Proteases are enzymes that cleave proteins into smaller components. They are widely involved in biological activity such as gene expression, immunological defense, migration, and cell death. Protease inhibitors play a role in suppressing this unwanted biological activity that could benefit the host. In this chapter, we have discussed the importance of proteases and how the inhibitors interact with the protease to block the activity. By looking in to the interaction of these proteases and inhibitors, we could design and create suitable small molecule or drug, targeting the substrate binding site. Additionally, the existing inhibitors can be further modified to increase the binding potential and to improve the inhibitory effects.

References

Bachovchin, W. W., Plaut, A. G., Flentke, G. R., Lynch, M., & Kettner, C. A. (1990). Inhibition of IgAl proteinases from *Neisseria gonorrhoeae* and *Haemophilus influenzae* by peptide prolyl boronic acids. *Journal of Biological Chemistry*, *265*, 3738–3743.

Blow, D. M., Birkthoft, J. J., *et al.* (1969). Role of a buried acid group in the mechanism of action of chymotrypsin. *Nature*, *221*, 337–340.

Burton, J., Wood, S. G., Lynch, M., & Plaut, A. G. (1988). Substrate analogue inhibitors of the IgA1 proteinases from *Neisseria gonorrhoeae*. *Journal of Medicinal Chemistry*, *31*, 1647–1651.

Culp, E., & Wright, G. D. (2017). Bacterial proteases, untapped antimicrobial drug targets. *The Journal of Antibiotics*, *70*, 366–377.

De Francesco, R., & Steinkühler, C (2000). Structure and function of the hepatitis C virus NS3-NS4A serine proteinase. *Current Topics in Microbiology and Immunology*, *242*, 149–169.

Giri, P. K., *et al.* (2010). Modifying the substrate specificity of *Carcinoscorpius rotundicauda* serine protease inhibitor domain 1 to target thrombin. *PLoS One*. doi:10.1371/journal.pone.0015258

Harper, E., & Berger, A. (1972). On the size of the active site in proteases: Pronase. *Biochemical and Biophysical Research Communications*, *46*, 1956–1960.

Heutinck, K. M., ten Berge, I. J. M., Hack, C. E., Hamann, J., & Rowshani, A. T. (2010). Serine proteases of the human immune system in health and disease. *Molecular Immunology*, *47*, 1943–1955.

Holwerdas, B. C., *et al.* (1994). Activity of two-chain recombinant human cytomegalovirus protease. *Journal of Biological Chemistry*, *269*, 25911–25915.

Jashni, M. K., *et al.* (2015). Synergistic action of a metalloprotease and a serine protease from *Fusarium oxysporum* f. sp. *lycopersici* cleaves chitin-binding tomato chitinases, reduces their antifungal activity, and enhances fungal virulence. *Molecular Plant-Microbe Interactions*, *28*, 996–1008.

Jiang, N., *et al.* (2009). A novel serine protease inhibitor acts as an immunomodulatory switch while maintaining homeostasis. *Journal of Innate Immunity*, *1*, 465–479.

Jobichen, C., *et al.* (2018). Structure of ScpC, a virulence protease from *Streptococcus pyogenes*, reveals the functional domains and maturation mechanism. *The Biochemical Journal*, *475*, 2847–2860.

Jobichen, C., Prabhakar, M. T., Loh, S. N., & Sivaraman, J. (2020). Structural basis for the inhibition mechanism of ecotin against neutrophil elastase by targeting the active site and secondary binding site. *Biochemistry*. doi:10.1021/acs.biochem.0c00493

Jobichen, C., Ying Chong, T., Hui Ling, T., & Sivaraman, J. (2021). The autocatalytic cleavage domain is not required for the activity of ScpC, a virulence protease from *Streptococcus pyogenes*: A structural insight. *Biochemistry*, *60*, 1564–1568.

Kobayashi, H., *et al.* (2009). Structural basis for the kexin-like serine protease from *Aeromonas sobria* as sepsis-causing factor. *Journal of Biological Chemistry*, *284*, 27655–27663.

Lesk, A. M., & Fordham, W. D. (1996). Conservation and variability in the structures of serine proteinases of the chymotrypsin family. *Journal of Molecular Biology*, *258*, 501–537.

Li, Q., & Kang, C. (2020). Insights into structures and dynamics of flavivirus proteases from NMR studies. *International Journal of Molecular Sciences*, *21*, 2527.

Lin, C., Thomson, J. A., & Rice, C. M. (1995). A central region in the hepatitis C virus NS4A protein allows formation of an active NS3-NS4A serine proteinase complex in vivo and in vitro. *Journal of Virology*, *69*, 4373–4380.

Loveland, A. N., Chan, C.-K., Brignole, E. J., & Gibson, W. (2005). Cleavage of human cytomegalovirus protease pUL80a at internal and cryptic sites is not essential but enhances infectivity. *Journal of Virology*, *79*, 12961.

Matusick-Kumar, L., *et al.* (1994). Phenotype of the herpes simplex virus type 1 protease substrate ICP35 mutant virus. *Journal of Virology*, *68*, 5384–5394.

Murakami, Y., *et al.* (2012). Inhibition of *Aeromonas sobria* serine protease (ASP) by α2-macroglobulin. *Biological Chemistry*, *393*, 1193–1200.

Pierson, T. C., & Kielian, M. (2013). Flaviviruses: Braking the entering. *Current Opinion in Virology*, *3*, 3–12.

Rao, M. B., Tanksale, A. M., Ghatge, M. S., & Deshpande, V. V. (1998). Molecular and biotechnological aspects of microbial proteases. *Microbiology and Molecular Biology Reviews*, *62*, 597.

Reiling, K. K., *et al.* (2003). Structure of human pro-chymase: A model for the activating transition of granule-associated proteases. *Biochemistry*. doi:10.1021/bi020594d

Rohr, K. B., *et al.* (2006). X-ray structures of free and leupeptin-complexed human αI-tryptase mutants: Indication for an α→β-tryptase transition. *Journal of Molecular Biology*, *357*, 195–209.

Runswick, S., Mitchell, T., Davies, P., Robinson, C., & Garrod, D. R. (2007). Pollen proteolytic enzymes degrade tight junctions. *Respirology*, *12*, 834–842.

Sharma, A., & Gupta, S. P. (2017). Fundamentals of viruses and their proteases. In *Viral proteases and their inhibitors* (1st ed.). doi:10.1016/B978-0-12-809712-0.00001-0

Shenoy, R. T., *et al.* (2011). Structural basis for dual-inhibition mechanism of a non-classical kazal-type serine protease inhibitor from horseshoe crab in complex with subtilisin. *PLoS One*, *6*, e18838.

Sivaraman, H., Er, S. Y., Choong, Y. K., Gavor, E., & Sivaraman, J. (2021). Structural basis of SARS-CoV-2-and SARS-CoV-receptor binding and small-molecule blockers as potential therapeutics. *Annual Review of Pharmacology and Toxicology*. doi:10.1146/annurev-pharmtox-061220-093932

Stroud, R. M. (1974). A family of protein-cutting proteins. *Scientific American*, *231*, 74–88.

Tanji, Y., Hijikata, M., Satoh, S., Kaneko, T., & Shimotohno, K. (1995). Hepatitis C virus-encoded nonstructural protein NS4A has versatile functions in viral protein processing. *Journal of Virology*, *69*, 1575–1581.

Tschesche, H., Kolkenbroac, H., & Bode, W. (1987). The covalent structure of the elastase inhibitor from anemonia sulcata — A "non-classical" kazal-type protein. *Biological Chemistry Hoppe-Seyler.* doi:10.1515/bchm3.1987.368.2.1297

van Maarseveen, N., & Boucher, C. (2006). Resistance to protease inhibitors. In *Antiretroviral resistance in clinical practice.* Mediscript.

Vinhas, R., *et al.* (2011). Pollen proteases compromise the airway epithelial barrier through degradation of transmembrane adhesion proteins and lung bioactive peptides. *Allergy*, *66*, 1088–1098.

Yano, A., Suzuki, K., & Shinshi, H. (1999). A signaling pathway, independent of the oxidative burst, that leads to hypersensitive cell death in cultured tobacco cells includes a serine protease. *The Plant Journal*, *18*, 105–109.

Yano, A., Suzuki, K., Uchimiya, H., & Shinshi, H. (1998). Induction of hypersensitive cell death by a fungal protein in cultures of tobacco cells. *MPMI*, *11*, 115–123.

https://doi.org/10.1142/9789811254796_0006

6 *In Silico* Approaches for Understanding Antimicrobial Resistance in Bacterial Pathogens

Sudha Ramaiah, Sravan Kumar Miryala,
C.K. Hithesh Kumar and Anand Anbarasu*

*Medical & Biological Computing Laboratory,
School of Bio-Sciences & Technology,
Vellore Institute of Technology, Vellore 632014, India*

Abstract

Sustained antibiotic usage for the treatment of bacterial infections has resulted in alarming levels of antimicrobial resistance (AMR). Though bacteria were initially susceptible to the antibiotics, they have gradually developed high levels of resistance upon continuous exposure. Therapeutic options for such multidrug resistant (MDR) bacterial infections have become difficult and often result in higher mortality rates. Thus there is an urgent need to design and develop potent compounds to combat MDR bacterial infections. Conventional drug discovery process in the earlier days was time-consuming, expensive and laborious. The emergence of information technology has resulted in a new field of bioinformatics, and now *in silico* approaches are used extensively in drug design, development and discovery, resulting in saving valuable time, money and resources. Even though researchers are trying to develop newer antimicrobial

*Corresponding author: e-mail: aanand@vit.ac.in

compounds, bacteria are evolving at much higher rates and the emergence of resistance to the newer anti-bacterial compounds is also higher. Hence, it is important to understand the mechanism of AMR during the process of drug design and development. The *in silico* approaches can be employed to unravel the resistance patterns by studying both at the genotypic and phenotypic levels. In the present chapter we discuss the *in silico* methods using relevant examples that our group has researched upon to understand the mechanisms of AMR in the context of structural and systems biology. We hope that the readers will find the contents useful and can employ the suggested methods to study and understand the mechanisms of AMR in other bacterial pathogens as well.

1. Introduction

The emergence of rapidly increasing multidrug resistance (MDR) among the pathogenic bacteria is a major clinical and public health problem. The major concern is in the case of acquired resistance, where susceptible bacteria develop resistance to an antibiotic agent and then proliferate and spread under the selective pressure of the antibiotic. β-Lactam antibiotics have been extensively used in the treatment of infectious diseases, even though their use has been mystified by the development of resistance mechanisms. The most common mechanism of resistance to β-lactam antibiotics is the production of β-lactamases and alteration in the binding site of penicillin-binding proteins (PBPs). Therefore it is important to explore the role of stabilizing interactions in the stability and specificity of β-lactamases and PBPs.

Hydrophobic effects, hydrogen bonds, disulfide bridges and van der Waals interactions all play considerable role in stabilizing biological systems. Apart from the regular hydrogen bonds that stabilize the protein structure, there are several weak hydrogen bonds which provide significant amount of energy to stabilize the protein structure (Dougherty, 1996; Gallivan & Dougherty, 2000;

Gromiha, 2003). Weak hydrogen bonds include cation–π interactions, C–H$\cdots\pi$ interactions, C–H$\cdots$O interactions and N–H$\cdots\pi$ interactions. Even though these non-conventional interactions are weak in nature, they are still important because of their higher occurrence in proteins and cumulatively they provide significant energy for protein folding and stability (Acceptors *et al.*, 1988). Thus it is important to systematically analyze the contribution of cation–π interactions, C–H$\cdots\pi$ interactions, C–H$\cdots$O interactions, N–H$\cdots\pi$ interactions and the role of metal ions in the stability and functional specificity of β-lactamases and PBPs.

Conventional drug discovery process involves large capital investments and usually takes a long time for drug development. Since there are several limitations for drug development, there is a need for newer approaches in the drug discovery process. Various *in silico* methods such as molecular modeling, molecular docking, virtual screening, pharmacophore modeling, molecular dynamics simulations (MDS) and ADMET prediction are used to understand the mechanisms of antimicrobial resistance (AMR).

The advent of systems biology and its toolsets, integrative models that combine experimentally known features with computational gene and protein networks, have significantly improved our understanding of the emergence and evolution of the antibiotic resistant phenotypes. Computational gene/protein networks present a graphical model of associated genes and help us to understand the complexity of interactions in a meaningful manner. However, to the best of our understanding there are only a few reports on the use of gene networks in predicting potential drug targets and in understanding the virulence and resistance mechanisms.

In the present chapter, we discuss the different *in silico* approaches using suitable well-studied models that our research team has analyzed to understand the mechanisms of AMR and to identify potential compounds that could be exploited for new drug discovery. We hope this chapter will be interesting to researchers and they might find the open source tools and databases suggested suitable for exploring AMR and for new drug discovery.

Table 1 Mechanism of action of various antibiotics.

S. No.	Mechanism of Action	Antibiotics
1	Inhibition of cell wall synthesis	Penicillin Cephalosporins Bacitracin Vancomycin Ampicillin
2	Inhibition of cell membrane function	Cinnamycin Clotrimazole Salinomycin Surfactin Valinomycin
3	Inhibition of nucleic acid synthesis	Actinomycin Cinoxacin Ciprofloxacin Enrofloxacin Sulfamethazine
4	Inhibition of protein synthesis	Azithromycin Chloramphenicol Erythromycin Josamycin Tetracycline
5	Inhibition of other metabolic processes	Actinonin Sulfanilamide Ciprofloxacin Enrofloxacin Ofloxacin

2. Mechanism of Action of Antibiotics

There are five mechanisms of antibiotic action against bacteria and they are presented in Table 1.

3. *In silico* Techniques to Understand the Mechanism of AMR

We have systematically analyzed the contribution of cation–π interactions, C–H$\cdots\pi$ interactions, C–H$\cdots$O interactions, N–H$\cdots\pi$ interactions and the role of metal ions in the stability and functional specificity of β-lactamases and PBPs.

3.1. Computing Non-covalent Interactions

Nonredundant set of β-lactamases and PBPs were selected from the protein data bank (PDB) (Berman *et al.*, 2000). The criteria used for the selection of the nonredundant data set are as follows:

i) Structures were solved with less than 2.5 Å resolution.
ii) Sequence identity among the proteins in the data set was less than 40%. If the protein contained more than one chain, then chain A was considered for analysis.

3.1.1. *Cation–π interactions*

We computed the energetic contribution of cation–π interactions for each protein in the data set using the cation–π trends using realistic electrostatics program (CAPTURE; Gallivan & Dougherty, 1999). It calculates the distance between ammonium nitrogen (NZ) in Lys or the guanidine carbon (CZ) in Arg and the centers of all aromatic rings, phenol, indole and benzene in Tyr, Trp and Phe, respectively, which has implemented a subset of OPLS force field (Jorgensen & Rives, 1988) to estimate the energetic contribution of cation–π interactions. Only cation–π interactions with binding energies that rise above a certain threshold are retained (Anbarasu *et al.*, 2009).

3.1.2. *Non-conventional interactions (C–H···π interactions, N–H···π interactions, C–H···O interactions)*

Non-conventional interactions were computed using the program Hydrogen Bond Analysis Tool (HBAT) (Tiwari & Panigrahi, 2007). The criteria used for C–H···O interactions were d (H–O) ≤ 3.0 Å and θ (C–H···O) ≥ 90°, where d was the distance between the H and the acceptor O and θ was the angle between C–H bond and center of the acceptor atom. The criteria for X–H···π (where X = C, N) were P1 ≤ 5.0 Å, P2 ≤ 4.0 Å, P3 ≥ 90 Å and P4 ≤ 40°. In π-electron acceptor, the distances were usually measured to the centroid (M) of multiple bonds or phenyl rings (Panigrahi & Desiraju, 2007). P1 and P2 were distances from X and H, respectively, to M, P3 was the angle between vectors C–H and H–M, and P4 was the angle between CM and MN.

3.2. Computing Environmental Preferences

3.2.1. *Secondary structure*

Secondary structure assignment of interacting residues was done based on the information available from PDB. Proteins were categorized according to the manually assigned classes of α-helix, β-strand and coil.

3.2.2. *Solvent accessibility*

Analysis of hydrophobicity of interacting residues was indispensable to predict the conformation of amino acid residues on a protein backbone (Eyal *et al.*, 2004). Solvent accessibility pattern of interacting residues has been calculated by using ASA-View (Ahmad *et al.*, 2004).

3.2.3. *Inter-residue contacts*

The α-carbon atoms were generally used to represent the amino acid residues in protein. The distances between the residues involved in non-conventional interactions were computed by calculating the distance between the α-carbon of the first residue and the corresponding residues in protein. Composition of the amino acids correlated with this residue was calculated within a sphere of 8 Å, the range which was adequate for local and non-local interactions (Lavanya *et al.*, 2013a). The contribution from $<\pm 4$ with respect to α-carbon atom was represented as short range contact, ± 4 to ± 10 as medium-range contact, and $>\pm 10$ were treated as long-range contact.

3.2.4. *Conservation patterns*

Importance of interacting residues in the function of β-lactamases and PBPs was calculated using ConSurf algorithm (Glaser *et al.*, 2003).

3.2.5. *Stabilization centers*

Stabilization centers are residues involved in cooperative long-range contacts, which are likely to play an important role in ensuring stability of the protein structure and preventing its unfolding. For locating stabilization center in the interacting residues, we employed SCide server (Dosztányi *et al.*, 2003).

3.3. Computational Modeling

Over the last few decades, computational modeling has become increasingly relevant in biochemical and biomolecular sciences. Today, we can easily scan virtual libraries of millions of compounds for possible new inhibitors and run simulations of huge biomolecular complexes in microsecond or millisecond timescales. Molecular modeling is a collection of (computer-based) methods for calculating, describing and manipulating the structures and reactions of molecules, as well as the properties that are influenced by these three-dimensional (3D) structures. Here we present the hierarchy of computational modeling methods used as standard tools by organic chemists for searching, rationalizing and predicting the structure and reactivity of small molecule and bio-macromolecule (Urhahne *et al.*, 2009).

Protein–ligand binding is critical in structure-based drug design, for which 3D structure of the protein is required. To begin our computational drug discovery process, we look for the protein's 3D structure in an appropriate PDB (Berman *et al.*, 2000). The PDB is a database that contains all of the recognized 3D structures of proteins (http://www.rcsb.org/). Two main techniques, X-ray crystallography and nuclear magnetic resonance spectroscopy (NMR), are used to determine 3D structures. Structure determination using these experimental methods is laborious and expensive, and the PDB database may not have all known protein structures for all available sequences. As a result, a protein must be modeled using existing data and sequence (Forster, 2002). This *in silico* technique uses a method known as "homology-based modelling" to model proteins. This method of modeling is based on the sequence similarity of evolutionarily equivalent proteins. Homology modeling techniques may be used to build 3D representations of the protein coding sequence. When there is no simple sequence homology, threading methods that use specialized schemes to link protein sequences to a library of known structures have been shown to classify the probable protein fold (Malathi & Ramaiah, 2018).

3.3.1. *Template identification and sequence homology*

Template identification is the first step in homology modeling. This involves comparing unknown amino acid sequences to those already in the PDB to find homologous sequences whose structure has already been determined. Similarity searches using programs like BLAST for amino acid sequence alignment identify these homologue sequences. The BLAST (Altschul *et al.*, 1997) and FASTA (Pearson & Lipman, 1988) families of programs use the former method, which involves scanning a query sequence against a database of template sequences and scoring the alignments using broad-spectrum matrices like BLOSUM (Henikoff & Henikoff, 1993) or PAM (Dayhoff *et al.*, 1978). Using information from protein families (represented as position-specific scoring matrices or hidden Markov models) as family-specific matrices and using intermediate sequence searching procedures can improve sensitivity (Contreras-Moreira *et al.*, 2002).

3.3.2. *Model building*

The model can be constructed in a number of ways: (a) spatial restraint, (b) rigid-body assembly, (c) segment matching and (d) artificial evolution (Malathi & Ramaiah, 2018).

3.3.3. *Refinement modeling*

Amino acid residues are added, deleted and substituted in model-building methods. Loop and side-chain modeling are used in this model refinement. Molecular dynamics (MD), Monte Carlo methods and genetic algorithms are used to refine the model. Certain force fields, such as OPLS, AMBER, MM3 and CHARMM22 are used to reduce the energy of the modeled structures (Malathi & Ramaiah, 2018).

3.3.4. *Loop modeling*

Loops, which appear to be the variable portion of the protein, are formed by the insertion and substitution of amino acid residues into the sequences of homologous proteins. The missing loop region sequence segment is searched for in template proteins for modeling in template-based loop modeling. The loop is modeled using non-template-based methods (*De novo* methods) if that particular sequence is not available in the template (Malathi & Ramaiah, 2018).

3.3.5. *Side chain modeling*

The replacement of side chains on the backbone structure is used to model side chains. The root mean square deviation values of the modeled side chains are examined (Malathi & Ramaiah, 2018).

3.3.6. *Model validation*

Validation of the protein is needed after homology modeling to ensure that the model is accurate. WHATCHECK, WHAT IF, VADAR and PROCHECK can be used to look at the stereochemical nature of a protein. The torsion angles of the main chain are tested using the Ramachandran plot evaluation. When a higher percentage of residues are present in the permitted zone than in the disallowed zone in a scatter plot, it indicates that the protein is structurally feasible. MODELLER, SWISS PDB VIEWER, SWISS MODEL and COMPOSER are some of the programs available for homology modeling (Sali & Blundell, 1993). With the aid of the prototype OXA-24 carbapenem hydrolyzing class D β-lactamase (CHDL), the homology modeling method, MODELLER 9.16 was used to construct the OXA-143 CHDL and validated. The OXA-143 CHDL structure was established in this study to investigate the imipenem resistance mechanism in OXA-143 CHDL expressing *Acinetobacter baumannii* (Malathi *et al.*, 2017; Wei *et al.*, 2016).

3.4. Molecular Docking

Molecular docking studies are used to understand the interaction between a ligand and a target protein at the atomic level. These molecular docking studies have two goals: prediction of protein–ligand binding orientation and the estimation of the interaction. Before the start of the docking process, it is necessary to identify the active site of the protein where the ligands can bind. For the prediction of active sites, many online programs are available like

CASTp, Q-SiteFinder, LigA Site and MetaPocket (Laurie & Jackson, 2005). A molecular docking study without the prediction of the active site is known as "blind docking" (Malathi *et al.*, 2016).

The aim of ligand–protein docking is to predict the most common binding models of a ligand with a three-dimensionally known protein. Successful docking procedures effectively search high-dimensional spaces and use a scoring function that ranks candidate dockings correctly. Docking can be used to conduct virtual screening on large libraries of compounds, rank the effects and suggest structural hypotheses about how the ligands inhibit the target, which is extremely useful in lead optimization. The configuration of the docking input structures is just as important as the docking itself and evaluating the results of stochastic search methods can be difficult at times (Schleinkofer *et al.*, 2006). **Figure 1** illustrates the multiple docking flowcharts from different tools.

3.5. Virtual Screening

Virtual screening is a popular *in silico* method for the lead identification process that scans the chemical database for an active lead. There are two types of virtual screening approaches: structure-based and ligand-based. Via molecular docking tests, the 3D structure of the target protein is used to screen against the compounds present in the chemical libraries in structure-based virtual screening (Malathi & Ramaiah, 2018). Hundreds of thousands of compounds can be synthesized and tested thanks to the widespread use of emerging technologies like combinatorial chemistry and high-throughput screening in drug discovery. Furthermore, the number of potential therapeutic targets emerging from functional genomics is rapidly increasing. All of these factors placed further pressure on researchers to devise a useful virtual screening strategy for prioritizing screening compounds. Virtual screening has been applied to various stages of the drug discovery process, including hit discovery and lead optimization, thanks to recent advances and improvements in automated computational

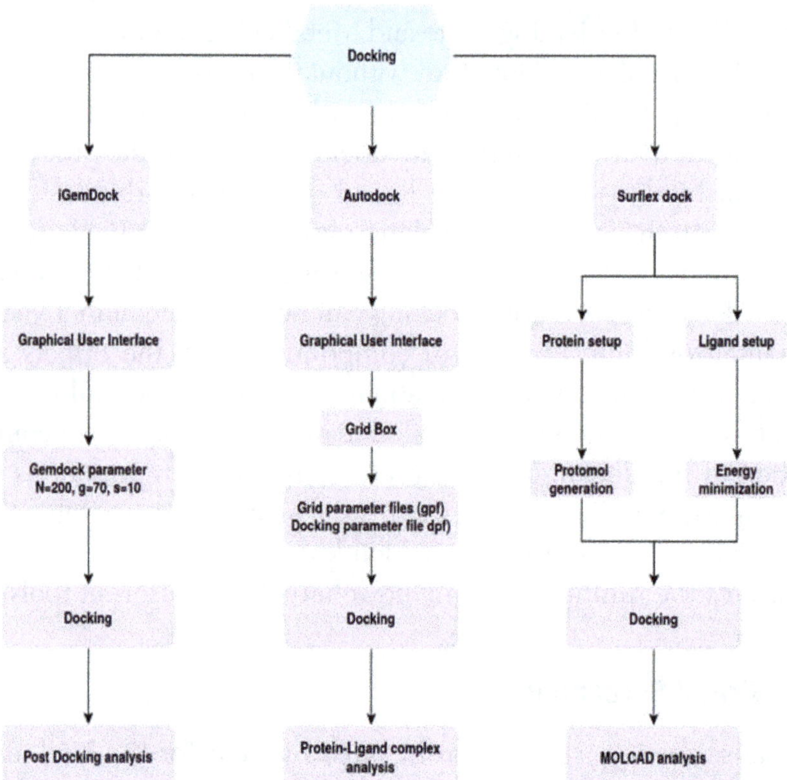

Fig. 1 Standard docking workflow. This is an example of a standard docking workflow. This flowchart depicts the main steps that are shared by all docking protocols. The 3D structures for the target macromolecule and small molecule are selected first, and then each structure must be processed in accordance with the docking method's requirements. Following docking, the results must be evaluated in order to select the binding modes with the highest scores.

methods. Virtual screening encompasses a wide range of analytical techniques (Edward & Sabharwal, 2017).

The docking technique is used in structure-based virtual screening methods to classify the active lead based on the binding affinity of the compound with the target and the functional scores. We used the structure-based virtual screening technique to test possible inhibitors for OXA-10 ESBL-expressing *Pseudomonas aeruginosa* against the millions of compounds in the ZINC

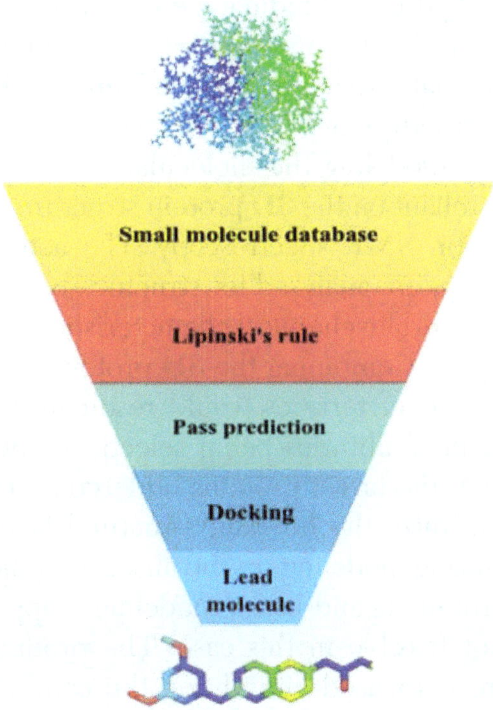

Fig. 2 Methodologies of virtual screening.

database (Malathi & Ramaiah 2016). It was also used to find new inhibitors for the ceftaroline-resistant methicillin-resistant *Staphylococcus aureus* penicillin-binding protein 2a (PBP2a). Digital screening was carried out on the Dock blaster server (Irwin *et al.*, 2009; Lavanya *et al.*, 2016). **Figure 2** depicts various methodologies used in the virtual screening procedure.

3.6. Pharmacophore Modeling

The molecular characteristics that are important for the macromolecular recognition of biologically reactive ligands are called pharmacophore modeling. Pharmacophores are modeled with the characteristics including the hydrophobic, aromatic, anionic and cation residues hydrogen binding agent. Pharmacophore models are used to determine the molecules in the chemical library as a query during virtual screening. The modeling of pharmacophores is focused on structure and ligand in two groups. In pharmacophore structural modeling the molecular structure of the target protein is fully reliant on the 3D protein structure solved by X-ray crystallography or NMR spectroscopy. The active location and space relationships are analyzed for structure-based pharmacophore modeling for certain chemical characteristics that complement the binding ligand. Combining the 3D protein conformation and the ligand's key characteristics would result in expected effects from large chemical libraries being selectively identified. When ligand is binding, the target proteins undergo structural changes. In order to maximize the hit rate, structural flexibility must be incorporated during modeling. In the absence of the 3D structure of the target protein, ligand-based modeling is applied. Structural screening is not feasible in this case. The production of ligand pharmacophore is focused entirely on the common characteristics of the pharmacophore and the QSAR generation. Two distinct chemical structures share the same characteristics in the common characteristics pharmacophores. These chemical properties are obtained from the known structures of the ligand. Hydrophobic interactions, hydrogen connections and electrostatic interactions are typical features. The design of pharmacophore models in ligand-based pharmacophore has two main steps: (1) ligands are arranged in the training set with a conformation space for ligand-conformational versatility, and (2) ligands are aligned in the training to identify common chemical characteristics from all ligands (Malathi & Ramaiah, 2018).

Software used for pharmacophore modeling are HipHop, DISCO, HypoGen and PHASE (Martin, 2000). The ligand-based pharmacophore search was carried out in a study to find non-ATP competitive inhibitors for the mechanistic or mammalian target of rapamycin (mTOR). The spatial arrangement of ligand and protein model was generated with hydrophobic interactions of residues C5, C19, C21, C43, C45 and C49 of rapamycin to construct a model by the ZINCPharmer platform. It has resulted in eight new inhibitors with better activity (Kistet *et al.*, 2018).

3.7. Molecular Dynamics

MD is a technique that allows for a greater radius of convergence than normal energy minimization. However, only modest progress was achieved in refining some of the models closer to the native state in a recent analysis on a small number of protein models using state-of-the-art explicit solvent MD and implicit solvent for energy calculations (Lee *et al.*, 2001). It is the study of simulating the motion of a system of particles using Newton's classical equations. It is a fascinating field that sits at the intersection of mathematics, biology, chemistry, physics and computer science, not just at the interface of theory and experiment, but also at the intersection of mathematics, biology, chemistry, physics and computer science.

The ability to observe and predict motion, whether of the solar system or biological systems, provides a connection between the past and the future, as Laplace pointed out. Clearly, while an X-ray crystallographic image of a biomolecule is extremely useful, it is inadequate for understanding a broad spectrum of biological activity. It only provides a summary of a complex structure, but molecules are living things, with their constituent atoms constantly interacting with one another and with their surroundings. As a result, MD is needed to explain a system's broad range of thermally accessible states and to link structure and function. We can learn a lot about mean atomic fluctuations, heat capacities, rates of configurational changes, enzyme–substrate binding, different forms of coordinated motion and, maybe, protein folding by studying the dynamics of a molecular system over time (Schlick, 1996).

Currently, the PDB contains approximately 177,200 entries, including over 155,200 proteins and 12,900 nucleic acids, alone or in complexes. The understanding of basic biological phenomena such as enzyme mechanisms and regulation, transport across membranes, the construction of large structures such as ribosomes or viral capsids, or how DNA is read and transcription is regulated is aided by molecular recognition rules established by such structural information. One of the burgeoning areas of modern systems biology is the analysis and prediction of protein–protein interaction networks (Hospital *et al.*, 2015). *Figure 3* describes the schematic representation of MD simulations.

3.8. QSAR Studies

Computer drug design applies two techniques, namely the pharmaceutical design or the drug design based on the ligand. As structural and molecular biology grows dramatically, scientists aim to develop a structural drug design approach to innovate new molecules for different diseases. Only because of the docking score, the highly efficient ligands are highly challenging for further growth; this is overcome by the generation and it is more realistic to produce a statistically validated model that results in a high capacity for prediction. This can be obtained by the use of CoMFA to analyze the relationships between quantitative structural behavior in three dimensions and to provide statistically demonstrated models. CoMFA has the most predictive models (Thillainayagam *et al.*, 2019).

3.9. Systems Biology Approaches

Systems biology approaches help in acquiring enormous amount of biological information produced by experimental procedures and process it to explain how the systems work. Gene network analysis is another emerging field where the biological systems are studied at molecular level by understanding the interactions

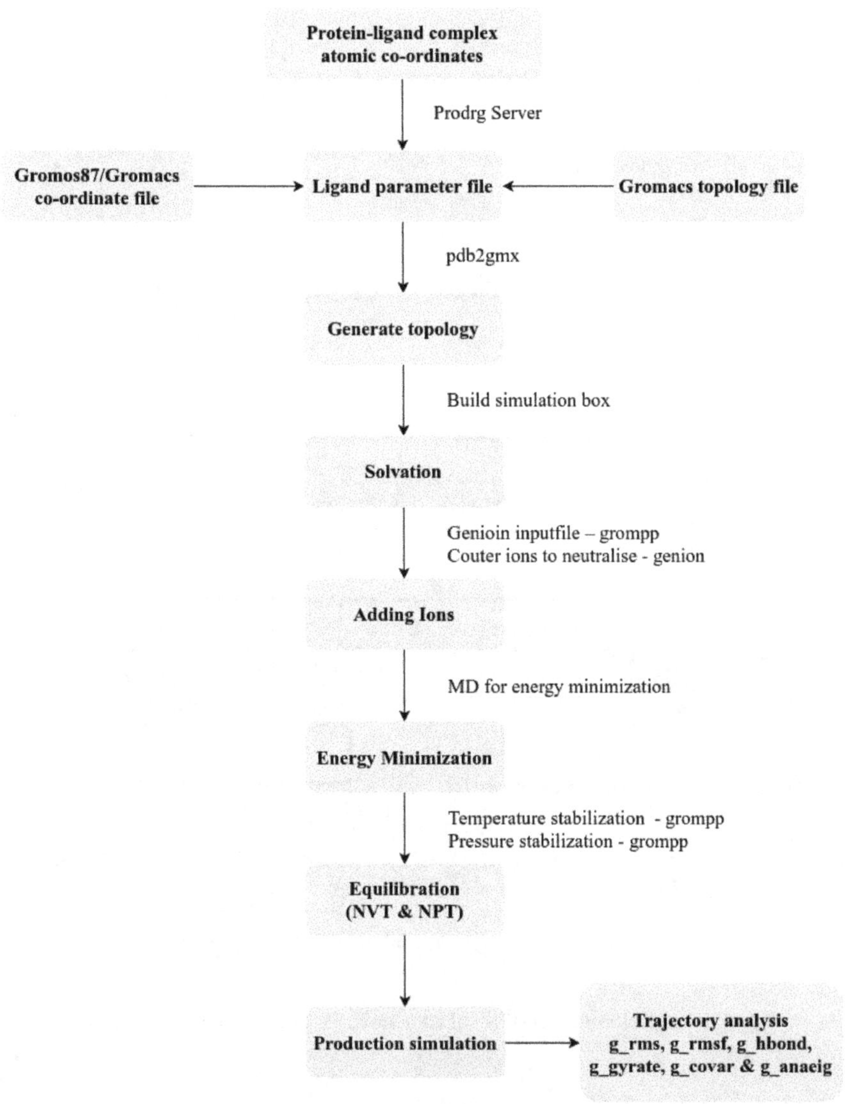

Fig. 3 Molecular dynamics simulations.

between the important genes to address the functional relationship and evolutionary conservation. A schematic representation of molecular interaction network analysis is shown in **Fig. 4** (Miryala *et al.*, 2018).

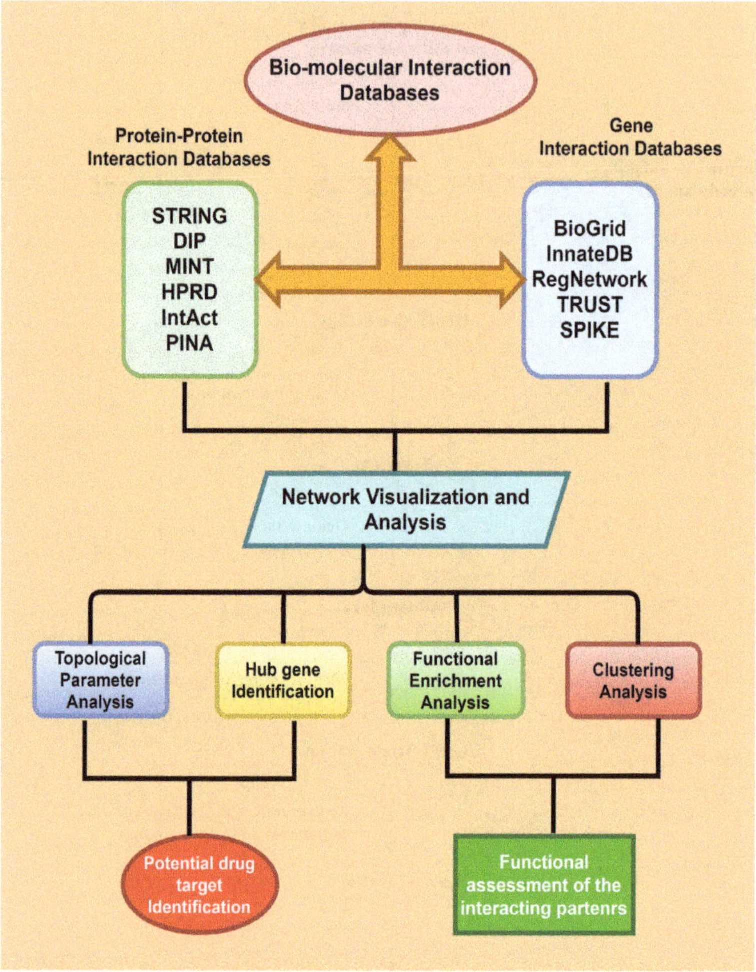

Fig. 4 A systematic workflow of molecular interaction network analysis.

4. Revealing the Mechanism of AMR by *in silico* Methods: Classical Examples

4.1. Penicillin-binding Proteins and β-lactamases

We explored the role of non-conventional interactions in the stability and functional specificity of β-lactamases and PBPs. Around 40% of interacting residues have more than one stabilizing regions in β-lactamases. The stabilization centers are higher in C–H$\cdots\pi$ interacting residues followed by cation–π, C–H$\cdots$O and N–H$\cdots\pi$ interacting residues. In PBPs around 25% of interacting residues have more than one stabilization centers. More than 60% of C–H$\cdots$O, C–H$\cdots\pi$ and N–H$\cdots\pi$ interacting residues and above 40% of cation–π interacting residues are highly conserved which reveals the functional importance of these residues in β-lactamases. In PBPs around 58% of residues are conserved in C–H$\cdots$O interactions, whereas 50% of residues are conserved in C–H$\cdots\pi$ interactions. Our analysis shows that cation–π, C–H$\cdots\pi$ and N–H$\cdots\pi$ interacting residues contribute to the global conformational stability of β-lactamases, whereas C–H$\cdots$O interactions contribute to the local conformational stability of β-lactamases. Similar to β-lactamases, in PBPs C–H$\cdots$O interactions contribute to the local conformational stability, whereas C–H$\cdots\pi$ contribute to the global conformational stability of PBPs. Solvent accessibility pattern of interacting residues shows that these residues contribute to the overall stability of β-lactamases and PBPs as the interacting residues preferred to be in both core and terminus region. Secondary structure preference of interacting residues shows that most amino acids have a clear preference to participate in a certain secondary structure type. The results obtained from this study will be useful in understanding the stability patterns of β-lactamases and PBPs (Lavanya *et al.*, 2013a, 2013b, 2013c, 2014a, 2014b, 2015a).

4.2. ampC

The *ampC* gene codes for β-lactamase cephalosporinase, which confirms the drug resistance against most of all the existing β-lactamases, although carbapenems are exceptional. Due to the mutation the gene can express more in the presence of β-lactam antibiotics, which in turn helps the bacterium to exhibit drug resistance. In our study, we have explored the functional association of *ampC* gene and the role of these potential interactions in inducing the β-lactamase synthesis. We have identified various genes based on their role in regulatory mechanism of β-lactamase through different gene ontology (GO) terms such as biological processes (BP), cellular components, molecular function (MF) and KEGG pathways. Especially, the genes *ampR*, *ampD*, *frdD* and *gcvA* along with *ampC* regulate the level of transcription in the presence or absence of the β-lactam inducers such as cefoxitin and imipenem. We have also performed the multiple sequence alignment (MSA) of *ampC* proteins to understand the amino acid variation. The MSA results reveal that the *ampC* is conserved in all bacterial species. The mutations mainly observed via the amino acid substitution occurred mainly in the active site regions. From our study, we observed that within the active site (amino acid residues from 91 to 98) the two amino acid residues Phe and Lys are conserved in *ampC* β-lactamase. The amino acid residues Lys and Ser play a critical role in orientating the active site by electrostatic interaction that creates a net positive potential in the catalytic site, which is predicted as the binding site of β-lactam antibiotics (Anitha *et al.*, 2014).

4.3. Metallo-β-lactamase

Metallo-β-lactamases (MBL) are class of bacterial enzymes which are metal-dependent and hydrolyze the β-lactam antibiotics and thus help the bacterium to exhibit drug resistance against the antibiotics used for the treatment. In our study we have curated 37 MBL proteins and 751 interactions from various bacterial species. Gene network analysis has shown dense interactions between the functional partners. The functional enrichment analysis has shown that the interacting functional partners are mainly involved in cell wall synthesis and other associated pathways. The mutation in gene *FmtA* can affect the cell wall structure and there is an enhancement of the expression during the presence of β-lactam antibiotics. The genes *fibA* and *fibB* involve in the formation of inter-peptide bridges in peptidoglycan biosynthesis pathway which helps in resistance against the antibiotics. The other functional partners DAPB and ASD are observed to have role in lysine biosynthesis pathway which is important as it provides the essential amino acids and also for the bacterial cell wall components. Another important observation is enrichment of *de novo* UMP biosynthetic process, which is essential for bacteria not only in cell wall synthesis but also in virulence and biofilm formation. The genes Bla1 and Bla2 are enriched with molecular function two-component system and β-lactamase activity. The genes *gerC*, *ispA*, *fni* and *mvk* are mainly involved in critical pathways essential for bacterial cell survival, isoprenoid biosynthesis process and also in terpenoids backbone biosynthesis pathways. It is also observed that these genes are involved in early stages of the cell wall synthesis. The proteins reported from the study are mainly present in cytoplasm, periplasmic space and membrane that are critical for bacterium in arranging the rigid cell wall. With their important role in bacterial machinery and major roles in bacterial antibiotic resistance, these genes could be exploited for designing new anti-bacterial compounds (Anitha *et al.*, 2016).

4.4. OXA β-lactamase

OXA type β-lactamases hydrolyses most of the antibiotics including the carbapenem group of antibiotics. The cleavage of antibiotic by the enzyme renders the antibiotic ineffective and the increased binding affinity of the OXA β-lactamase and the substrate should be studied to understand the resistance mechanism. In this study, we have explored the resistance mechanism of imipenem in *A. baumannii* by OXA-143 and OXA-231 CHDL. We employed *in silico* approaches to explore the binding affinity of imipenem with OXA-143 and its variant OXA-231. From our results, we observed that the high binding affinity of imipenem with OXA-143 leads to the hydrolysis of the antibiotic and thus makes the antibiotic ineffective, whereas the weak binding of imipenem with OXA-231 implies that the antibiotic will not undergo hydrolysis and it will be effective. Molecular dynamics and simulation studies also confirmed that the OXA-143 and imipenem complex showed much stability when compared with the OXA-231 and imipenem complex (Malathi *et al.*, 2017).

4.5. Carbapenamase

We explored the antibiotic resistance caused by carbapenamase in *Klebsiella pneumoniae*. The major reason for the β-lactam resistance is the enzyme *K. pneumoniae* carbapenamase (KPC). The secretion of KPC-2 and KPC-3 by the *K. pneumonia* strains exhibit resistance against imipenem and also for β-lactam inhibitors. In our study, we have performed molecular docking and dynamics simulation studies to analyze the resistance mechanism of KPC-2 with imipenem and KPC-3 with imipenem at structural level. We found that the KPC-3-imipenem complex has the highest c-score values and greater stability than the KPC-2-imipenem complex. It is believed that the greater the interaction between the substrate and the β-lactamase enzyme, the higher the chances of hydrolysis of the substrate. From our results, we have observed that the increased H-bond interaction and strong binding affinities may have emanated the hydrolysis of imipenem by KPC-3 enzyme. It is also observed that the weak binding affinity for KPC-3-tazobactam inhibitor results in resistance mechanism. Various reports stated that the available β-lactam inhibitors are ineffective in KPC-3 expressing pathogenic strains. We have also performed virtual screening to identify more effective inhibitors for KPC-3 and found that the chemical compounds ZINC48682523, ZINC50209041 and ZINC50420049 showed higher binding affinities when compared with the KPC-3-tazobactam complex. Molecular dynamics and simulation studies confirmed that these newly identified inhibitors displayed more stability and they might prevent KPC-3 enzyme from cleaving imipenem. Thus these inhibitors can be exploited in designing novel β-lactamase inhibitors (Malathi *et al.*, 2019a, 2019b).

4.6. Enterococcus Faecalis

Enterococcus faecalis is an opportunistic, nosocomial bacterial strain which exhibits resistance to the antibiotics chloramphenicol, tetracycline, vancomycin, linezoid, ampillicin and other known antibiotics. The drug resistance displayed by *E. faecalis* strains is mainly due to the exogenous AMR genes, and there is an urgent need to understand the role of these AMR genes at molecular basis in drug resistance. We employed gene interaction network approach to explore the role of AMR genes along with the functional partners in drug resistance acquired by the *E. faecalis* V583 strain. From our results, we have observed that the AMR genes mainly involved in three resistance mechanisms where 19 genes were characterized displaying alteration of drug target (pbps, mur and van genes), eight genes were corresponded to complete replacement/bypass of target sites (van genes) and seven genes portrayed ABC transporter MDR efflux pumps (msrA, EF_1680, EF_1682 and pbps). The major antibiotic resistance obstructions were displayed to β-lactams (penicillin, ampicillins and cephalosporins), glycopeptide (vancomycin), erythromycin and MLSB antibiotics by various genes, making the treatment of this strain a challenge. The network analysis of the AMR gene interactions showed that the genes *mraY*, *pbpC*, *murE*, *mrtG* and *murD* have maximum number of interactions. These genes with more number of direct interactions considered as the hub genes and can be exploited for new drug discovery (Naha *et al.*, 2020).

4.7. Staphylococcus Aureus

The MDR exhibited by the *S. aureus* strains renders the treatment worse and new therapeutics needs to be developed to fight against these drug resistant *S. aureus* strains. It is necessary to understand the functional relationship between the AMR genes with their functional partners to understand the drug resistance patterns and by which we can design successful drugs to combat against the drug resistance. We have identified the key genes which play a major role in drug resistance mechanism such as alterations in drug target (ant, ble, llm, gyrB, fosB, knt and blaZ), multidrug efflux pump (arlR, arlS, sepA, semB, sigB, sbtA, norB, mepA and tet38) and enzymatic inactivation (aac, aacAaphD, ermA, folA, grlA, gyrA, knt, msrA1, PBP, qacA, res, SAV0052, tetM) (Anitha *et al.*, 2016).

4.8. Klebsiella Pneumoniae

The rapid emergence of β-lactam resistance in Gram-negative bacteria is a major problem in the treatment of infections caused by pathogenic bacterial strains, in particular *K. pneumoniae.* In our study we have presented a systems biology approach to understand the role of SHV-ll gene in drug resistance mechanism patterns in *K. penumoniae* strain. An interaction network of 51 functional partners along with 256 edges was constructed using Cytoscape. We observed that SHV-11 gene has a role in drug resistance mechanism along with its functional partner genes *gyrA*, *parC*, *glsA*, *osmE*, *yjhA*, *yhdT*, *rimI*, *pepB*, *KPN_00437* and *KPN_01875*. The clustering analysis of gene interaction network has resulted the involvement of genes in important KEGG pathways, GO terms such as biological processes (BP) and molecular functions (MF). The genes *gyrA*, *parC*, *gyrB*, *parE* and *recA* with more number of direct interactors serve as the hub nodes in the network. These active functions lead to β-lactam resistance in *K. pneumonia* and the *acrB* gene; the genes acrA and tolC play an important role in the exclusion of the drug by multidrug efflux pumps (Miryala *et al.*, 2020).

4.9. Mycobacterium Tuberculosis

Capreomycin and bedaquiline are currently used for MDR TB treatment. To understand the impact of these antibiotics on *Mycobacterium tuberculosis* (Mtb) genes, we have curated the gene expression data where the Mtb cultures were exposed on the bedaquiline and capreomycin. Based on the *P*-value cut-off (<0.05) and logFC values (≤0.5 and ≥0.5), we have selected the top differentially expressed Mtb genes during the antibiotic exposures. We observed that the top differentially expressed Mtb genes were related to universal stress genes, two-component regulatory systems and drug efflux pumps. We have also curated the Mtb gene data sets and carried out the functional over-representation analysis using the individual gene expression values. FOA resulted with the positive enrichment of the pathways acetyl CoA, histidine and sigG regulons during both the drug exposures. During bedaquiline drug exposure the operons dihydropteroate synthase, ATP synthase subunit, cytochrome c and cytochrome c oxidase are positively enriched, whereas, during the capreomycin exposure the operons CRISPER-associated protein-related operon, tRAN methyltranferase activity and 50S ribosomal protein-related operons are positively enriched. We further constructed the gene interaction networks of antibiotic resistance genes and virulence genes of Mtb to understand the impact of the antibiotics at the molecular level and thus to understand the AMR and virulence patterns. From the obtained results, we observed that the virulence genes mdtB, nrp Rv3673c, fabG4 and eccB5 have shown the highest number of direct interactions, whereas in AMR interaction data gyrA, gyrB, Rv1747, rpsL and poB genes showed the highest number of interactions. These genes with more number of direct interactions can be exploited for new drug discovery; by targeting these genes we can restrict the association of these genes with the corresponding functional partners (Miryala *et al.*, 2020).

4.10. Pseudomonas Aeruginosa

We have used a computational approach to understand various drug resistance mechanisms which contribute to MDR in *P. aeruginosa.* The interaction network of 60 AMR genes along with the 337 functional interactions was analyzed. Functional enrichment analysis of AMR genes has shown that the genes in the network are mainly associated with efflux pump mechanisms, alginate biosynthesis, biofilm formation and *ampC* β-lactamase biosynthesis. Interestingly, the genes phoP, phoQ and cat are observed to have roles in more than one drug-resistant mechanism. The interaction network analysis has shown that the AMR genes *oprJ*, *oprM*, *oprN*, *ampC*, *gyrA*, *mexA*, *oprD*, *mexB* and *nfxB* have higher number of direct interactions and they are considered as the hub nodes in the network; these genes can be used as the potential drug targets for developing new drugs (Miryala *et al.*, 2019).

4.11. *Salmonella Enterica* Serovar Typhi

Salmonella enterica is a well-known human enteric pathogen which causes typhoid fever. The MDR acquired by the *S. enterica* strains made the treatment difficult. In our study we have explored the MDR mechanisms displayed by *S. enterica* strains and also identified potential drug targets that can be exploited in new drug discovery. Initially we have curated 44 AMR genes with 275 functional interactions and constructed the interaction network. The clustering analysis has shown three highly interconnecting clusters. Functional enrichment analysis has shown that AMR genes are mainly involved in drug resistance mechanisms such as the drug targ*et al*ternation and multidrug efflux pumps. Especially, seven genes *arnA*, *arnB*, *arnC*, *arnD*, *arnE*, *arnF* and *arnT* are observed to have critical role in cationic antimicrobial polypeptide molecule resistance. The genes *mdtH*, *mdtM*, *mdtG*, *emrD* and *mdtA* play a crucial role in major facilitator superfamily efflux systems, and the genes *acrA* and *acrB* play an important role in acrAB-tolC efflux pump. The genes *tolC*, *macB*, *acrA*, *acrB* and *mdfA* were observed in multiple drug resistance pathways. The results obtained from the study will be helpful for the experimental biologists to understand various drug resistance mechanisms and the new drug targets can be used to explore new drug leads in the treatment of *S. enterica* infections (Reetika *et al.*, 2020).

5. *In silico* Approaches to Design Antiviral Compounds

5.1. Dengue Viruses

Around 50% of the world's population is at the risk of dengue, a viral infection. Presently, there are not many drugs and prophylactic measures available to control dengue viral infection and hence there is an urgent need to develop effective anti-dengue compound from natural sources. We explored the antiviral properties of the medicinal plant *Vetiveria zizanioides* against dengue virus. Initially, the antiviral properties of active compounds were examined using docking analysis along with reference ligand. The enzyme–ligand complex which showed higher binding affinity than the reference ligand was employed for subsequent analysis. The stability of the top scoring enzyme–ligand complex was further validated using molecular simulation studies. On the whole, the study reveals that the compound ethyl 4-(4-methylphenyl)-4-pentenoate has an effective antiviral property, which can serve as a potential lead molecule in drug discovery process (Lavanya *et al.*, 2016).

Extracts from the leaves of *Azadirachta indica* has been traditionally used in folk medicine for viral infections. We explored the antiviral potency of nimbin, the active compound from the neem leaf extract against the envelope protein of dengue virus. Progression of viral entry into the host cell is facilitated by the envelope protein of dengue virus, suggesting it as an effective antiviral target. Nimbin is found to be effective against the envelope protein of all four types of dengue virus (Dengue 1–4), which is evident from our *in silico* analysis. Our findings suggest the clinical importance of nimbin, which can serve as effective lead compound for further analysis (Lavanya *et al.*, 2015b).

5.2. Hepatitis C Virus

Presently, there are no effective vaccines and antivirals for the prevention and treatment of Hepatitis C virus infections and hence there is an urgent need to develop potent HCV inhibitors. We carried out molecular docking, MD and 3D-QSAR on heteroaryl 3-(1,1-dioxo-2H-(1,2,4)-benzothiadizin-3-yl)-4-hydroxy-2(1H)-quinolinone series using NS5B protein. A total of 41 quinolinone derivatives are used for molecular modeling study. The binding conformation and hydrogen bond interaction of the docked complexes were analyzed to model the inhibitors. We identified the molecule XXXV that had a higher affinity with NS5B. Compound XXXV with c-score 4.98 was identified as the best fit ligand from the molecular docking studies. The simulation graph examination indicates high stability of the compound XXXV-NS5B when compared with free NS5B protein. The high-energy compound XXXV was used for the alignment of test and training set compounds as well as for the generation of CoMFA descriptors. The constructed models indicate good external and internal predictive capability. The steric contour plots reveal that substitution of non-bulky group in quinolinone and bulky group in thiadiazine system as probable reasons for high inhibition. The electrostatic contour plots indicate that substitution with charged groups at thiadiazine system of quinolinone has increased the inhibitory action. The MD study confirmed the stability of the compound XXXV-NS5B complex. The developed CoMFA descriptors parameters, which were calculated using a test set of 13 compounds, were statistically significant. We believe that the generated models will be useful for designing of HCV inhibitors. Our results will provide useful insights and leads to design potent anti-Hepatitis C virus molecules (Malathi *et al.*, 2019a, 2019b).

5.3. SARS-CoV-2 (Novel Corona Virus)

No commercially available drug candidate has yet been devised which is unique to and not repurposed against SARS-CoV-2 and has high efficacy or safe toxicity profile or both. Taking curcumin as a reference compound, we identified a new commercially available cyclohexanone compound, ZINC07333416 with binding energy (−8.72 kcal/mol) better than that of popularly devised anti-Covid-19 drugs like viral protease inhibitor lopinavir, nucleoside analogue remdesivir and the repurposed drug hydroxychloroquine when targeted to the active-site of SARS-CoV-2 Main protease (Mpro) through docking studies. The ligand ZINC07333416 exhibits crucial interactions with major active site residues of SARS-CoV-2 Mpro viz. Cys145 and His41 involving in the protease activity, as well as GLU-166 and ASN-142 which play the pivotal role in the protein dimerization. The protein–ligand stable interaction was further confirmed with MDS studies. Based on virtual assessment, ZINC07333416 also has significant values in terms of medicinal chemistry, pharmacokinetics, synthetic accessibility and antiviral activity that encourage its experimental applications against Covid-19 (Basu *et al.*, 2020).

6. *In silico* Approaches to Design Anti-*Plasmodium Falciparum* Compounds

As there is high level of resistance to all the classes of anti-malarial compounds, including artemisinin derivatives, there is an urgent need for the design and development of novel and potent anti-malarial drugs particularly against the *Plasmodium falciparum* which causes severe malaria. Considering the immediate need of effective anti-malarial drugs, this current work is carried out. In our study, the molecular docking and 3D-QSAR CoMFA analyses have been effectively carried out to a set of novel quinolinyl chalcone derivatives. These studies are performed to analyze the structural requirements for the design and development of highly potent inhibitors against PfLDH. The outcome of the docking study suggests that the hydrogen bonding interactions are the major interaction which could be considered as vital in the modification of inhibitory activities of quinolinyl chalcone derivatives.

Based on the best docked alignments, highly predictive CoMFA model is developed. The model shows statistically significant results in terms of cross-validated coefficient q^2 of 0.850, conventional coefficient r^2 of 0.912, $r^2_{(pred)}$ of 0.855 and small *SEE* of 0.280 specifying the existence of better statistical relationship between the descriptors and inhibitory activity. Both 3D-QSAR CoMFA model and docking studies have provided the information which is complementary to each other. The 3D contour plots derived from the CoMFA rendered crucial details for the augmented activity for the quinolinyl chalcone derivatives such as substitution of electronegative and bulky groups at the dioxolyl group of prop-2-en-1-one side chain and quinolinyl group of quinolinyl chalcone derivatives which could be applied in the design and development of highly successful active analogues of quinolinyl chalcone derivatives against *P. falciparum*. These models could be used as a tool in the design of effective anti-malarial compounds to combat malaria (Mahalakshmi *et al.*, 2019b).

7. Conclusion

The MDR exhibited by the pathogenic bacteria is alarming and poses a threat to the mankind. There is an urgent need to be taken to develop new therapeutics to combat against these pathogenic bacteria. The traditional drug discovery process requires huge investments and lot of time for the new drug development. Various systems biology approaches help in functional assessment and identification of new potential drug targets. The new *in silico* techniques such as virtual screening, molecular modeling, pharmacophore modeling, molecular docking, dynamics and simulation help in drug discovery. To conclude, we have presented a detailed workflow of various *in silico* and systems biology approaches helpful in drug discovery. We have also discussed the important factors to be taken into account while designing the new drugs and the reports published using the approaches discussed in the chapter. Our reports on PBPs, β-lactamases, carbapenamases and on important pathogenic bacteria namely *E. faecalis*, *S. aureus*, *K. pneumoniae*, *M. tuberculosis*, *P. aeruginosa* and *S. enterica* serover Typhi can be used as models for researchers to explore AMR in resistance genes/protein as well as in other pathogenic bacteria. In addition, these models can also be used to explore new antiviral and antibacterial compounds. We hope that the contents of the chapters will be useful for researchers exploring AMR and those involved in new drug discovery.

Acknowledgments

We would like to thank VIT for providing us the necessary facilities to carry out the research presented in this chapter. We would also like to thank Dr K.M. Kumar, Dr P. Lavanya, Dr P. Anitha, Dr T. Mahalakshmi, Dr Malathi, Mr Somuya Basu, Mr Aniket Naha, and Ms Reetika Debroy for their research contributions that we have presented in this chapter.

Funding Statement

The authors thank the Indian Council of Medical Research (ICMR), the Government of India agency for the research grants: SR: ICMR-IRIS ID: 2014-0099 and ICMR-IRIS ID: 2020-0690; MSK: ICMR-IRIS ID: 2020-7788; AA: ICMR-IRIS ID: 2011-03260 and ICMR-IRIS ID: 2019-0810.

References

Acceptors, B., Levitt, M., & Perutz, M. F. (1988). Rings act as hydrogen. *Journal of Molecular Biology*, *201*(4), 751–754.

Ahmad, S., Gromiha, M. M., Fawareh, H., & Sarai, A. (2004). ASAView: Database and tool for solvent accessibility representation in proteins. *BMC Bioinformatics*, 5, 1–5.

Anbarasu, A., Anand, S., Babu, M. M., & Sethumadhavan, R. (2007). Investigations on C–H$\cdots\pi$ interactions in RNA binding proteins. *International Journal of Biological Macromolecules*, *41*(3), 251–259.

Anitha, P., Anbarasu, A., & Ramaiah, S. (2016). Gene network analysis reveals the association of important functional partners involved in antibiotic resistance: A report on an important pathogenic bacterium. *Staphylococcus aureus*. *Gene*, *575*(2), 253–263.

Anitha, P., Bag, S., Anbarasu, A., & Ramaiah, S. (2015). Gene and protein network analysis of AmpC β lactamase. *Cell Biochemistry and Biophysics*, *71*(3), 1553–1567.

Basu, S., Veeraraghavan, B., Ramaiah, S., & Anbarasu, A. (2020). Novel cyclohexanone compound as a potential ligand against SARS-CoV-2 main-protease. *Microbial Pathogenesis*, *149*(July), 104546.

Berman, H. M., Battistuz, T., Bhat, T. N., Bluhm, W. F., Bourne, P. E., Burkhardt, K., Feng, Z., Gilliland, G. L., Iype, L., Jain, S., Fagan, P., Marvin, J., Padilla, D., Ravichandran, V., Schneider, B., Thanki, N., Weissig, H., Westbrook, J. D., & Zardecki, C. (2002). The protein data bank. *Acta Crystallographica Section D: Biological Crystallography*, *58*(6 I), 899–907.

Contreras-Moreira, B., Fitzjohn, P. W., & Bates, P. A. (2002). Comparative modelling: An essential methodology for protein structure prediction in the post-genomic era. *Applied Bioinformatics*, *1*(4), 177–190.

Dayhoff, M. O., Schwartz, R. M., & Orcutt, B. C. (1978). A model of evolutionary change. In *Atlas of protein sequence and structure* (pp. 345–352).

Debroy, R., Miryala, S. K., Naha, A., Anbarasu, A., & Ramaiah, S. (2020). Gene interaction network studies to decipher the multi-drug resistance mechanism in *Salmonella enterica* serovar Typhi CT18 reveal potential drug targets. *Microbial Pathogenesis*, *142*(February), 104096.

Dosztányi, Z., Magyar, C., Tusnády, G. E., & Simon, I. (2003). SCide: Identification of stabilization centres in proteins. *Bioinformatics*, *19*(7), 899–900.

Dougherty, D. A. (1996). Cation-π interactions in chemistry and biology: A new view of benzene, Phe, Tyr, and Trp. *Science*, *271*(5246), 163–168.

Edward, S. G., & Sabharwal, N. (2017). MongoDB, *Encyclopedic Reference of Genomics and Proteomics in Molecular Medicine*, (D), 22–25.

Eyal, E., Najmanovich, R., Mcconkey, B. J., Edelman, M., & Sobolev, V. (2004). Importance of solvent accessibility and contact surfaces in modeling side-chain conformations in proteins. *Journal of Computational Chemistry*, *25*(5), 712–724.

Forster, M. J. (2002). Molecular modelling in structural biology. *Micron*, *33*(4), 365–384.

Gallivan, J. P., & Dougherty, D. A. (1999). Cation-π interactions in structural biology. *Proceedings of the National Academy of Sciences of the United States of America*, *96*(17), 9459–9464.

Gallivan, J. P., & Dougherty, D. A. (2000). A computational study of cation-π interactions vs salt bridges in aqueous media: Implications for protein engineering. *Journal of the American Chemical Society*, *122*(5), 870–874.

Glaser, F., Pupko, T., Paz, I., Bell, R. E., Bechor-Shental, D., Martz, E., & Ben-Tal, N. (2003). ConSurf: Identification of functional regions in proteins by surface-mapping of phylogenetic information. *Bioinformatics*, *19*(1), 163–164.

Gromiha, M. M. (2003). Influence of cation-π interactions in different folding types of membrane proteins. *Biophysical Chemistry*, *103*(3), 251–258.

Henikoff, S., & Henikoff, J. G. (1993). Performance evaluation of amino acid substitution matrices. *Proteins: Structure, Function, and Bioinformatics*, *17*(1), 49–61.

Hospital, A., Goñi, J. R., Orozco, M., & Gelpí, J. L. (2015). Molecular dynamics simulations: Advances and applications. *Advances and Applications in Bioinformatics and Chemistry*, *8*(1), 37–47.

Kilpeläinen, T., Shahgholian, H., & Zhong, X. (2014). Growth estimates through scaling for quasilinear partial differential equations. *Annales Academiae Scientiarum Fennicae Mathematica*, *32*(1), 595–599.

Kist, R., Timmers, L. F. S. M., & Caceres, R. A. (2018). Searching for potential mTOR inhibitors: Ligand-based drug design, docking and molecular dynamics studies of rapamycin binding site. *Journal of Molecular Graphics and Modelling*, *80*, 251–263.

Laurie, A. T. R., & Jackson, R. M. (2005). Q-SiteFinder: An energy-based method for the prediction of protein-ligand binding sites. *Bioinformatics*, *21*(9), 1908–1916.

Lavanya, P., Ramaiah, S., & Anbarasu, A. (2013a). Non-canonical H-bonds in β-lactamases: Importance of C-H···π interactions. *Journal of Biological Inorganic Chemistry*, *18*(5), 539–545.

Lavanya, P., Ramaiah, S., & Anbarasu, A. (2013b). Influence of C–H.O interactions on the structural stability of β-lactamases. *Journal of Biological Physics*, 39(4), 649–663.

Lavanya, P., Ramaiah, S., & Anbarasu, A. (2013c). Cation-π interactions in β-lactamases: The role in structural stability. *Cell Biochemistry and Biophysics*, *66*(1), 147–155.

Lavanya, P., Ramaiah, S., & Anbarasu, A. (2014a). Binding site residues in β-lactamases: Role in non-classical interactions and metal binding. *Journal of Coordination Chemistry*, *67*(17), 2898–2910.

Lavanya, P., Ramaiah, S., & Anbarasu, A. (2014b). Computational analysis of N–H···π interactions and its impact on the structural stability of β-lactamases. *Computers in Biology and Medicine*, *46*(1), 22–28.

Lavanya, P., Ramaiah, S., Singh, H., Bahadur, R., & Anbarasu, A. (2015a). Investigations on the role of CH···O interactions and its impact on stability and specificity of penicillin binding proteins. *Computers in Biology and Medicine*, *65*, 85–92.

Lavanya, P., Ramaiah, S., & Anbarasu, A. (2015b). Computational analysis reveal inhibitory action of nimbin against dengue viral envelope protein. *VirusDisease*, *26*(4), 243–254.

Lavanya, P., Ramaiah, S., & Anbarasu, A. (2016). Ethyl 4-(4-methylphenyl)-4-pentenoate from *Vetiveria zizanioides* inhibits dengue NS2B-NS3 protease and prevents viral assembly: A computational molecular dynamics and docking study. *Cell Biochemistry and Biophysics*, *74*(3), 337–351.

Lee, M. R., Tsai, J., Baker, D., & Kollman, P. A. (2001). Molecular dynamics in the endgame of protein structure prediction. *Journal of Molecular Biology*, *313*(2), 417–430.

Malathi, K., Anbarasu, A., & Ramaiah, S. (2016). Ethyl iso-allocholate from a medicinal rice Karungkavuni inhibits dihydropteroate synthase in *Escherichia coli*: A molecular docking and dynamics study. *Indian Journal of Pharmaceutical Sciences*, *78*(6), 780–788.

Malathi, K., Anbarasu, A., & Ramaiah, S. (2017). Exploring the resistance mechanism of imipenem in carbapenem hydrolysing class D beta-lactamases OXA-143 and its variant OXA-231 (D224A) expressing *Acinetobacter baumannii*: An in-silico approach. *Computational Biology and Chemistry*, *67*, 1–8.

Malathi, K., & Ramaiah, S. (2018). Bioinformatics approaches for new drug discovery: A review. *Biotechnology and Genetic Engineering Reviews*, *34*(2), 243–260.

Malathi, K., Anbarasu, A., & Ramaiah, S. (2019a). Identification of potential inhibitors for *Klebsiella pneumoniae* carbapenemase-3: A molecular docking and dynamics study. *Journal of Biomolecular Structure and Dynamics*, *37*(17), 4601–4613.

Malathi, K., Ramaiah, S., & Anbarasu, A. (2019b). Comparative molecular field analysis and molecular docking studies on quinolinone derivatives indicate potential Hepatitis C virus inhibitors. *Cell Biochemistry and Biophysics*, *77*(2), 139–156.

Miryala, S. K., Anbarasu, A., & Ramaiah, S. (2018). Discerning molecular interactions: A comprehensive review on biomolecular interaction databases and network analysis tools. *Gene*, *642*, 84–94.

Miryala, S. K., Anbarasu, A., & Ramaiah, S. (2019). Impact of bedaquiline and capreomycin on the gene expression patterns of multidrug-resistant *Mycobacterium tuberculosis* H37Rv strain and understanding the molecular mechanism of antibiotic resistance. *Journal of Cellular Biochemistry*, *120*(9), 14499–14509.

Miryala, S. K., Anbarasu, A., & Ramaiah, S. (2020). Role of SHV-11, a class A β-lactamase, gene in multidrug resistance among *Klebsiella pneumoniae* strains and understanding its mechanism by gene network analysis. *Microbial Drug Resistance*, *26*(8), 900–908.

Naha, A., Kumar Miryala, S., Debroy, R., Ramaiah, S., & Anbarasu, A. (2020). Elucidating the multi-drug resistance mechanism of *Enterococcus faecalis* V583: *A gene interaction network analysis. Gene*, *748*, 144704.

Parimelzaghan, A., Anbarasu, A., & Ramaiah, S. (2016). Gene network analysis of metallo beta lactamase family proteins indicates the role of gene partners in antibiotic resistance and reveals important drug targets. *Journal of Cellular Biochemistry*, *117*(6), 1330–1339.

Pearson, W. R., & Lipman, D. J. (1988). Improved tools for biological sequence comparison. *Proceedings of the National Academy of Sciences of the United States of America*, 85(8), 2444–2448.

Sanchez, G. (2013). Las instituciones de ciencia y tecnología en los procesos de aprendizaje de la producción agroalimentaria en Argentina. El Sistema Argentino de Innovación: Instituciones, Empresas y Redes. *El Desafío de La Creación y Apropiación de Conocimiento*, *141*, 128–141.

Schleinkofer, K., Wang, T., & Wade, R. C. (2006). Molecular docking. *Encyclopedic Reference of Genomics and Proteomics in Molecular Medicine*, *443*, 1149–1153.

Thillainayagam, M., Malathi, K., Anbarasu, A., Singh, H., Bahadur, R., & Ramaiah, S. (2019). Insights on inhibition of *Plasmodium falciparum* plasmepsin I by novel epoxyazadiradione derivatives–molecular docking and comparative molecular field analysis. *Journal of Biomolecular Structure and Dynamics*, 37(12), 3168–3182.

Tiwari, A., & Panigrahi, S. K. (2007). HBAT: A complete package for analysing strong and weak hydrogen bonds in macromolecular crystal structures. *In Silico Biology*, 7(6), 651–661.

Urhahne, D., Nick, S., & Schanze, S. (2009). The effect of three-dimensional simulations on the understanding of chemical structures and their properties. *Research in Science Education*, 39(4), 495–513.

Wei, L., Chintala, S., Ciamporcero, E., Ramakrishnan, S., Elbanna, M., Wang, J., & Pili, R. (2016). Genomic profiling is predictive of response to cisplatin treatment but not to PI3K inhibition in bladder cancer patient-derived xenografts. *Oncotarget*, 7(47), 76374–76389.

Zhuang, Y., Zhou, X., & Wang, S. (2012). Gapped BLAST and PSI-BLAST: A new generation of protein database search programs. *Plant Systematics and Evolution*, 298(7), 3389–3402.

https://doi.org/10.1142/9789811254796_0007

7 An Integrative Approach to Explore Potent Therapeutic Protein Targets in Multidrug-resistant Nosocomial Pathogen *Acinetobacter Baumannii*

Jeyaraman Jeyakanthan*,†, Chitra Jeyaraj Pandian‡, Jeba Mercy Jeyaseelan‡, Sundarraj Rajamanikandan†, Dhamodharan Prabhu†, Ravi Guru Raj Rao†, Mutharasappan Nachiappan† and Jemima Kingsley§

†*Structural Biology and Bio-Computing Lab, Department of Bioinformatics, Science Block, Alagappa University, Karaikudi, Tamil Nadu, India*

‡*Department of Biotechnology, Dr. Umayal Ramanathan College for Women, Karaikudi, Tamil Nadu, India,*

§*Orbito Asia Diagnostics, Puliakulam Rd, Coimbatore, Tamil Nadu, India*

Abstract

Acinetobacter baumannii is one of the multidrug resistant (MDR) pathogens responsible for nosocomial infection causing bacteremia, urinary tract infection, and surgical wound infection. Moreover, *A. baumannii* forms biofilms and survives for several days in a dry environment contributing to its endemic infections in hospital installations. Therefore, the occurrence of extreme

*Corresponding author: e-mail:jjkanthan@gmail.com and jjeyakanthan@algappauniversity.ac.in

drug-resistant or MDR strains of *A. baumannii* due to biofilm formation and quorum sensing (QS) is posing a foremost challenge to the medical community. In this regard, an integrative approach including protein crystallography of therapeutic targets in *A. baumannii*, *in vitro* evaluation of bacterial adhesion for biofilm formation, *in vivo* QS activity, and structure-based drug design targeting the therapeutic proteins will provide the alternative options to combat *A. baumannii* infections. The chapter will provide a complete overview of all potential therapeutic protein targets in *A. baumannii* that aid in designing novel drugs or inhibitors.

1. Introduction

Acinetobacter baumannii is a nonmotile, Gram-negative, glucose nonfermentative, catalase-positive, and oxidase-negative coccobacilli associated with nosocomial infections. The recent emergence of multidrug resistance (MDR) in *A. baumannii* has imposed a serious threat to public health causing infections in blood, skin, urinary tract, and soft tissues. *A. baumannii* is also called as "Iragibacter," since several *A. baumannii* infections were reported suddenly among soldiers and veterans who served in Iraq war. MDR *A. baumannii*-mediated cross-infections spread in civilian hospitals through injured military soldiers repatriated from war zones. Most of the *A. baumannii* infections occur in immunocompromised patients, and spreads within intensive care units (ICUs). This especially impacts patients who have prolonged hospital stays in ICUs, and it represented about 20% of infection in ICU setting. Since then, several virulence factors have been identified in *A. baumannii*, namely, capsular polysaccharides, outer membrane proteins, lipopolysaccharides, proteases, protein secretion system, iron chelating agents, and phospholipases. Several studies have reported the rapid emergence of *A. baumannii* strains that are resistant to many of the antibiotics already in use. World

Health Organization has listed *A. baumannii* as one of the global priority 1: critical pathogen among antibiotic-resistant ESKAPE pathogens, namely *Enterococcus faecium*, *Staphylococcus aureus*, *Klebsiella pneumoniae*, *A. baumannii*, *Pseudomonas aeruginosa*, and *Enterobacter* species. Several antibiotic resistance strategies such as multidrug efflux pump, target modifications, permeability defects, and enzymatic degradation have been adopted by *A. baumannii* to escape from the lethal effects of antibiotics. In this chapter, we review the protein crystallographic approaches, *in vitro* and *in vivo* characterization techniques and computational methods to explore the potent drug targets in *A. baumannii*.

2. Protein Crystallography in Structural Analysis of Therapeutic Targets in *Acinetobacter baumannii*

Information about the three-dimensional (3D) structure of proteins is essential to understand the biological processes. X-ray crystallography is the most versatile technique that provides detailed structural information of protein molecule at the atomic level without any size limitation. Several technological advances in protein crystallography have made tremendous progress and now about 1,80,000 crystal structures have been deposited in the Protein Data Bank (PDB). The structural information provided in the PDB has significantly enhanced the elucidation of several biological processes besides facilitating the structure-based drug discovery. Protein crystals are composed of about 50% solvent (can vary between 25% and 95%) in which protein or nucleic acid occupies the remaining volume. Therefore, the individual molecules in protein crystals are surrounded by high water layers that sustain the protein structure in accordance with biological environment. Therefore, the parameters like binding of ligand, biochemical requirement, spectroscopic and enzymatic characteristics of protein crystals are same as the fully solvated molecules. Crystalline proteins exhibit hydrogen bonds, salt bridges, and hydrophobic bonds in proportion to its molecular weight with their neighboring atoms. Mother liquors for growing protein crystals should be aqueous in nature to which the target protein is tolerant. Protein crystals are generally soft, limited in size, easily crushable, can disintegrate on dehydration, diffract X-rays weekly, are temperature-sensitive and radiation-sensitive with poor optical properties when compared to conventional small molecules. Due to protein polymorphism, multiple crystal forms sometimes coexist in the same mother liquor sample. Many proteins assume several kinetically favored characteristic solid states. Very high levels of supersaturation, about two or three times higher than required for sustenance of crystal growth, are generally required for protein crystal to nucleate (Chernov, 2003). Moreover, the kinetics of protein crystal nucleation is slower due to the low diffusivity, poor association, and large size of the protein crystals. The major steps involved in the crystallographic detection of protein structure are shown in **Fig. 1**.

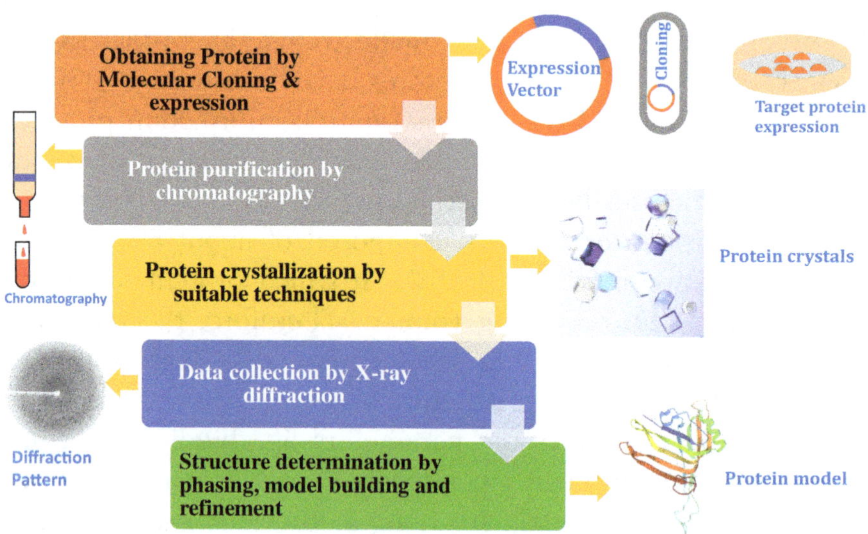

Fig. 1 Flowchart representing basic steps involved in protein crystallography.

Detection of protein crystals in the X-ray diffraction method involves two phases: (i) identification of physical, chemical, and biochemical conditions to yield good protein crystals; and (ii) modifications in initial conditions to get optimal protein crystals for diffraction analysis. The approaches to screen crystallization conditions involve (i) systemic variation in temperature, pH, type of precipitant, or concentration of precipitant; and (ii) shotgun approach.

Protein crystallization includes two basic steps: nucleation and growth. Nucleation is a first-phase transition in which molecules move to an ordered state from disordered state. Surface free energy, supersaturation, and molecular dimensions of nuclei obtained by nucleation process should be considered during crystallization. Protein crystals predominantly grow by dislocation mechanism, two-dimensional (2D) nucleation, and normal growth with 3D-nucleation occasionally. Supersaturation of mother liquor is the significant factor that determines the occurrence, magnitude, kinetics of nucleation, and crystal growth. Supersaturation is a non-equilibrium condition in which the protein quantity needs to be more than the solubility limit under specific conditions. Once the saturation limit is attained, the equilibrium can be reestablished by the formation of crystals. Therefore, few properties of the protein have to be modified to decrease their solubility and to increase the attraction between protein molecules. The supersaturation can be promoted by different approaches such as (i) modifying the protein itself by shifting the ionization state of amino acids found in protein surface, (ii) modifying the chemical activity of water by adding salt, (iii) modifying the degree of intramolecular attraction by altering the pH or by adding bridging ions, and (iv) modifying nature of protein–solvent interaction by adding ions or polymers. Crystal growth can be performed in physical apparatus to modify the protein solubility and mother liquor properties (McPherson *et al.*, 2003). Recent micro-techniques for crystallization employ plexiglass buttons for microdrops or oils, while multichambered plastic trays are also used for hanging drop or sitting drop methods.

Precipitants or crystallizing agents for protein crystallization can be classified into four types: (i) organic solvents, (ii) salts, (iii) long-chain polymers, and (iv) low-molecular-weight polymers or organic compounds (nonvolatile). Examples of the above categories include ethanol, ammonium sulfate, polyethylene glycol (PEG) 4000, and methyl pentanediol or PEG with molecular weight of less than 1000 for organic solvents, salts, long-chain polymers, and low-molecular-weight polymers, respectively. During the salting-in and salting-out process, the competition of salt ions (especially the anions) with proteins for binding water molecules is necessary for the maintenance of protein stability (McPherson & Gavira, 2014). The pH is also a significant variable that affects protein solubility.

Additives used in protein crystallization can be classified into the following eight categories:

1. Physiologically relevant molecules (coenzymes, metal ions, substrate, inhibitors, and prosthetic groups) that bind to enzyme active sites and induce stable homogenous conformation;
2. Chemical protectants or reducing agents (β-mercaptoethanol, dithiothreitol), heavy metal scavengers (ethylenediaminetetraacetic acid, ethylene glycol-bis(β-aminoethyl ether)-N,N,N′,N′-tetraacetic acid), and antimicrobial agents (It is Phenol, sodium azide, chlorobutanol);
3. Solubilizing agents and detergents (sulfobetaines, chaotropes like urea, ammonium salts);
4. Compounds that reduce twinning at concentrations less than 1%–5% (w/v) (ethanol, acetone, butanol, dimethyl sulfoxide, and dioxane);
5. Stabilizing agents that alter the interaction of protein surface with a water molecule and stabilize the protein's native conformation generally at a concentration of 1 M or more (trehalose,

proline, glycine, sucrose, taurine, sarcosine, and trimethylamine N-oxide);
6. Cross-linking multivalent molecules that cross-link charged amino and carboxyl groups on protein surface or by forming intra-hydrogen bonds between the polar groups on the protein surface (dicarboxylic acid or diamino containing molecules or aliphatic molecules with charged groups);
7. Multivalent charged compounds promoting lattice interactions; and
8. Nucleation-enhancing compounds with unique surfaces such as PEG and other polymeric substances can be used in low concentrations.

Growth of the protein crystal can be induced directionally at a low supersaturation level by seeding a metastable supersaturation solution with protein crystals obtained from earlier trials. Seeding is the widely used technique to initiate crystal growth, induce nucleation, and enhance crystal growth at a lower supersaturation level. Seeding can be performed when poor protein crystals have been obtained previously that can be used to serve as seeds. This process of seeding can be of two categories: (i) use of microcrystals as seeds and (ii) use of large macromolecular seeds. In case of the microcrystal seeding, stock solutions are serially diluted to a broad range under optimal crystal growth conditions so that the seeding yields microcrystals if the solution contains many seeds (Derewenda & Vekilov, 2005).

Therefore, the following important principles are essential in protein crystallography:

- *Homogeneity*: To obtain pure protein with a uniform molecular species population
- *Solubility*: High protein concentration can be dissolved without aggregates or precipitates

- *Stability*: Reducing modifications in protein to maintain its stability
- *Supersaturation*: Solution properties altered by appropriate supersaturation
- *Association*: Induce orderly association of protein thereby preventing aggregation
- *Nucleation*: Enhance controlled formation of critical nuclei
- *Variety*: Identify all possibilities in physical, chemical, and biochemical properties
- *Control*: Maintain the optimal state of the system during crystallization
- *Impurities*: Prevent impurities in mother liquor and lattice
- *Preservation*: Preserve and maintain grown crystals without disruption

2.1. Molecular Recognition of Protein and Structure-based Drug Discovery

The target bacterial proteins can be obtained through molecular cloning and expression of its gene by using polymerase incomplete primer extension and ligation-independent cloning of polymerase chain reaction (PCR) products. In the case of cloning multi-protein complexes, co-expression and co-folding approaches can be employed. The expressed proteins can then be purified using high-performance liquid chromatography. Further, the purified bacterial proteins were characterized for their mass, mono-disperse property, protein folding, peptide bond formation, and confirmation of reconstituted complexes using a variety of methods including mass spectrometry (MS), dynamic light scattering, circular dichroism (CD), proton nuclear magnetic resonance spectroscopy, and surface plasmon resonance or isothermal titration calorimetry. Good-quality protein crystals are essential for protein structure determination through X-ray diffraction analysis. Based on the suitable conditions for crystallization listed in the commercially available crystallization screens, the protein crystals can be optimized to yield good quality large crystals by seeding into any crystallization setup or by incorporating any modifications specified above. Crystallization of bacterial protein is followed by data collection through an X-ray diffraction experiment. Recently, third-generation synchrotrons are widely used for protein crystallography due to their high-quality data collection and speed which uses anomalous scatterers and CCD or pixel array detectors for crystal screening and structural data collection. The structure of bacterial proteins is determined through the suitable phasing techniques such as model building by conventional molecular replacement method and heavy-atoms-based method for obtaining electron density maps. These phasing methods are however being replaced with advanced protein structure determination approaches, namely, selanomethionine solved by MAD/SAD method using anomalous scatterers for signal (Schmidt *et al.*, 2014).

Structure determination of therapeutic protein targets in MDR nosocomial pathogens is essential to screen and identify suitable drugs to impede their antibiotic resistance and pathogenesis. For example, the outer membrane protein 33 (Omp33) protein is a porin implicated in carbapenem resistance in MDR *A. baumannii*. Omp33 prevents internal antibiotic concentration in *A. baumannii* and plays a vital role in virulence, adhesion, and biofilm formation. Omp33 is also known to induce apoptosis in immune cells and connective tissues, by activating the caspases and modulating autophagy. Therefore, Omp33 overproduction could substantially increase the mortality rate due to *A. baumannii*-induced nosocomial bacteremia and pneumonia. Therefore, the feasibility of considering Omp33 as a potent therapeutic target in *A. baumannii* is emphasized, and characterizing the crystal structure of Omp33 protein provides therapeutic strategies for treating *A. baumannii* infections. The X-ray crystal structure of Omp33 protein at 2.1 Å resolution comprises 14-β stranded barrels lacking stable extracellular loop constrictions with unusual periplasmic turns linking β-strands that fold into lumen pore and block the aqueous channel. The Omp33 monomers are packed through lateral contacts in the "ab" plane, while the "bc" plane does not show any monomeric association which results in layers of Omp33 monomers and presumes floating appearance in crystal. Omp33 contains about 300 amino acids including the first 26 residues as signal peptides, and cleaving this signal sequence leads to formation of mature polypeptide. Another important feature in the Omp33 crystal structure is 21 amino acid residues long-small periplasmic turn (T1 turn) which links β-strands 2 and 3. Among 21 residues, seven amino acids form α-helix structure and the loop folds back into barrel lumen without extending into periplasmic space that subsequently forms periplasmic constriction and closes the aqueous channel. The crystal structure of Omp33 protein was reported to function as a gated channel and reduce the permeability of bacterial envelope (Ruiz *et al.*, 2018).

Another example for novel therapeutic target in *A. baumannii* is the hemolysin co-regulated protein (hcp) which is responsible for the formation of hcp tube in the type VI secretion system (T6SS). Therefore, hcp acts as a virulence factor, as a chaperon, and as a transporter of effector molecules into human host cells. T6SS is also implicated in biofilm formation that was found to be substantially correlated with MDR activity. Ruiz *et al.* (2015) have reported the crystal structure of hcp protein in *A. baumannii* with β-barrel domains of 12 Å diameter formed by two β-sheets which are made up of five or five strands each. The barrel's hydrophobic core includes amino acid residues like valine, phenylalanine, leucine, isoleucine, methionine, and tryptophan. Ten residues in α-helix from Ser70 to Gly80 flank the barrel, while a 25 Å loop with His34 to Asp59 protrudes from the core. Therefore, 1.55 Å resolution of hcp protein crystal structure was reported to exhibit two β-sheets forming a β-barrel flanked by a short α-helix at one side, besides six hcp proteins interacting in both head-to-tail and head-to-head geometry to form a donut-shaped hexamer with 40

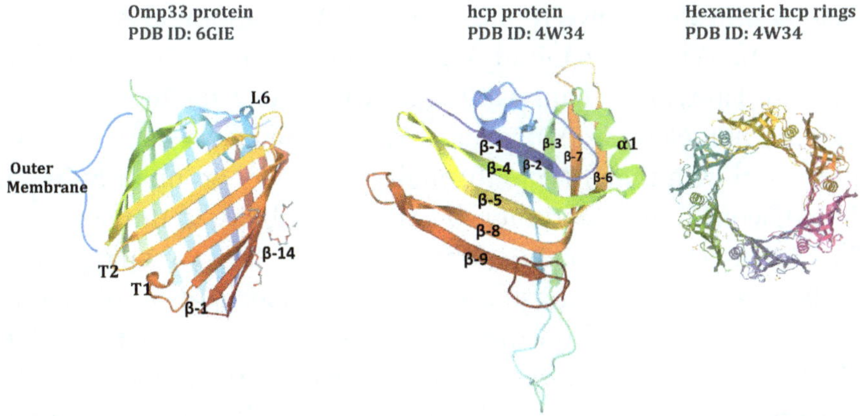

Fig. 2 Three-dimensional X-ray crystal structures of Omp33 and hcp proteins from *Acinetobacter baumannii*.

Å inner diameter (Ruiz *et al*., 2015). This structural data provides insights into the T6SS in *A. baumannii*. The number of crystal structures of therapeutic protein targets deposited in PDB for different *A. baumannii* strains includes 221, 60, 17, 15, 15, 14, 7, 6, 6, 5, and 4 proteins for *A. baumannii* strains ATCC 19606, AYE, AB307-0294, ATCC 17978, ACICU, AB0057, MRSN 3527, MRSN 3527, AB5075, SDF, and TCDC-AB0715, respectively.

2.2. Mechanism of Action and Catalysis of Enzymes

X-ray crystallographic analysis of protein targets also provides detailed information on the mechanism of action of protein and catalysis of enzymes, and evaluates the thermodynamics of ligand binding. For example, epimerase *Ab*-WbjB in *A. baumannii* is a dehydrogenase enzyme belonging to the family of short-chain dehydrogenases and reductases (SDR) that is reported to catalyze the conversion of UDP-N-acetyl-d-glucosamine to UDP-N-acetyl-fucosamine. *A. baumannii* utilizes this enzyme to produce capsule and lipo-oligosaccharides to evade the host immune response.

Shah *et al.* (2018) have reported a 2.65 Å resolution crystal structure of *Ab*-WbjB enzyme in *A. baumannii* as a hexamer, which is organized as trimer chain pair bound with coenzyme nicotinamide adenine dinucleotide phosphate ($NADP^+$) in each chain. $NADP^+$ interacted with the enzyme through quaternary group of lysine in the adjacent dimers and thereby offered stability to the hexamer. This structural information obtained from the crystallographic studies facilitates understanding of the mechanism of action of an enzyme. Based on these observations, it is evidenced that *Ab*-WbjB enzyme in *A. baumannii* is specific for substrate UDP-N-acetyl-d-glucosamine with binding equilibrium association constant (Ka) value of 0.23 µ/mol, and the variation in *Ab*-WbjB sequence compared to other SDR enzymes confirms the catalytic role of threonine residue (alternative to tyrosine) in the active site (Shah *et al.*, 2018). Hence the characterization of 3D structure of the *Ab*-WbjB enzyme in *A. baumannii* infers that the N-terminal side chains in SDR consensus catalytic motifs can act as an alternate participant in the active site of these epimerases. Moreover, binding of UDP-N-acetyl-d-glucosamine to *Ab*-WbjB in crystallographic analysis evidenced that this epimerase has a catalytic role in the conversion of UDP-N-acetyl-d-glucosamine to UDP-N-acetyl-fucosamine which is the precursor for the synthesis of surface glycoside in *A. baumannii.* Understanding the mode of action of *Ab*-WbjB enzymes which is responsible for core sugar synthesis in *A. baumannii* glycostructures will potentiate the use of *Ab*-WbjB as a future immunogenic therapeutic target. The catalytic reaction of the *Ab*-WbjB enzyme to convert UDP-N-acetyl-d-glucosamine to UDP-N-acetyl-fucosamine through several intermediates is shown in **Fig. 3a**.

Similarly, the catalysis of enzymes can be determined from the crystallographic analysis of protein targets. For example, pyrophosphatases are hydrolytic enzymes that cleave pyrophosphate (PPi) and release energy. This reaction shows that two divalent cations can activate water molecules in the catalytic center and thereby hydrolyze the pyrophosphate molecules through S_N2 mechanism. Si *et al.* (2019) have solved the co-crystal structure

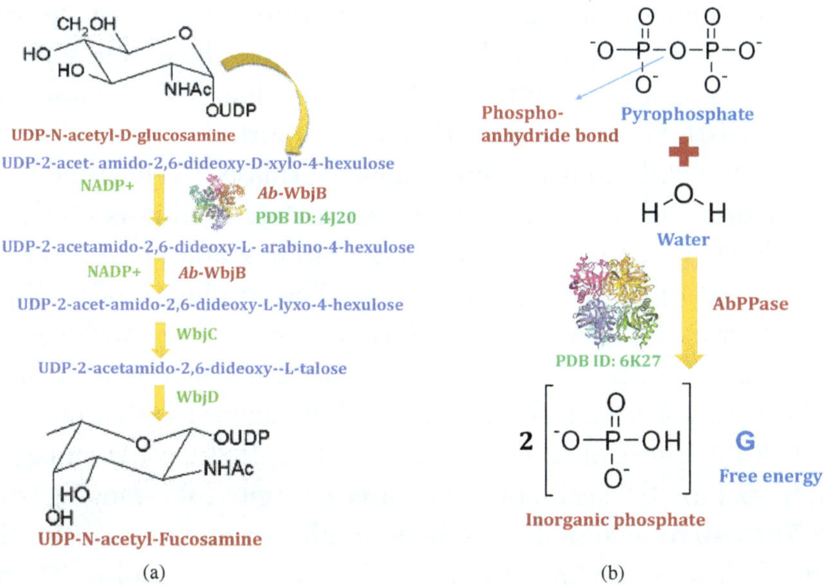

Fig. 3 (a) Mechanism of action of *Ab*-WbjB epimerase and (b) catalysis of *Ab*PPase.

of pyrophosphatases in *A. baumannii* (*Ab*PPase) along with water and reported that the solvent water molecule can act as catalytic water. Moreover, it has been reported that binding of sodium ions or monovalent cations to amino acid residues inside the loop found near the catalytic center of apo-*Ab*PPase can inhibit the enzyme reaction. Phosphorylated conserved lysine residue (K30) was reported to be the catalytic intermediate in PPi hydrolysis. Therefore, the structural data of *Ab*PPase derived from crystallographic analysis evidence new aspects of *Ab*PPase catalysis and could facilitate in designing of specific drugs to impede the growth of *A. baumannii*. **Figure 3b** explains the catalysis of *Ab*PPase in *A. baumannii.*

2.3. Relating 3D Protein Structure to Thermodynamics of Ligand Binding

Contribution of protein side chains involved in ligands or inhibitors binding can be evaluated by thermal stability and thermodynamic studies. The affinity between a protein or enzyme with its ligand can be optimized by evaluating the changes in entropy (ΔS) and changes in enthalpy (ΔH) of binding energy (Kanaujia *et al.*, 2010). Powers *et al.* (2014) have reported the crystal structure of *Acinetobacter*-derived cephalosporinases (ADCs) and their interaction with boronic acid transition state inhibitors (BATSI), namely S02030 and SM23, with high binding affinity of about 21 and 44 nM of Ki values, respectively. The resolution of an X-ray crystal structure of ADC in apo-form and in complex with ligands was reported to be 1.73 and 2.0 Å, respectively, with many canonical interactions. Thermodynamic analysis suggested that both the BALTI inhibitors of ADCs had favorable enthalpies (ΔH) ranging from −5.4 to −9.3 kcal/mol and relative energies (ΔG) ranging from −8.51 to −9.61 kcal/mol. This higher enthalpy compensates for the loss of entropy (ΔS) ranging from −2.7 to −14 cal/mol/K. Therefore, the crystallographic data of ADC enzyme in *A. baumannii* relate the 3D structural information to thermodynamics of BATSI binding, and the enthalpy-driven inhibitors can be optimized by introducing conformational constraints or hydrophobic groups.

3. *In vitro* and *in vivo* Functional and Molecular Characterization of Drug Targets in *Acinetobacter Baumannii*

MDR *A. baumannii* were reported to form biofilms and the bacterial cells in biofilms are resistant to antibiotics, phagocytosis, dehydration, exposure to acids, and ultraviolet light when compared to their planktonic stage. This evidences the modified metabolic activity of bacterial cells within the biofilm. The proteins that are upregulated and downregulated in *A. baumannii* biofilm cells can be analyzed by proteomic analysis. The following steps are involved in the identification of specific protein or proteins responsible for MDR especially the biofilm-associated proteins in *A. baumannii* (**Fig. 4**):

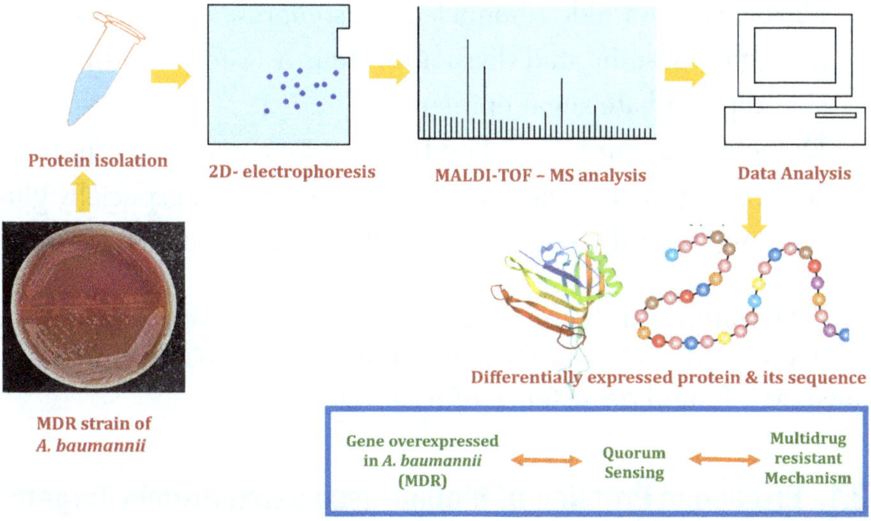

Fig. 4 Proteomic analysis of *Acinetobacter baumannii* by two-dimensional gel electrophoresis and MALDI analysis for identification of differentially expressed proteins.

1. Cultivating the clinical isolates of the *A. baumannii* under planktonic and biofilm formation conditions;
2. Separation of outer membrane enriched proteins by 2D gel electrophoresis;
3. Identifying the differentially expressed proteins by MALDI-TOF MS;
4. Screening and categorization of the upregulated proteins or the proteins that are expressed only in *A. baumannii* by reverse transcription-PCR;
5. Obtaining the protein-processing environmental data like sensors (histidine kinase or response regulator), iron transport proteins, and specific domain in diguanylate cyclase;
6. Identifying the proteins involved in bacterial metabolism, namely N-acetylmuramoyl-l-alanine amidase, NAD-linked malate dehydrogenase, Phosphoribosylformimino-5-aminoim-

idazole carboxamide ribonucleotideisomerase (ProFARisomerase), glucose-inhibited division protein A (GidA), and nucleoside-diphosphate sugar epimerase;

7. Detecting the proteins related to antibiotic resistance; and
8. Identifying the proteins involved in gene repair, especially glucose-inhibited division protein and exodeoxyribonuclease III.

Therefore, proteomic analysis of *A. baumannii* provides an essential platform to identify the significance of biofilms in tolerance, MDR, and persistence of bacteria.

3.1. Proteomic Profiling of Biofilm-associated Protein Targets

Biofilms can be defined as the assemblage of microbes wrapped in a matrix that acts as a cooperative association to render a protected mode for bacteria and empowering resistance to diverse antibiotics. This biofilm formation involves several factors such as substance for aggregation, collagen adhesion, acquisition of iron, and pili expression. Biofilm-associated protein (Bap) genes play a crucial role in intracellular adhesion, bacterial cell accumulation, and biofilm formation. The biofilm-forming ability of *A. baumannii* makes it to survive in abiotic and biotic surfaces including hospital environments and medical devices. *A. baumannii* also forms biofilms on the air–liquid interface of pellicles and surfaces of solids. The extracellular appendages involved in biofilm formation in *A. baumannii* are capsular polysaccharides, alginate, poly-β-(1–6)-N-acetylglucosamine and pili. In case of *A. baumannii*, the chaperone-usher pathway synthesized pili (Csu pili), CsuE adhesin in pilus tip, Type IV pili with PilA subunits, chaperone-usher pathway synthesized P pili, Ata auto transporter, transmembrane anchor domain, flexible passenger domain, and biofilm-associated protein (Bap and Bap-like BLP1, BLP2) are involved in stabilizing the 3D structure of biofilm on the abiotic surface as well as enhancing the bacterial adhesion to host. Biofilm development in *A. baumannii* is affected by resistance nodulation division efflux pumps, namely

AdeABC, AdeFGH, and AdeIJK. AdeFGH that are involved in the transport of quorum sensing (QS) molecules. OmpA protein is involved in the attachment of A. *baumannii* to abiotic surfaces or epithelial cells. Porins in A. *baumannii*, namely CarO, OprD, and OprCare are found to involve in metabolite uptake for siderophore synthesis in pellicles. Acinetobactin and enterobactin receptors in A. *baumannii* are involved in iron acquisition systems. Biofilm and pellicle formation are regulated by QS system, second messengers, and signal transduction systems. Cyclic di-guanosine monophosphate (GMP) and GacSA/BfmRS systems are involved in Csu pili synthesis, while CheA/Y regulatory systems regulate the Csu pili and acinetin expression through QS. Iron(III) ions are necessary for the development of pellicle. AdeABC or AdeFGH and ppGpp efflux pumps participate in biofilm formation and inhibit the production of AbaR as well as acinetin-505, respectively. Proteins in A. *baumannii*, namely outer membrane protein-A proteins coded by csuE genes enhance the formation of biofilm by A. *baumannii*. The biofilm reduces the diffusion of drugs through the microbial cell that thereby leads to antibiotic resistance and persistent survival of A. *baumannii* in a harsh environment. Therefore, formation of biofilms and antibiotic resistance in A. *baumannii* can be significantly correlated. Biofilm-associated proteins in A. *baumannii* code for a large surface protein containing about 8620 amino acids which is made of arrays of modules with 80–110 residues appearing similar to antibody-like motifs. Shin *et al.* (2009) have reported that the following few proteins were present only in the biofilms of A. *baumannii* cells.

1. UDP-galactose 4-epimerase that catalyze the formation of UDP-glucose from UDP-galactose essential for the synthesis of extracellular or capsular polysaccharides necessary for biofilm formation especially on abiotic surfaces.
2. ProFAR isomerase is involved in the biosynthesis of histidine which is essential for *de novo* purine synthesis, in nitrogen metabolism, and in biofilm formation.

3. Highly conserved GidA or tRNA uridine 5-carboxymethylaminomethyl modifying enzyme that alters tRNA in errors during gene expression is involved in virulence, antibiotic resistance, swarming, and biofilm persistence in *A. baumannii*.
4. Phosphodiesterase or diguanylate cyclase with EAL, GGDEF, and PAS domains that are involved in cyclic-di-GMP phosphodiesterase, cyclic-di-GMP-synthesizing diguanylate cyclase, and light/oxygen/redox sensing activities, respectively, and play a key role in bacterial motility, extra-polysaccharide synthesis, and biofilm formation.
5. N-acetylmuramoyl-l-alanine amidase hydrolyzes the peptidoglycan layer in bacterial cell wall with autocatalytic activity, besides enhancing extracellular DNA production that favors attachment of bacterial population to biofilms.

Similarly, the two outer membrane proteins, namely OmpW and OprE3 were found to be significantly downregulated in biofilm of *A. baumannii* (Lee *et al.*, 2017) and are involved in iron storage (bacterioferritin) or signal peptide and Lipoate-protein ligase activity, respectively. MALDI-TOF MS analysis evidenced two or more folds change in expression levels of aforesaid proteins. The upregulated proteins in biofilms of *A. baumannii* are also involved in metabolism, gene repair, processing information from the environment, biofilm formation, and antibiotic resistance.

3.2. Proteomic Analysis of QS-dependent Proteins

QS can be defined as the regulatory mechanism involved in bacterial cell communication mediated by signal molecules or autoinducers that have a hormone-like function to regulate population density and stimulate adaptation. QS relies on cell density which depends on the concentration of signaling molecule for cell-to-cell communication. The autoinducers alter the expression of many proteins in the entire bacterial population by binding specifically to the QS transcriptional regulators. The QS has been reported to have a strong correlation with the virulence factor production, plasmid transfer, motility, biofilm formation, and antibiotic resistance which enhances the bacterial cells to survive and proliferate in a favorable environment with efficient intracellular communication. In *A. baumannii*, QS has been found to act as signal molecules in influencing the formation of biofilm that is a significant factor essential for its extreme antibiotic resistance and survival characteristics. Drugs inhibiting either QS or causing premature QS-regulated gene expression can offer wide-spectrum control of *A. baumannii*-mediated infections. Furthermore, QS signals that regulate biofilm production and other virulence proteins expression are considered as potential drug targets for novel drug design. For example, natural and synthetic small molecules/compounds or acyl-homoserine lactone (AHL)-degrading enzymes can lead to misregulation or inhibition of QS in *A. baumannii*. Autoinducer antagonists also interrupt cell-to-cell communication by impeding the coordinated expression of genes in QS networks. AbaI and AbaR are the two proteins in *A. baumannii* that are homologous to the LuxI/LuxR system in other Gram-negative pathogens. This system has an autoinducer or signal molecule, namely AHLs which synthesize the signal molecule AbaI and the QS receptor activator AbaR. Therefore, AbaI and AbaR are the two components of QS machinery in *A. baumannii* which comprises the sensor proteins autoinducer synthase and receptor protein AHLs, respectively (Shin *et al.*, 2009). Aba regulates the biofilm formation, virulence, mobility, and competence of bacteria by forming a complex with N-(3-hydroxydodecanoil)-l-homoserine lactone (3-OH-C12-HSL) which on reaching threshold concentration, transports AHL molecules to its receptors and thereby increases the synthesis of AHL molecules. However, the QS mechanism acts under stress conditions induced by the environment like the presence of hydrogen peroxide and bile salts in respiratory and gastrointestinal tracts, respectively. Other QS-related enzymes in *A. baumannii* includes

AidA enzyme which acts as quorum quenching agent by degradation of N-dodecanoyl-l-homoserine lactone and N-(3-oxo-dodecanoyl)-l-homoserine lactone signal molecules (Lopez *et al.*, 2017). Another enzyme MomL was found to decrease biofilm formation as well as increase biofilm susceptibility to different antibiotics in *A. baumannii.* Therefore, *A. baumannii* QS system consists of AbaI inducer and its receptor AbaR that has autoinducer synthase function synthesizing AbaR-AHL molecules. The formed AbaR–AHL complex activates AbaI synthesis and QS-dependent gene expression that further triggers synthesis of Csu pili and acinetin-505 production (Monem *et al.*, 2020).

3.3. Characterization of Virulence and Drug-resistance-Associated Proteins

A. baumannii has become extreme drug resistant (XDR) to almost 22 antimicrobial agents belonging to nine categories, namely aminoglycosides, anti-pseudomonal fluoroquinolones, anti-carbapenems, polymixins, beta-lactamase, penicillin inhibitors, cephalosporins, tetracyclines, and folate pathway inhibitors. This resistance mechanism of *A. baumannii* to several antibiotics is mediated by intrinsic and acquisition processes. Oxacillinase enzyme is a class of D-beta-lactamases that are the prime cause for carbapenem resistance in *A. baumannii*. Other classes of beta-lactamase present in *A. baumannii* include class A, ampC, and metallo-beta-lactamase (MBL) like imipenemases, MBL from New Delhi (NDM), and verona integron-encoded MBL. Overexpression of ampC gene regulated by insertion sequence (ISAba1) produces an increased amount of class C-beta lactamases which is responsible for the resistance of *A. baumannii* to third-generation antibiotics, namely cephalosporins. Aminoglycoside-modifying enzymes like acetyltransferase, nucleotidyltransferases, and phosphotransferases that alter amino or hydroxyl groups of aminoglycosides are other examples of therapeutic targets in *A. baumannii*. It has been reported that the outer membrane protein (Omp) in *A. baumannii* especially OmpA is associated with adhesion to epithelial cells, biofilm formation, modification of cellular permeability, and drug resistance. The variation in the permeability of cells results in increased expression of efflux pumps. Moreover, mutations in the genes producing gyA/parC topoisomerases and rpsJ proteins in *A. baumannii* lead to resistance against fluoroquinolones and tigecycline, respectively. Mutations in the two-component system PmrAB in *A. baumannii* can increase the production of phosphoethanolamine leading to colistin resistance. In the case of efflux pumps in *A. baumannii*, overexpression of AdeFGH pump confers resistance against diverse antibiotics or chemicals like clindamycin, trimethoprim, fluoroquinolones, sulfamethoxazole, safranin O, acridine orange, ethidium bromide, and tetracycline-tigecycline. AdeIJK pump in *A. baumannii* induces resistance to folates and fusidic acid (Monem *et al.*, 2020).

4. Computational Multi-omics Approach Toward Identification of Drug Targets in *Acinetobacter Baumannii*

The proteome is the entire set of proteins present or expressed in a cell, tissue, organism or species. This proteome data generally translated from the completely sequenced and annotated genome. Pan-proteome is the total set of proteins that are expressed by closely related strains of the same microbe, and it comprises (i) proteome common for all strains, (ii) dispensable proteome that are not present in more than two strains, and (iii) unique proteins found only in a particular strain providing identity to it. Therefore, the availability of annotated genomes enhances the analysis of pan-genomics and comparative genomics for further understanding the mechanism of MDR. Elucidation of protein structures and its interactions plays a crucial role in understanding the physiological and pathological functions of a cell (Jeyakanthan *et al.*, 2005). A protein interacting with various protein partners are called as hub proteins, which can be predicted by PPI network. These interaction information facilitate the validation of predicted protein function, role of specific protein in metabolic pathways, and identification of functional association of proteins. All available strains of *A. baumannii* having complete genome and latest assembly can be considered for analysis of core proteome, and FTP NCBI Refseq server is widely used in the retrieval of proteome of different strains. The following steps are involved in core proteomics analysis: (i) clustering of similar proteins by CD-HIT program, (ii) selecting cluster of proteins (COP) commonly present in all *A. baumannii* strains, (iii) retrieval of proteins in selected *A. baumannii* strain from common COPs and analysis of metabolic pathway using Kyoto Encyclopedia of Genes and Genomes (KEGG) database. Subtractive genomics involves BLASTp against human proteome, Database of Essential Genes (DEG), and Drug Bank Database to retrieve nonhomologous protein, to functionally characterize hypothetical proteins, and to identify suitable drug targets along with physicochemical parameters, respectively (Solanki & Tiwari, 2018). The druggable score of the selected protein can be predicted using fpocket. The identification and visualization of protein–protein interactions can be performed using STRING database and Cytoscape, respectively. The hub proteins can be identified based on the node degree.

4.1. Comparative Proteomic and Subtractive Genomic Analysis to Identify Drug Targets

In recent years, subtractive genomics is considered as a versatile tool to identify the therapeutic targets for designing of new antibiotics against drug-resistant pathogens. Currently, vast information about proteomic and genomic data of *A. baumannii* strains allows to extensively use the computational methods for the identification of the promising drug and vaccine candidates. Subtractive genomics is an approach that subtracts bacterial pathogenic genes that

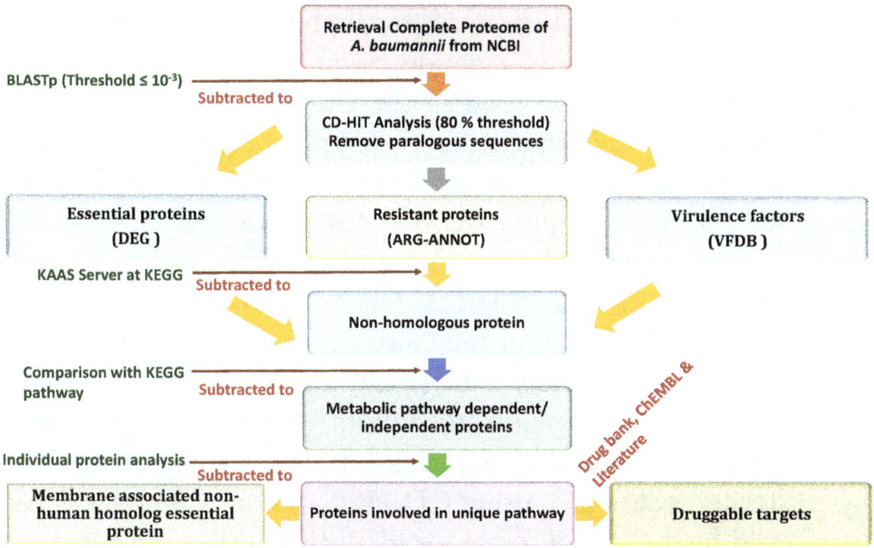

Fig. 5 The basic steps involved in subtractive genomics for druggability analysis.

are necessary for its survival, which are not present in the host. The shortlisted proteins can be further cloned, overexpressed, and purified in affinity chromatography followed by validation of drug candidates in *in vivo* animal models. The steps involved in subtractive genomics (**Fig. 5**) are (i) retrieval of proteome or genome data and phylogenetic analysis, (ii) CD-HIT analysis, (iii) screening of essential proteins, (iv) analysis of virulence factors, (v) analysis of resistance proteins, (vi) selection of nonhomologous proteins to host, (vii) identification of pathogen-specific pathway, and (viii) druggability analysis.

Bacterial proteome redundancy is a barrier for effective use of dataset and removal of redundant sequences which is necessary to avoid repetitive search results. Therefore, all the searched strains of *A. baumannii* have to be separated according to their non-redundancy and redundancy levels. All the selected proteomes including the reference proteome can be downloaded from the UNIPROT database and subjected to BLASTp against the reference strain of *A. baumannii* SDF (Kaur *et al.*, 2013). Genome data of selected *A. baumannii* strains can be obtained from NCBI, and the International Nucleotide Sequence Database Collaboration numbers can be used in the case of complete genome, while whole genome sequencing number can be applied for draft sequence. RNAmmer can be used to search whole genome DNA sequence for rRNA sequences. One 16s rRNA gene can be randomly sampled per *A. baumannii* strain as only slight sequence difference exists among 16srRNA genes within the same genome of the species. MEGA6 tool and ClustalW are widely employed in the construction of phylogenetic tree using 16srRNA sequence of all *A. baumannii* strains and for multiple sequence alignment of the sequence, respectively. Duplicate proteins can be identified by clustering techniques using CD-HIT and the amino acids can be aligned by the global sequence identity algorithm (Kaur *et al.*, 2013).

The target proteins with homologous matches in database of essential genes are considered as potential drug targets. BLASTp search against DEG bacterial proteins with cut-off parameters like *E*-value and bit score identifies the essential proteins in *A. baumannii* proteome. The virulence factors enable bacteria to alter or degrade defense mechanism of host which is mediated by various steps, namely, adhesion, colonization, and invasion. Virulence factor database can be used to classify the proteins in four categories, namely, offensive, defensive, nonspecific, and virulence-associated proteins. Antibiotic resistance gene-ANNOTation database can be used to detect putative and existing novel antibiotic resistance gene or proteins in *A. baumannii.* BLAST search of *A. baumannii* proteome against the Antibiotic resistance gene-ANNOTation database predicted the proteins responsible for antibiotic resistance. Manual comparative analysis of virulence, essential, and resistance proteins for identifying nonhomologous to host proteins are the key steps to identify drug targets to design pathogen-specific drugs. KEGG database can be used to identify the metabolic pathways of nonhomologous proteins. Metabolic pathway of host can also be enlisted with a K number and compared to *A. baumannii* metabolic pathways to find the pathways that are found only in the pathogen and not in human. The proteins can further be grouped based on their role such as common pathways found in both pathogen and host as well as in pathogen-specific unique pathways. The druggability of the target proteins in unique pathway can then be searched against all possible therapeutic targets in Drug Bank database. The selected proteins with bit score greater than 100 and *E*-value less than 0.005 are considered as the potential therapeutic targets that can be further categorized based on the consensus location identified by using online servers such as PSORTb and CELLOv2.5. The proteins with low molecular weight around 100–110 kDa can enhance the accessibility value of therapeutic protein targets. Then, the proteins playing vital role in specific biosynthetic pathway can be selected for further *in silico* analysis. The metabolic functional interaction between the proteins has to be performed for all the identified target proteins using protein interaction database STRING to provide critical evaluation and integration of protein–protein association including direct or indirect interactions.

Homology modeling technique can be adopted to construct the 3D structural models of the drug targets in *A. baumannii*. The query protein sequences can be subjected to BLASTp analysis in PDB to identify the appropriate template with more than 30% identity for modeling. The models can be generated using software like MODELLER and the coordinates of the bound ligand or lead molecules can be transferred to homology model through ligand modeling (Rajamanikandan & Srinivasan, 2017). The designed model with top Discrete Optimized Protein Energy score and Molpdf score can be subjected to further validation. Stereochemical quality of crude homology model can be evaluated to access the overall structural geometry of the drug targets using Ramachandran plot. ERRAT plot can be employed to check the steric hindrances in the amino acid side chains that can be validated by PROCHEK and ERRAT plot. CastP can be employed to identify amino acid residues in active site. The amino acid sequence of target proteins can be aligned with other bacterial proteins using ClustalX to identify the conserved amino acid residues. A literature search can be carried out to identify the ligands with higher minimum inhibitory activity reported against the same targets of different bacteria. 3D structure of selected lead molecules can be constructed by molecular modeling. Geometry optimization and minimization of 3D structures can be assessed by Gastieger–Huckel partial charges and Tripos force field, respectively. Molecular docking can then be applied to dock lead molecules in binding site or active site of the protein, and the ligands can be ranked based on their interaction in the active site with good binding energy. Three essential steps are involved in molecular docking: (i) ligand and protein preparation, (ii) grid generation, and (iii) ligand docking. The best docked lead compound can be studied for their ADME properties. The ADME properties and drug-likeliness can be studied using QikProp module of Schrodinger. Molecular dynamics (MD) simulation can be carried out to predict the stability of the refined homology model of target proteins. The particular trajectories obtained from MD simulation of protein–ligand complex were used for analysis of hydrogen bond and binding free energy estimation using molecular mechanics generalized Boltzmann surface area method (Choubey & Jeyaraman, 2016).

5. Other Possible Drug Targets Involved in Metabolic Pathways of *Acinetobacter Baumannii*

Earlier studies on *A. baumannii* strain AB5075 showed the presence of 438 essential genes in transposon mutagenesis. However, in a recent study by Tillery *et al.* (2020) from Seattle Structural Genomics Center for Infectious Disease reported that 342 essential genes are found in *A. baumannii* strain AB5075, out of which 306 genes have been successfully cloned, 192 proteins have been expressed, 165 soluble proteins screened, 121 proteins purified,

52 crystallized, and 29 protein structures were deposited in PDB. The following proteins are considered as therapeutic targets in *A. baumannii* strain AB5075, which are involved in various metabolic pathways such as protein synthesis, fatty acid synthesis, glycolysis, and cell wall or lipid synthesis.

1. **Therapeutic protein targets in A. *baumannii* involved in amino acid or protein synthesis**
   a. Tetrahydrodipicolinate N-succinyltransferase is a promising drug target in A. *baumannii*, as the mammals lack this biosynthetic enzyme that is involved in the synthesis of L-2-succinylamino-6-oxopimelate during synthesis of lysine and therefore can have reduced mammalian toxicity (Schnell *et al.*, 2012).
   b. 2,6-Diaminoheptanedioate (DAP) is the potent target in A. *baumannii*, as it is involved in the synthesis of both cell wall and protein by catalyzing pathways in peptidoglycan and l-lysine synthesis, respectively (Hor *et al.*, 2013).
   c. 3-Dehydroquinate synthase is an attractive target in A. *baumannii* with low toxicity, as the mammals lack this synthetic enzyme that is involved in shikimate pathway during dehydroquinate synthesis in the presence of NAD and zinc (De Mendonca *et al.*, 2011).
   d. Translation elongation factor P that is used for development of specific inhibitors without imposing toxicity to human and is required for impeding ribosomal stalling involved in elongating polypeptides with successive proline residues (He *et al.*, 2019).
   e. Methionine aminopeptidases are potential drug targets in A. *baumannii* that remove N-terminal methionine from nascent proteins before post-translational modification (Yuan *et al.*, 2011).

f. Methionine—tRNA ligase are alternate therapeutic targets in *A. baumannii* that is involved in binding of amino acid residues to their respective tRNA during protein synthesis in ribosomes, and its specific inhibitors block protein synthesis (Cvetesic & Gruic-Sovulj, 2017; Faghih *et al.*, 2017).
g. Tyrosyl-tRNA synthetase that catalyzes tRNAaminoacylation in *A. baumannii* can be used as selective target (Sun *et al.*, 2017; Xiao *et al.*, 2011).

2. Therapeutic protein targets in *A. baumannii* involved in fatty acid synthesis

a. Alpha subunit of malonate decarboxylase in a multienzyme complex is a potent therapeutic target in *A. baumannii* since it is involved in malonate synthesis using acetate and carbon dioxide as substrates (Chohnan *et al.*, 2003).

3. Therapeutic protein targets in *A. baumannii* involved in glycolysis pathway

a. Selective inhibition of phosphoglycerate mutase independent of 2,3-bisphosphoglycerate in *A. baumannii* impedes the interconversion of phosphoglycerates (Hallows *et al.*, 2012).
b. Fructose-bisphosphate aldolase in *A. baumannii* is a promising therapeutic target involved in synthesis of dihydroxyacetone phosphate and glyceraldehyde-3-phosphate (Daher & Therisod, 2010; Tran *et al.*, 2016).
c. Thiamine monophosphate kinase in *A. baumannii* is a significant drug target, as it is absent in mammalian cells and is involved in thiamine phosphate synthesis (Begley *et al.*, 1999).

Therapeutic protein targets in A. *baumannii* involved in synthesis of cell wall and lipid synthesis including membrane proteins are as follows:

1. UDP-N-acetylmuramoylalanyl-d-glutamyl-2,6-DAP-d-alanyl-d-alanyl ligase (Elamin *et al.*, 2017)
2. UDP-N-acetylmuramate:alanine ligase (Baum *et al.*, 2009)
3. 2-Dehydro-3-deoxyphosphooctonate aldolase (Harrison *et al.*, 2012)
4. Lipoprotein-releasing transmembrane protein (Mcleod *et al.*, 2015)
5. UDP-N-acetylglucosamine diphosphorylase (Bos *et al.*, 2007)
6. Lipid A export permease (Di Somma *et al.*, 2019)

Other possible ungrouped targets involved in metabolic pathways in A. *baumannii* are 1-deoxy-d-xylulose 5-phosphate reductoisomerase, coproporphyrinogen III, and glutamine-dependent NAD^+ synthetase.

6. Conclusion

Sequence information of all the bacterial species is mostly available due to the advancement in the molecular biology and sequencing techniques. Integration of sequence data obtained from next-generation sequencing and comparative genomics along with *in vivo* or *in vitro* analysis can be employed for identification of novel targets for development of antimicrobial agents. Therapeutic targets are proteins that are necessary for bacterial survival, and their inhibition would result in hindrance to bacterial metabolism and growth. Based on this consideration, this chapter provides an overview about the structural information, antimicrobial resistance, and genomic information obtained from protein crystallographic technique, *in vivo* methods, and computational analysis, respectively, along with the future options available for treatments. *A. baumannii* infections are associated with nosocomial infections, such as bacteremia, urinary infection, and endocarditis. *A. baumannii* is one of the major pathogens involved in hospital-acquired infection. Synergistic combination of cell wall active agents with antibiotics was employed as therapeutics for *A. baumannii* infections. However, extensive use of different antibiotics has led to the emergence of MDR and XDR strains of *A. baumannii* that have posed major challenge in treatment. Therefore, there is an utmost need to identify potent therapeutic targets that are involved in the major metabolic pathways, survival, and pathogenesis of *A. baumannii*. Many enzymes in *A. baumannii* infections are also known as choke point enzymes that do not show similarity to human analogs. Hence inhibition of these choke points impedes key metabolic pathways, namely amino acid or protein metabolism, or peptidoglycan biosynthesis or metabolism of nucleotide sugar, and thereby poses challenge for survival of *A. baumannii*. The specified potent drug targets can be exploited for development of wide-spectrum antibiotics. This detailed integrative information facilitates in rational drug design to combat infections caused by *A. baumannii*.

6.1. Summary

X-ray crystallography is a widely adopted technique in structure biology to provide detailed information about protein targets without any size limit. Structural analysis of therapeutic targets using protein crystallography in *A. baumannii* provides detailed information regarding molecular recognition of protein, enzyme catalysis, mode of protein action, and relating 3D protein structure to thermodynamics of ligand binding, which will enhance structure-based drug discovery process. *In vitro* and *in vivo* analyses of therapeutic targets in *A. baumannii* provide a complete picture of proteome as well as characteristics of biofilm-associated protein targets, QS-dependent proteins, virulence factors, and antibiotic resistance proteins. Computational multi-omics approach toward identification of drug targets in *A. baumannii* can be achieved by comparative proteomic and subtractive genomic strategies to identify potent drug targets. This wealth of structural data and proteome analysis would significantly enhance the elucidation of several biological processes and lead to development of potent therapeutics against *A. baumannii*.

Acknowledgment

JJ thank the DST INDO-TAIWAN (GITA/DST/TWN/P-86/2019), Board of Research in Nuclear Sciences (BRNS) (35/14/February 2018 BRNS/35009), DST-Fund for Improvement of S&T Infrastructure in Universities & Higher Educational Institutions (FIST) (SR/FST/LSI-667/2016) (C), and DST-Promotion of University Research and Scientific Excellence (PURSE) (No. SR/PURSE Phase 2/38 (G), 2017). JJ greatly acknowledges Tamil Nadu State Council for Higher Education (TANSCHE), (File No. RGP/2019-20/ALU/HECP-0049) JJ and SR acknowledge MHRD-RUSA 2.0, New Delhi [F.24e51/2014-U, Policy (TNMulti-Gen), Dept. of Edn., Govt. of India, dated October 09, 2018] for facilities and funding. JJ Thank Bioinformatics and Computational Biology Centre (DBT-BIC)–Ref No.BT/PR40154/BTIS/137/34/2021 for funding.

References

Baum, E. Z., Crespo-Carbone, S. M., Foleno, B. D., Simon, L. D., Guillemont, J., Macielag, M., & Bush, K. (2009). MurF inhibitors with antibacterial activity: Effect on muropeptide levels. *Antimicrobial Agents and Chemotherapy*, *53*, 3240–3247.

Begley, T. P., Downs, D. M., Ealick, S. E., McLafferty, F. W., Van Loon, A. P. G. M., & Taylor, S. (1999). Thiamin biosynthesis in prokaryotes. *Archives of Microbiology*, *171*, 293–300.

Bos, M., Robert, V., & Tommassen, J. (2007). Biogenesis of the gram-negative bacterial outer membrane. *Annual Review of Biochemistry*, *61*, 191–214.

Chernov, A. A. (2003). Protein crystals and their growth. *Journal of Structural Biology*, *142*(1), 3–21.

Chohnan, S., Akagi, K., & Takamura, Y. (2003). Functions of malonate decarboxylase subunits from *Pseudomonas putida. Bioscience*, *Biotechnology*, and *Biochemistry*, *67*, 214–217.

Choubey, S. K., & Jeyaraman, J. (2016) A mechanistic approach to explore novel HDAC1 inhibitor using pharmacophore modeling, 3D-QSAR analysis, molecular docking, density functional and molecular dynamics simulation study. *Journal of Molecular Graphics and Modelling*, *70*, 54–69.

Cvetesic, N., & Gruic-Sovulj, I. (2017). Synthetic and editing reactions of aminoacyl-tR-NAsynthetases using cognate and non-cognate amino acid substrates, *Methods*, *113*, 13–26.

Daher, R., & Therisod, M. (2010). Highly selective inhibitors of class II microbial fructose bis-phosphate aldolases. *ACS Medicinal Chemistry Letters*, *1*, 101–104.

De Mendonca, J. D., Adachi, O., Rosado, L. A., Ducati, R. G., Santos, D. S., & Basso, L. A. (2011). Kinetic mechanism determination and analysis of metal requirement of dehydroquinate synthase from *Mycobacterium tuberculosis* H37Rv: An essential step in the function-based rational design of anti-TB drugs. *Molecular Biology*, *7*, 119–128.

Derewenda, Z. S., & Vekilov, P. G. (2005). Entropy and surface engineering in protein crystallization. *Acta Crystallographica Section*, *D62*, 116–124.

Di Somma, A., Caterino, M., Soni, V., Agarwal, M., Pasquale, P., Zanetti, S., Molicotti, P., Cannas, S., Nandicoori, V. K., & Duilio, A. (2019). The bifunctional protein GlmU is a key factor in biofilm formation induced by alkylating stress in *Mycobacterium smegmatis*. *Research in Microbiology*, *170*, 171–181.

Elamin, A. A., Steinicke, S., Oehlmann, W., Braun, Y., Wanas, H., Shuralev, E. A, Huck, C., Maringer, M., Rohde, M., & Singh, M. (2017). Novel drug targets in cell wall biosynthesis exploited by gene disruption in *Pseudomonas aeruginosa*. *PLoS One*, *12*(10), 1–18.

Faghih, O., Zhang, Z., Ranade, R. M., Gillespie, J. R., Creason, S. A., Huang, W., Shibata, S., Barros-Álvarez, X., Verlinde, C. L., Hol, W. G., Fan, E., & Buckner, F. S. (2017). Development of methionyl-tRNA synthetase inhibitors as antibiotics for Gram-positive bacterial infections. *Antimicrobial Agents and Chemotherapy*, *61*(11), e00999-17.

Hallows, W. C., Yu, W., & Denu, J. M. (2012). Regulation of glycolytic enzyme phosphoglycerate mutase-1 by Sirt1 protein-mediated deacetylation. *Journal of Biological Chemistry*, *287*, 3850–3858.

Harrison, A. N., Reichau, S, & Parker, E. J. (2012). Synthesis and evaluation of tetrahedral intermediate mimic inhibitors of 3-deoxy-D-manno-octulosonate 8-phosphate synthase. *Bioorganic & Medicinal Chemistry Letters*, *22*, 907–911.

He, C., Liu, N., Li, F., Jia, X., Penh, H., Liu, Y., & Xiao, Y. (2019). Complex structure of *Pseudomonas aeruginosa* arginine rhamnosyltransferase EarP with its acceptor elongation factor P. *Journal of Bacteriology*, *201*(13), e00128-19.

Hor, L., Dobson. R., Downton, M., Wagner, J., Hutton, C., & Perugini, M. (2013). Dimerization of bacterial diaminopimelate epimerase is essential for catalysis. *Journal of Biological Chemistry*, *288*, 9238–9248.

Jeyakanthan, J., Inagaki, E., Kuroishi, C., & Tahirov, T. H. (2005). Structure of PIN-domain protein PH0500 from *Pyrococcus horikoshii*. *Acta Crystallographica Section F: Structural Biology and Crystallization Communications*, *61*(5), 463–468.

Kanaujia, S. P., Jeyakanthan, J., Nakagawa, N., Balasubramaniam, S., Shinkai, A., Kuramitsu, S., Yokoyama, S., & Sekar, K. (2010). Structures of apo and GTP-bound molybdenum cofactor biosynthesis protein MoaC from *Thermus thermophilus* HB8. *Acta Crystallographica Section D: Biological Crystallography*, *66*(7), 821–833.

Kaur, N., Khokhar, M., Jain, V., Bharatam, P. V., Sandhir, R., & Tewari, R. (2013). Identification of druggable targets for *Acinetobacter baumannii* via subtractive genomics and plausible inhibitors for MurA and MurB. *Applied Biochemistry and Biotechnology*, *171*(2), 417–436.

Lee, C. R., Lee, J. H., Park, M., Park, K. S., Bae, I. K., Kim, Y. B., Cha, C. J., Jeong, B. C., & Hee, S. (2017). Biology of *Acinetobacter baumannii*: Pathogenesis, antibiotic resistance mechanisms, and prospective treatment options. *Frontiers in Cellular and Infection Microbiology*, 7(55), 1–35.

Lopez, M., Mayer, C., Laura, F. G., Blasco, L., Muras, A., Federico, M. R., Bou, G., Otero, A., & Tomas, M. (2017). Quorum sensing network in clinical strains of *A. baumannii*: AidA is a new quorum quenching enzyme. *PLoS One*, *12*(3), e0174454.

Mcleod, S., Fleming, P. R., MacCormack, K., McLaughlin, R. E., Whiteaker, J. D., Narita, S., Mori, M., Tokuda, H., & Miller, A. A. (2015). Small-molecule inhibitors of gram-negative lipoprotein trafficking discovered by phenotypic screening, *Journal of Bacteriology*, *197*, 1075–1082.

McPherson, A., Cudney, R., & Patel, S. (2003). The crystallization of proteins, nucleic acids and viruses for X-ray diffraction analysis. *Biopolymers*, *8*, 427–468.

McPherson, A., & Gavira, J. A. (2014). Introduction to protein crystallization. *Acta Crystallographica Section F*, 70, 2–20.

Monem, S., Blaszk, B. F., Lupkowska, A., Kuczy, D., Karolina, S., & Ewa, L. (2020). Mechanisms protecting *Acinetobacter baumannii* against multiple stresses triggered by the host immune response, antibiotics and outside-host environment. *International Journal of Molecular Sciences*, *21*(15), 5498.

Powers, R. A., Swanson, H. C., Taracila, M. A., Florek, N. W., Romagnoli, C., Caselli, E., Prati, F., Bonomo, R. A., & Wallar, B. J. (2014). Biochemical and structural analysis of inhibitors targeting the ADC-7 cephalosporinase of *Acinetobacter baumannii*. *Biochemistry*, *53*(48), 7670–7679.

Rajamanikandan, S., & Srinivasan, P. (2017). Exploring the selectivity of auto-inducer complex with LuxR using molecular docking, mutational studies and molecular dynamics simulations. *Journal of Molecular Structure*, *1131*, 281–293. https://doi.org/10.1016/j.molstruc.2016.11.056

Ruiz, F. M., Santillana, E., Spinola-Amilibia, M., Torreira, E., Ulebras, E., & Romero, A. (2015). Crystal structure of Hcp from *Acinetobacter baumannii*: A component of the type VI secretion system. *PLoS One*, *10*(8), e0136978.

Ruiz, J. A, Zahn, M., Basle, A., & Berg, B. V. D. (2018). Crystal structure of the *Acinetobacter baumannii* outer membrane protein Omp33. *Acta Crystallographica Section D*, *74*(9), 852–860.

Schmidt, T., Bergner, A., & Schwede, T. (2014). Modelling three-dimensional protein structures for applications in drug design. *Drug Discovery Today*, 19, 890–897.

Schnell, R., Oehlmann, W., Sandalova, T., Braun, Y., Huck, C., Maringer, M., Singh, M., & Schneider, G. (2012). Tetrahydrodipicolinate N-succinyltransferase and dihydrodipicolinate synthase from *Pseudomonas aeruginosa*: Structure analysis and gene deletion. *PLoS One*, *7*(2), e31133.

Shah, B. S., Ashwood, H. E., Harrop, S. J., Farrugia, D. N., Paulsen, I. T., & Mabbutt, B. C. (2018). Crystal structure of a UDP-GlcNAc epimerase for surface polysaccharide biosynthesis in *Acinetobacter baumannii*. *PLoS One*, *13*(1), e0191610.

Shin, J. H., Lee, H. W., Kim, S. M., & Kim, J. (2009). Proteomic analysis of *Acinetobacter baumannii* in biofilm and planktonic growth mode. *Journal of Microbiology*, *47*, 728–735.

Si, Y., Wang, X., Yang, G., Yang, T., Li, Y., Ayala, G. J., Li, X., Wang, H., & Su, J. (2019). Crystal structures of pyrophosphatase from *Acinetobacter baumannii*: Snapshots of pyrophosphate binding and identification of a phosphorylated enzyme intermediate. *International Journal of Molecular Sciences*, *20*(18), 4394.

Solanki, V., & Tiwari, V. (2018). Subtractive proteomics to identify novel drug targets and reverse vaccinology for the development of chimeric vaccine against *Acinetobacter baumannii. Scientific Reports*, *8*, 9044.

Sun, J., Lv, P., & Zhu, H. (2017). Tyrosyl-tRNA synthetase inhibitors: A patent review. *Expert Opinion on Therapeutic Patents*, *27*, 557–564.

Tillery, L., Barrett, K., Dranow, D.M., Craig, J., Shek, R., Chun, I., Barrett, L. K., Phan, I. Q., Subramanian, S., Abendroth, J., Lorimer, D. D., Edwards, T. E., & Voorhis, W. C. (2020). Towards a structome of *Acinetobacter baumannii* drug targets. *Protein Science*, *29*, 789–802.

Tran, H. T, Lee, S. H, Ho, T. H., Hong, S., Huynh, K., Ahn, Y., Oh, D., & Kang, L. (2016). Crystallographic snapshots of active site metal shift in *E. coli* fructose 1,6-bisphosphate aldolase. *BMB Reports*, *49*, 681–686.

Xiao, Z. P., Ma, T. W., Liao, M. L., Feng, Y., Peng, X., Li, J., Li, Z., Wu, Y., Luo, Q., Deng, Y., Liang, X., & Zhu, H. (2011). Tyrosyl-tRNA synthetase inhibitors as antibacterial agents: Synthesis, molecular docking and structure–activity relationship analysis of 3-aryl-4-arylaminofuran-2(5H)-ones. *European Journal of Medicinal Chemistry*, *46*, 4904–4914.

Yuan, H., Chai, S., Lam, C., Howard, X. H., & Ye, Q. (2011). Two methionine aminopeptidases from *Acinetobacter baumannii* are functional enzymes. *Bioorganic and Medicinal Chemistry Letters*, *21*, 3395–3398.

https://doi.org/10.1142/9789811254796_0008

8 Peptides as Antiviral Drugs

Pachaiappan Raman*,†, Vinduja Vasudevan†,
Vrithi Sundararaman†, Samantha Prathab†,
Ineya Madhavan† and Velmurugan Devadasan‡

†*Department of Biotechnology, School of Bioengineering,
SRM Institute of Science and Technology,
Kattankulathur Campus, Chennai 603 203, Tamil Nadu, India*
‡*Office of the Dean Sponsored Research,
Publications and Collaborations, AMET University,
Kanathur, ECR Road, Chennai, P.C.-603 112*

Abstract

Viral disorders like hepatitis, HIV-AIDS, and diseases like the recent SARS-CoV-19, are becoming the major reasons for morbidity and mortality of humans as well as animals. The massive differences between virus and its pathogenesis and epidemiology indicate that there is really no simple panacea to this problem. As an alternative treatment for viral diseases, the growing desire for natural products has prompted research into the pharmacological significance of biologically active substances from diverse natural sources. This mini review is intended to focus on the natural peptides with antiviral properties against a variety of viruses that can be further developed into potential antiviral drugs. It may lead us to develop a wide range of therapeutics that can prevent, control, and also help in eradicating such viral diseases.

*Corresponding author: e-mail: pachaiar@srmist.edu.in

1. Introduction

While viral infections have been known from ancestral periods, it was not until the 19th century that researchers were able to understand the "filterable particles," later named viruses. Ever since, significant scientific advances in the regulation of viral replication, infection, and vaccine development have led to impressive developments in human–virus associations, like for instance, eradication of smallpox, control and management of measles, as well as transmission of polio. However, viruses continue to stay as one of the major causal factors of human diseases, largely because the development and production of quality vaccines are difficult and time consuming (Boas *et al.*, 2019; Mahmoud, 2016). The effectiveness of viruses in evolution has been ensured by four general characteristics: genetic variation, variety of means of transmission, effective replication inside host cells, and the ability to thrive in host cells (Mulder *et al.*, 2013).

A peptide is derived from a larger precursor protein and has a well-defined biological activity on its own. Peptides play a significant role in therapeutics due to their anti-inflammatory, anti-aging, and muscle binding properties. So far these therapeutic peptide products have been used for treating metabolic disorders, respiratory disease, hematological disorders, and deficiency of the immune system. Peptides are known to possess high potency and selectivity as well specific binding affinity toward their targets in comparison with other bioactive molecules. Peptides can be biodegraded by peptidases, reducing their tissue retention, leading to reduced toxicity. They are expected to impact a wide activity on various microorganisms. In this brief review, we will be reporting few of the natural peptides that possess virucidal activity against various viruses.

2. Mode of Action of Peptides Against Viruses

Antiviral peptides exhibit their potency against viruses by three ways: (i) disruption of attachment of virus and also its fusion with the cell membrane, (ii) damaging the envelope of the virus, and (iii) suppressing of multiplication by interfering with the polymerase enzyme of virus (Skalickova *et al.*, 2015). Antimicrobial peptides (AMPs) hinder the viral proliferation cycle of influenza virus by the above-mentioned mechanisms:

1. The peptides blocking viral attachment and fusion with cell membrane: There are two means for inhibiting the virus entrance. The peptides can interfere with sialic acid attachment by obstructing the receptor site of hemagglutinin (HA). The second process entails the intrusion with HA with the conformational change imperative for the viral fusion by which the fusion of virus with the membranes of the endosomes are hindered along with the obstruction of release of RNA to host cell (Skalickova *et al.*, 2015).
2. The peptides that interrupt the viral envelope: The principle of antiviral activity in virus resistance attacks the membrane of virus or the cholesterol-rich lipid rafts. The latter triggers instability of the proteins present on the surface of the virus that is rich in lipid raft domains (Rajendran *et al.*, 2010). Cathelicidins are human antiviral peptides capable of disrupting the viral envelope and they have been reported to produce a variety of host-protective pathways, like promoting repairs of the barriers, production of cytokine and chemokine, modulating the differentiation of dendritic cells, polarization of T-cells, and also showing powerful anti-sepsis as well as anti-inflammatory properties (Choi *et al.*, 2012). Melittin is a popular and widely known membrane-disrupting peptide obtained from European honeybee's (*Apis mellifera*) venom (Raghuraman *et al.*, 2007). It seems to have various implications on lipid bilayer membranes, like vesicular deformation, artificial pores formation, disruption, and lysis (Ladokhin *et al.*, 2001). As of now, the

destruction of virion envelopes caused by peptides is loosely documented. Two of the most explored membrane disruption mechanisms invoked to describe the secretion of bilayer lipid contents are: (i) rupture formation (Gordon-Grossman *et al.*, 2009, 2012) and/or (ii) destruction/solubilization of lipid bilayer (Benachir *et al.*, 1995; Oren & Shai, 1998).

3. The peptides that impede the viral replication: Viral RNA-dependent RNA polymerase (RdRp) comprises three subunits, which are PA, PB1, and PB2. PB1 takes care of polymerization reaction and the cleavage of the endonuclease (Ruigrok *et al.*, 2010). PB2 is in charge of recognizing along with the binding the host mRNA cap structure (Fechter, 2003), while PA endonuclease manages cleavage of host pre-mRNA (Dias *et al.*, 2009; Yuan *et al.*, 2009). Disruption of the RdRp assembly is a tremendous possibility in order to stop enzyme activity and also replication of viruses (Skalickova *et al.*, 2015).

3. Techniques for Identification and Verification of Antiviral Peptides

3.1. Computational Approach

Identification of peptides from computational approach includes two techniques, namely, docking and peptidomimetics. Using molecular docking via *in silico* screening, the peptides can be detected computationally in which a docking program is used to predict the target site named as pocket or protusion. Eventually, library of peptides profiled with these protusions results as highest binding site (Nevola & Giralt, 2015). Peptidomimetics is another method which mimics the target which is designed, thus preventing the interactvity of proteins by competitive binding (Sen *et al.*, 2019).

3.2. Biological Approach

Techniques using biological approach involve phage display, mRNA display, ribosome display, and yeast display. Phage display involves using phages to display foreign peptides. It is an appropriate system for delivering small peptides, that is, peptides with less than 20 amino acids. This technique is also effective in selecting peptides that are organ-specific (Fukunaga & Taki, 2012; Matsubara, 2012). The mRNA display technique utilizes the prokaryotic/eukaryotic cell-derived transcription as well as translation machinery (Wang & Liu, 2011). Ribosome display method uses non-covalent polypeptide ribosome-mRNA compounds for display system (Dreier & Pluckthun, 2011). In yeast display method, peptides are normally merged with the Aga2 subunit of the yeast protein (Linciano *et al.*, 2019).

3.3. Advanced Approach

There are further advanced technical approaches like surface plasmon resonance (SPR), bio-layer interferometry, and fluorescence resonance energy transfer (FRET), which are used in validating the identified peptides. SPR is a label-free detection technique which examines the binding kinetics of two bimolecular associations in real time (Patching, 2014). Biolayer interferometry is an optical analytical system with real-time monitoring and label-free detection (Shah & Duncan, 2014). FRET is a distance-dependent technique that involves radiation-less transfer of energy from the donor to the acceptor (Rogers *et al.*, 2012).

4. AMPs

The salient feature of peptides in therapeutics is the capability to hydrolyze the peptidase enzymes found in the body that reduces the harmful side effects by avoiding pile up in certain organs (Ali *et al.*, 2013). Those which reveal immunomodulatory and inhibitory properties that protect against infection induced by fungi, bacteria, viruses, or protozoa are termed as naturally occurring AMPs. These have been used as replacement for many antibiotics to treat bacterial infections but nowadays they are also used as antiviral therapeutics (Ahmed *et al.*, 2019). AMPs are almost smaller than 10 kDa and are hydrophobic in nature (Hultmark, 2003). These AMPs are grouped according to their length, structure (secondary and tertiary), and whether or not they have disulfide bridges (Bals, 2000). The report from AMP database provides almost 3000 AMPs in which 189 possess antiviral effects (Wang *et al.*, 2016). The antiviral action of AMP is based on its adsorption on the surface of virus or its direct action on envelope of the virus (Belaid *et al.*, 2002). According to the type of pathogen, its expression can be continuous or inducible. The antiviral effect depends on its capability to arrest the spread of viral infection from one cell to other via compact junctions or to avoid the development of syncytium (Jenssen *et al.*, 2006).

Several AMPs are derived from various sources such as bacteria, insects, vertebrates, and invertebrates (Reddy *et al.*, 2004). *Drosophila melanogaster* is a good model for studying innate immune pathways by which its response to septic injury produces several AMPs like drosomycin, drosocin, cecropins, diptericin, and attacin (Hoffmann *et al.*, 1999). A species of ant called *Pachycondyla goeldii* produces about 15 varied peptides like ponericidins in its venom with antibacterial and insecticidal properties (Orivel *et al.*, 2001).

Acalolepta luxuriosa is a beetle which contains three AMPs from its hemolymph named as acaloleptin A1, A2, and A3 with molecular masses of 8 kDa. The venom of certain spiders like *Lycosa carolinensis* and *Cupiennius salei* contains peptides such as lycotoxins and cupiennin-1 (Kuhn-Nentwig *et al.*, 2002). Vertebrates like *Limulus polyphemus*, a similar horse shoe crab contains polyphemusin, an isoform of tachyplesin in its hemocytes (Miyata *et al.*, 1989). *Androctonus australis*, a scorpion produces a highly cationic peptide, droctonin effective in inhibiting Gram positive and also Gram negative bacteria (Ehret-Sabatier *et al.*, 1996). Vertebrates such as cattle and sheep have peptides like BMAP-28 and SMAP-29, respectively, with varied antimicrobial activities (Skerlavaj *et al.*, 1996, 1999).

5. Action of Peptides Against Specific Viruses

5.1. Plant Peptide Against Herpes Simplex Virus

A peptide was extracted from *Melia azedarach* L. leaves known as meliacine. It is a cyclic peptide containing only aliphatic amino acids. In a study by Villamil *et al.* (1995), it was shown that meliacine hindered the replication and hence the proliferation of herpes simplex virus (HSV) type-1 (HSV-1) was curbed. It was documented that meliacine forbids the proliferation of HSV-1 by repressing the antigen expression in affected cells. However, it did not show any effect on the viral adsorption and penetration phases of the viral cycle.

A 2 kDa peptide was extracted from the seeds of *Sorghum bicolor* L. by antiviral-guided fractionation. This peptide was reported to strongly hinder the replication of HSV-1 in Vero cells. The findings also stipulate that the 2 kDa peptide was not only able to prevent infection emergence and propagation but also had a prophylactic *in vitro* activity against HSV-1 illness (Camargo-Filho *et al.*, 2008).

5.2. Plant Peptide Against Junin Virus

Junin virus (Arenaviridae family) triggers a serious human illness termed as the Argentine hemorrhagic fever (AHF) (Weissenbacher *et al.*, 1987). The existing treatment for AHF patients is early immune plasma administration that lowered mortality rate from 15%–30% to 1%. Unfortunately, 11% of the cured patients were reported to suffer from late neurological problems (Enria & Maiztegui, 1994).

It was reported (Castilla *et al.*, 1998) that the replication of Junin virus in Vero cells was suppressed when the cells were treated with the meliacine prior to infection or shortly after the adsorption of the virus. The findings of the study also indicate that meliacine hinders two replicative phase events that affect fusion of membranes, which are uncoating and budding.

5.3. Plant Peptide Against Foot and Mouth Disease Virus

Foot and mouth disease virus (FMDV) belonging to the family Picornaviridae is a virus which attacks a huge variety of cloven-hoofed animals like cattle, pigs, goats, sheep, and so on, which are of agricultural importance as well as of commercial significance worldwide. Inactivated vaccines are used to treat the disease but the issue with vaccination is the antigenic variance of the virus (Wachsman *et al.*, 1998).

Meliacine, extracted from leaves of *M. azedarach* L. plant was reported to stifle the replication of the FMDV in BHK-21 cells. It is reported to inhibit and impede the mechanism of FMDV uncoating in BHK-21 cells by blocking vesicular acidification and this was found out by labeling the cells with acridine orange (Wachsman *et al.*, 1998).

5.4. Plant Peptide Against HIV

From the seeds of Ceylon spinach (*Basella rubra*), two antifungal peptides were derived (Wang & Ng, 2001). These antifungal peptides are known as α- and β-basrubins. These peptides were known to forestall the HIV-1 reverse transcriptase enzyme's activity by around 79% and 54%, respectively.

Another study by Wang and Ng (2005) reports yet another antifungal peptide of molecular weight 7 kDa, that was known to exhibit inhibitory effect on HIV-1 reverse transcriptase enzyme. It was extracted from coconut (*Cocos nucifera*). The IC_{50} value of its inhibitory impact was found to be 52.5 μM.

A research conducted by Wang and Ng (2000) indicated that a novel peptide extracted from the seeds of *Ginkgo biloba* had a virucidal effect on HIV. Ginkgobilobin was stated to disrupt of HIV-1 reverse transcriptase. It is a 13 kDa peptide and only its N-terminal sequence has been documented.

A natural antifungal peptide, Sesquin, was extracted from ground beans (*Vigna sesquipedalis*) (Wong & Ng, 2005). Ground beans are widely popular in the Chinese cuisine. The isolated peptide of molecular weight 7 kDa with an N-terminal sequence was reported to be very greatly similar to other plant defensins. Sesquin was also reported to demonstrate inhibition of HIV-1 reverse transcriptase enzyme, thereby blocking and impeding the proliferation of the virus.

Similarly, HIV-1 reverse transcriptase's function was also impeded by a 5.9 kDa antifungal peptide derived from the seeds of kale (*Brassica alboglabra*) (Lin & Ng, 2008). According to this study an IC_{50} value of 7.9 μM was recorded.

Ascalin like other antifungal peptides inhibited HIV-1 reverse transcriptase with an IC_{50} of 10 μM. This 9.5 kDa peptide was extracted from the *Allium ascalonicum* shallot bulbs (Wang & Ng, 2002).

5.5. Plant Peptide Against Poliovirus

Ussery *et al.* (1977) reported that an antiviral basic peptide extracted from Pokeweed (*Phytolacca americana*), called PAP, led to around 96% reduction of poliovirus in HeLa cells. It is proposed that the mechanism of the peptide's antiviral efficacy entails its delivery by the virus to viable cells assisted by suppression of host cell ribosomes.

6. Antiviral Peptides from Sources other than Plants

Table 1 illustrates a list of antiviral peptides from various sources along with the Uniprot id, peptide sequence, molecular mass, and

Table 1 Antiviral peptides from different sources.

S. No.	Uniprot Id	Name	Source	Peptide Sequence	Molecular Mass (Da)	Antiviral Activity	Reference
1	P49913	Cathelicidin (LL-37)	*Homo sapiens*	LLGDFFRKSKEK IGKEFKRIV QRIKDFLR NLVPRTES	19,301	Virucidal activity against HIV, respiratory syncytial virus (RSV), Zika virus, Kaposi's sarcoma-associated herpes virus	He *et al.* (2018)
2	P81180	Cyanovirin-N	*Nostoc ellipsosporum* (cyanobacteria)	LGKFSQTCYNSAI QGSVLTSTCE RTNGGYNTSSI DLNSVIENVDGSLKW QPSNFIETCRN TQLAGSSELA AECKTRAQQFVST KINLDDHIA NIDGTLKYE	11,014.2	It binds to a variety of glycans rich in mannose on HIV-1 gp120	Alexandre *et al.* (2013)
3	P82357	Spinigerin	*Pseudacanthotermes spiniger* (termite)	HVDKKVADK VLLLKQLRIM RLLTRL	3,001.8	HIV inhibitory, IC_{50} = 1.4 μM	Lamberty *et al.* (2001); Wang *et al.* (2010);

4	K0A7P3	Piscidin-1	*Epinephelus malabaricus* (fish)	FFHHIF RGIVHVGK TIHRLVTG	7,663	Inhibits channel catfish virus, frog virus 3 (FV3) as well as HIV-1	Chinchar *et al*. (2004); Silphaduang and Noga (2001); Wang *et al*. (2010)
5	Q1ELT9	Latarcin 1	*Lachesana tarabaevi* (spider venom)	SMWSGMW RRKLKKLRNA LKKKLKGE	10,038	Inhibits replication of dengue NS2B-NS3pro virus	Kozlov *et al*. (2006); Rothan *et al*. (2014)
6	P80711	Clavanin B	*Styela clava* (sea squirt)	VFQFLGRII HHVGNFV HGFSHVF	2,695	Anti-HIV effect	Lee *et al*. (1997); Wang *et al*. (2010)
7	O07623	Subtilosin A	*Bacillus subtilis*, *Bacillus amyloliquefaciens*, or *Bacillus atrophaeus*; *Bacillus tequilensis* FR9	NKGCATCS IGAACLV DGPIPDFEIA GATGLFGLWG	3,401.8	Antiviral effect against HSV-1 and HSV-2	Quintana *et al*. (2014)
8	P84272	Dahlein 5.6	*Litoria dahlia* (frog)	GLLASL GKVFGGYL AEKLKPK	2,187	Antiviral effect against HIV	Van Compernolle *et al*. (2005)
9	P83412	Alloferon 1	Blowfly, *Calliphora vicina*	HGVSGH GQHGVHG	1,265	Inhibits HSV multiplication	Chernysh *et al*. (2002); Kuczer *et al*. (2011)

(*Continued*)

Table 1 (*Continued*)

S. No.	Uniprot Id	Name	Source	Peptide Sequence	Molecular Mass (Da)	Antiviral Activity	Reference
10	P01501	Melittin	Honeybee venom, *Apis mellifera*	GIGAVLKVL TTGLPALISWI KRKRQQ	7,585	Inhibitory effect against HSV-1 and HSV-2	Yasin *et al*. (2000)
11	Q8QFQ4	Ranatuerin 2P	North American frog, *Rana pipiens*	GLMDTVKN VAKNLAGHML DKLKCKITGC	7,941	Virucial effect against HIV	Van Compernolle *et al*. (2005)
12	P33046	Indolicidin	Bovine neutrophils, *Bos taurus*	ILPWKWPWWPWRR	16,479	Inhibits HSV-1 and HSV-2	Selsted *et al*. (1992); Yasin *et al*. (2000)
13	P62568	Caerin 1.1	Australian green tree frog, *Litoria splendida*	GLLSVLGS VAKHVLPHV VPVIAEHL	2,585	Inhibits HIV infection with little adverse effect on T cells	Van Compernolle *et al*. (2005); Wong *et al*. (1997)
14	P51437	mCRAMP	*Mus musculus* (mouse)	GLLRKGGEK IGEKLKKIG QKIKNFFQ KLVPQPEQ	19,453	Active against RSV	Gallo *et al*. (1997)
15	P81534	Human beta-defensin-3	*H. sapiens*	GIINTLQKY YCRVRGG RCAVLSCL PKEEQIGK CSTRGRK CCRRKK	7,697	HIV virucidal effect through direct association with virions as well as modulation of CXCR4 co-receptor	Weinberg *et al*. (2006); Harder *et al*. (2001)

16	P82422	Ponericin L2	*Pachycondyla goeldii*, ants	LLKELW TKIKGAGK AVLGKIKGLL	2,578	Active against HIV	Orivel *et al*. (2001); Wang *et al*. (2010)
17	P84645	Palicourein	*Palicourea condensata*	GDPTFCG ETCRVIPV CTYSAALG CTCDDRS DGLCKRN	3,928	Inhibits the cytopathic effects of HIV	Bokesch *et al*. (2001)
18	Q6JWQ9	Epinecidin-1	Orange-spotted grouper, *Epinephelus coioides* (fish)	GFIFHII KGLFHAG KMIHGLV	7,663	Antiviral activity against non-enveloped, spherical virus (betanodavirus)	Pan *et al*. (2007); Wang *et al*. (2010)
19	P82022	Frenatin 2	*Litoria infrafrenata*, white-lipped tree frog	GLLGTL GNLLNGLGL	1,425	Active against yellow fever virus	Muñoz-Camargo *et al*. (2016); Raftery *et al*. (1996)
20	P84801	Griffithsin	*Griffithsia* sp. (strain Q66D336), Red alga	SLTHRKFGGSGGSPFS GLSSIAVRSGSYLD AIIIDGVHHGGSG GNLSPTFTFGSG EYISNMTIRSGDY IDNISFETNMGR RFGPYGGSGGSANT LSNVKVIQINGS AGDYLDSLDIYYEQY	12,731	It binds to the HIV envelope glycoprotein and prevents the virus from entering cells	Mori *et al*. (2005)

(*Continued*)

Table 1 (*Continued*)

S. No.	Uniprot Id	Name	Source	Peptide Sequence	Molecular Mass (Da)	Antiviral Activity	Reference
21	P86041	Scytovirin	*Scytonema varium*, cyanobacterium	GSGPTYC WNEANNPG GPNRCSNNKQC DGARTCSSSGFC QGTSRKPDP GPKGP TYCWDEAKN PGGPNRCSN SKQCDGARTCSSSG FCQGTAGHAAA	9,722	It binds multiple mannose-rich glycans on HIV-1 gp120	Alexandre *et al.* (2013); Bokesch *et al.* (2003)
22	P0DTB9	Urumin	*Hydrophylax bahuvistara*, frog	IPLRGAFINGR WDSQCHRF SNGAIACA	2,961	Virucidal activity against H1N1 influenza A virus	Holthausen *et al.* (2017)

the corresponding antiviral activity. The peptide sequence given in the table for each of the peptide was taken from the antimicrobial and antiviral peptide database (Database: Wang *et al.*, 2009). The molecular mass of these peptides was taken from https://www.uniprot.org/.

6.1. Bacterial Source

Locillomycin is an antiviral peptide derived from *Bacillus subtilis* which targets porcine epidemic diarrhea virus. The peptide decreased the number of virus copies by 300-fold at a dose of 10 μg/ml (Luo *et al.*, 2015). Surfactin is also a *B. subtilis*-derived lipopeptide, an amphiphilic antiviral peptide which targets some viruses like HSV (type 1 and 2), HIV, Newcastle disease virus, simian immunodeficiency virus, and Porcine epidemic diarrhea virus by disintegrating the envelope of the lipid and the capsid by forming ion channels (Huang *et al.*, 2006; Yuan *et al.*, 2019).

Enterococcus faecium CRL35 produces enterocin CLR35, an antibacterial polypeptide of molecular mass 3.5 kDa, which showed antiviral efficacy toward HSV-1 and -2 thymidine–kinase positive and deficient strains in BHK-21 cells as well as in Vero cells. The peptide was also able to inhibit the intracellular viral proliferation (Wachsman *et al.*, 1999).

Cyanobacteria (*Nostoc ellipsosporum*), possess a 11 kDa protein, Cyanovirin-N, which targets the N-linked glycans to bind to the glycoprotein gp120 of the HIV envelope and impedes chronic infection (Boyd *et al.*, 1997; Tsai *et al.*, 2004; Van Compernolle *et al.*, 2005).

Likewise, feglymycin is also a naturally derived peptide from *Streptomyces* species that is of a molecular weight of 1.9 kDa which shows an antiviral effect against HIV. Feglymycin is reported to possess the anti-HIV effect by targeting the gp120 viral envelope protein and thereby preventing the viral entry (Férir *et al.*, 2012).

6.2. Algal Source

Coxsackievirus B_3 ($CV\text{-}B_3$) is considered to be an important pathogen belonging to the genus Enterovirus and family Picornaviridae (Han *et al.*, 2019) and one of the most common human infections triggered by this virus is heart-muscle infection (Turner, 2001). Despite the fact that no potent antiviral treatments for the prevention or treatment of the viral infection have been authorized (Nakayama *et al.*, 1989), a particular alga was found to possess antiviral properties against this virus. *Scenedesmus obliquus* is a fresh-water green algae, whose protein hydrolysate is obtained by three different enzymes, namely, pepsin, trypsin, or papain (Afify *et al.*, 2018). Protein hydrolysate is a complex mixture of inactive and active peptides of varied chain lengths and composition of amino acids (Tao *et al.*, 2018). *S. obliquus* protein hydrolysates had an antiviral impact against $CV\text{-}B_3$ with an IC_{50} value 66.2% at 100 μg/ml (Afify *et al.*, 2018).

The extracts' bioactivity toward impeding Coxsackie B_3 was determined by the cytopathic effect inhibition assay. In this assay, the stock $CV\text{-}B_3$ (100 μl) was allowed to infect the Vero confluent. Later the virus was removed and the tested extracts (100 μl) and maintenance medium were added to the wells and allowed to incubate for 3 days (Reed & Muench, 1938).

6.3. Fungal Source

Polysaccharide peptide (PSP) was derived from *Coriolus versicolor* (COV-1 strain). It is a Chinese fungus (Yun Zhi). The 100 kDa polysaccharide-bound peptide (Wang *et al.*, 1999; Yang *et al.*, 1992) is comprised about 90% of polysaccharides and 10% of peptides (Yeung, 2012). In a study conducted by Zhao *et al.* (2015), the virucidal action of PSP against tobacco mosaic virus was reported. They documented that PSP could initiate oxidative burst in the tobacco leaves and also enhances the expression of PR-1a and PR-5 proteins. Another research by Rodríguez-Valentín *et al.* (2018)

reported that PSP downregulated the viral replication as well as initiated the upregulation of some specific antiviral chemokines like regulated on activation, normal T cell expressed and secreted (RANTES), stromal cell-derived factor 1 alpha and also macrophage inflammatory proteins 1 alpha and beta. These chemokine receptors play a major role in reducing the HIV-1 replication as they target the viral entry phase of the viral cycle.

LB-1b is a polysaccharide–peptide compound extracted from the sporocarp of the edible abalone mushroom *Pleurotus abalonus*. In the study by Li *et al.* (2012) it was established that LB-1b, at low concentrations, showed inhibitory effect on HIV-1 reverse transcriptase. The IC_{50} value was found to be 12.5 μM.

Wang *et al.* (2007) conducted a research on the anti-HIV activity of peptides derived from 16 species of mushrooms. Of them, the highest inhibitory action against HIV-1 was found to be from the crude peptide extracts of *Russula paludosa*. The virus inhibitory activity of this peptide, SU2, was found to be 97.6%. The molecular weight of SU2 was 4.5 kDa. It was also reported that the peptide helps in killing the virus by protein–protein interactions and not by hindering the activity of HIV-1 integrase.

6.4. Animal Source

Hepatitis C virus (HCV) (Flaviviridae family) is a positive-strand RNA virus which is globally regarded as the principal reason for chronic hepatitis, hepatic steatosis, cirrhosis, and hepatocellular carcinoma (Lindenbach & Rice, 2005). A novel natural α-helical peptide, Hp1090, derived from venom of scorpion *Heterometrus Petersii* was reported to attack and kill HCV. Yan *et al.* (2011) documented the IC_{50} value of the peptide to be 7.62 μg/ml. It was also delineated that Hp1090 reduced the HCV infection by interacting directly with the membrane of the virus.

Scorpine-like peptide, Smp76, was extracted and characterized from *Scorpio maurus palmatus* (El-bitar *et al.*, 2020). This peptide possessed antiviral properties against HCV and dengue viruses. Smp76 prohibits HCV infection via inhibiting extracellular infectious agents without impacting replication of virus.

It was reported that the rabbit neutrophil peptide-1 (NP-1), a cationic peptide, inhibits the entry as well as the intercellular transmission of HSV-2. This peptide is an α-defensin molecule that is found to block the movement of VP16 (a viral integument protein) into the nucleus of the cell (Sinha *et al.*, 2003).

Indolicidin is an amide tri-decapeptide, obtained from bovine neutrophils' cytoplasmic granules. This peptide was found to inhibit the HIV at an IC_{50} value of around 67–100 μg/mL (Robinson *et al.*, 1998).

Human neutrophil peptides (HNP-1, HNP-2, and HNP-3) are α-defensin peptides found in humans that are widely known to possess antiviral properties against HIV-1 and help in forestalling the infection. HNP-1 is the first α-defensin to be discovered. It was documented that that even low levels of defensins found in average healthy human serum are sufficient to bind more than half of the gp120 spikes to HIV-1 and a greater number of CD4 receptors on the surface of the cell (Wang *et al.*, 2004).

Lactoferrin (LF) is a peptide derived from the milk of mammals. It is an 80 kDa peptide found to possess antiviral effects against various DNA and RNA viruses. LF restricts the virus from entering the host cell by obstructing the receptors present on the cells or by directly interacting with the virus (Van der Strate *et al.*, 2001). LF binds to the envelope proteins of HCV, thereby aiding in the inhibition of the viral adsorption onto the target cells (Yi *et al.*, 1997). LF exhibits a strong inhibition against the simian SA11 rotavirus *in vitro*. It was reported that not only does LF mitigate infection but it also retains an antiviral efficacy even after virus has penetrated the cell (Grover *et al.*, 1997). LF's antiviral effect on cytomegalovirus *in vitro* was identified (Hasegawa *et al.*, 1994) which was verified by subsequent work (Clarke & May, 2000; Harmsen *et al.*, 1995; Swart *et al.*, 1998, 1999). LF is likely to tamper with virus entry into the target cell (Andersen *et al.*, 2001), as LF pre-incubation to host cell is necessary for its antiviral function.

Researches were conducted on extracting peptides from dorsal glands of Australian toadlets *Uperoleia mjobergii*. Out of the 20 peptides present, they documented amino acid sequences for around seven of the peptides. Among the seven peptides, Uperin 3.6 is a peptide that was found to be having 17 amino acid residues which exhibit inhibitory effect toward HIV and thereby prevent infection (Bradford *et al.*, 1996).

Marine sponges have a broad variety of structurally distinct, bioactive nonribosomal peptide derivatives (Faulkner, 2000; Fusetani & Matsunaga, 1993; Rashid *et al.*, 2001). Microspinosamide, a novel cyclic depsipeptide containing a few amino acid residues, was derived from extracts of the Indonesian marine sponge collection *Sidonops microspinosa*. The different amino acids present include D-alanine, L-threonine, L-proline, L-N-methylglutamine, L-â-methylisoleucine, D-tryptophan, L-arginine, D-tert-leucine, D-cysteic acid, D-valine, and D-aspartic acid residues. Microspinosamide was reported to impede the infection of HIV-1 by inhibiting the cytotoxic effect (Mulder *et al.*, 2013; Rashid *et al.*, 2001).

A natural anionic stylicin AMP was derived and purified from Kuruma shrimp (*Marsupenaeus japonicus*) (Liu *et al.*, 2015). The peptide was designated to be Mj-sty. The expression of Mj-sty peptide was found to be very high in the gills and hemocytes part of the shrimp. The molecular mass of Mj-sty was reported to be 8.7 kDa and it was also documented to be a major peptide involved in the immune processes against white spot syndrome virus (WSSV).

7. Peptides Against SARS-CoV

COVID-19 is presently believed as a menace to life. It is a viral infection caused by corona virus (Walls *et al.*, 2020). Corona viruses are zoonotic, enveloped, positive single-stranded RNA virus which is found to affect both humans and animals, causing respiratory, gastrointestinal, hepatic, and neurobiological ailments.

This virus sets foot into human cells through the receptor binding domain (RBD) of its spike protein (S) and binding to angiotensin-converting enzyme 2 (ACE2) (Yan *et al.*, 2020). The entry of the virus can possibly be averted by interrupting the binding of SARS-CoV-2-RBD to ACE2 with designer drugs (Wan *et al.*, 2020).

Molecular dynamics simulations showed that the ACE2 peptidase domain $\alpha 1$ helix is predominant for binding SARS-CoV-2-RBD (Hoffmann *et al.*, 2020). The synthetic peptide fragment 23-mer of the ACE2 $\alpha 1$ helix (IEEQAKTFLDKFNHEAEDLFYQS) has the potential of successfully blocking the SARS-CoV-2 spike protein interaction with ACE2. Hence it can possibly be a promising therapeutic drug for COVID-19 treatment. Zhang, Pomplun, Loftis, Loas, *et al.* (2020) and Zhang, Pomplun, Loftis, Tan, *et al.* (2020) demonstrated that RBD domain possesses less affinity with 3- and 4-mer natural peptides of distinct origin, whereas 8- and 10-mer peptides showed high affinity to a whole spike virus protein. The peptides that showed high affinity to RBD have favorable amino acids important for binding of SARS-CoV-2 spike protein with ACE2 receptor on the epithelial cells (Kit & Kit, 2020).

There are several natural peptides which can potentially be used for blocking SARS-COV-2- ACE2 interactions (Kit & Kit, 2020). LF that is found in several mucosal secretions is one of the AMPs which has a notable activity in the innate immune system. LF has been shown to have broad antimicrobial effects against bacteria, fungi, and many viruses (Vorland, 1999). LF is a component of breast milk. Studies have demonstrated that breast milk's antiviral effects have been attributed to LF's direct antiviral activity. It interrupts the virus entry into cells by binding directly to the virus or through hindering association with cellular receptors (Van der Strate *et al.*, 2001).

The activity of LF against SARS-CoV was reported as a result of an improved host immune system. LF interferes with virus adsorption by preventing the spike protein from binding to host cell receptors (Lang *et al.*, 2011). The remarkable bioactivity of

LF makes it a viable alternative as a vaccine or as a drug conjugate with traditional antivirals to avoid the adverse effects of antiviral drugs (Van der Strate *et al.*, 2001).

Recently, scientists have designed a new drug which may combat the inflammation caused by COVID 19. TAT CARMIL1 is a composition of two naturally occurring small proteins or peptides. CAMIL1 is a natural protein and when combined with a peptide vehicle, TAT brings CARMIL1 directly into the cell, and it is found to efficiently inhibit a family of cytokines known as interleukins1, thus reducing the inflammatory storm (Wang *et al.*, 2020).

8. Bioinformatics Studies on Antiviral Peptides

Bioinformatics is a field that brings together computer science, biology, mathematics, and statistical techniques for analyzing and interpreting biological facts. This field has therefore been used in analysis of biological data and has been implemented in the domains of proteomics and genomics (Valdés *et al.*, 2017).

In silico analysis, the other name of bioinformatics, includes analytical methods for the managing, curate as well as interpretation of knowledge related to biological processes (Li-Chan *et al.*, 2015). These *in silico* approaches cover databases, online tools, and software packages like I-TASSER, FlexX, BIOPEP, ICM-Docking, and so on (Tu *et al.*, 2018).

Human papilloma viruses (HPV) are the major sources for cervical cancer in which more over 99% of cervical cancer tissues were affected with the DNA of the HPV virus (Monie *et al.*, 2008; Yuan *et al.*, 2001). The cell morphology of HPV consists of circular dsDNA with roughly 8,000 bp (Clifford *et al.*, 2003). L1 is the principal protein in these viruses' capsid structure which plays a vital role in infection (Buck *et al.*, 2013; Chen *et al.*, 2000; Kirnbauer *et al.*, 1992). Production of an L1 protein vaccine will probably proceed to vaccination against HPV infection and to the prevention of associated forms of cancer (Roden & Wu, 2006). HPV vaccines available do not have adequate efficacy against all forms of HPV. Yazdani *et al.* (2020) reported the designing of a potential L1 protein-based HPV peptide vaccine (molecular weight: 29.96 kDa) which was developed using a variety of bioinformatics tools. This peptide vaccine was created using two specific immunodominant epitopes. LBtope and BepiPred were the servers that were used by the researchers for epitope prediction. ANTIGENpro and vaccijen 2.0 servers were used to determine the antigenic potential of selected epitopes. ProtParam server examined molecular structure as well as the physicochemical properties of the vaccine. This HPV vaccine was also reported to trigger cell-mediated and humoral immunities that are crucial to hinder infection caused by different varieties of HPV viruses.

In a study by Chiozzi *et al.* (2016) the endogenous peptides present in donkey milk were analyzed for its ACE inhibitory activities and also antioxidant activities, incorporating a 2D technique of fractionation of peptides with *in vitro* assays, high-resolution mass spectrometry as well as bioinformatics analysis. Peptide Ranker, BioPep, and PepBank were the *in silico* analytical tools that were used for validating the obtained peptides. The two innovative antioxidant endogenous peptides, EWFTFLKEAGQGAKDMWR and GQGAKDMWR, and two ACE-inhibitory peptides, REWFTFLK and MPFLKSPIVPF, were documented to possess nutraceutical and functional properties.

Influenza A viruses are enveloped, negative ssRNA viruses that can cause serious respiratory infections and diseases. But due to the emergence of drug-resistant varieties it was reported that there is a direct need of developing novel antiviral agents against influenza A virus. Around nine peptides were designed to possess antiviral properties against influenza A virus using bioinformatics tools (López-Martínez *et al.*, 2013). They were extracted from influenza A HA1 and HA2 subunits with the goal of inhibiting the infection. Various *in silico* analysis tools that were used include Parker's scale with the Hydrophilicity Prediction program, EMBOSS server. Protein docking studies were determined using ClusPro.2.0 server. The results of docking studies were analyzed using Chimera v1.6rc and PyMOL 1.3 program.

Over 50 peptides, believed to suppress SARS-CoV-1, have been computationally tested against RBD of the SARS-CoV-2 spike protein (Chowdhury *et al.*, 2020). Around 15 peptides were chosen depending on binding affinity and interaction, which displayed a higher affinity compared to the human ACE2 receptor helix. The CABS-Fold was used to construct the peptides and were docked to the RBD using Patchdock. Molecular dynamics simulation revealed that S2P25 and S2P26 were the suitable choices which could effectively obstruct SARS-CoV-2 entry. For MD simulations, YASARA Dynamics software was reported to be used and for calculations AMBER 14 force field was. Peptide SAR analysis was done by using the ProtParam tool.

It is reported that hemocyanin has immune-related properties other than its established respiratory function. Shrimp hemocyanin produces AMPs but no antiviral peptides have been identified. In the thesis by Zhan *et al.* (2019), 45 regularly down-regulated protein domains and 10 upregulated protein domains were identified by the serum of WSSV-infected *Litopenaeus vannamei* and this was analyzed using 2D gel electrophoresis. Among the five peptides, LvHcL48 was studied even more by C-terminal sequencing of its primary sequence along with Edman N-terminal sequencing and also amino acid sequence alignment. This peptide was further reported to bind to VP28 viral envelope of WSSV, thereby impeding the infection.

9. Cryptides

Cryptides are peptide sequences that are formed during the maturation and degradation of functional proteins, which demonstrate different biological activity from that of source (parental) proteins.

The name "cryptides" was coined by Mukai *et al.* (2008, 2009) after the identification of mitochondrial bioactive peptides called mitocryptide 1 and 2 (MCT-1, MCT-2) (Ueki *et al.*, 2007).

Cryptides derived from either variable or constant regions of antibodies are rather very uncommon. The killer peptide (KP), the main element of a group of Ab-derived segments prepared with various biological processes, in particular, has received extensive research. It is a decapeptide, originating from the variable region of the anti-idiotypic Ab, reflecting the functional internal picture of a yeast killer toxin, bestowed with a broad range of antimicrobial activity. KP has demonstrated outstanding function against several distinct infectious agents, especially HIV and influenza A viruses, via different modes of action (Magliani *et al.*, 2011). The influence of hydrophobic amino acids may be responsible for virulence factors suppression, which allows KP to interfere with the lipid bilayer envelope, thereby contributing to its destabilization (Sala *et al.*, 2018).

10. Conclusion

Viral diseases are the extremely widespread infections found to be highly contagious. Hence, it is difficult to completely eradicate a viral infection. However, natural peptides with antiviral properties were found to be effective in controlling this disease spread and in curbing the intracellular propagation of viruses. The usage of peptide drugs in antiviral therapy is very much in the preliminary stages. Nevertheless, therapeutic applications of these natural antiviral peptides are vast. Therefore, new strategies as well as advanced techniques are necessary to make a major addition in order to win the endless battle against viral infections.

References

Afify, A. E. M. M., El Baroty, G. S., El Baz, F. K., Abd El Baky, H. H., & Murad, S. A. (2018). *Scenedesmus obliquus*: Antioxidant and antiviral activity of proteins hydrolyzed by three enzymes. *Journal of Genetic Engineering and Biotechnology*, *16*(2), 399–408.

Ahmed, A., Siman-Tov, G., Hall, G., Bhalla, N., & Narayanan, A. (2019). Human antimicrobial peptides as therapeutics for viral infections. *Viruses*, *11*, 704.

Alexandre, K. B., Moore, P. L., Nonyane, M., Gray, E. S., Ranchobe, N., Chakauya, E., McMahon, J. B., O'Keefe, B. R., Chikwamba, R., & Morris, L. (2013). Mechanisms of HIV-1 subtype C resistance to GRFT, CV-N and SVN. *Virology*, *446*(1–2), 66–76.

Ali, R., Rani, R., & Kumar, S. (2013). New peptide based therapeutic approaches. In G. Md. Ashraf, & I. A. Sheikh (Eds.), *Advances in protein chemistry*. Jeddah: OMICS Group eBooks.

Andersen, J. H., Osbakk, S. A., Vorland, L. H., Traavik, T., & Gutteberg, T. J. (2001). Lactoferrin and cyclic lactoferricin inhibit the entry of human cytomegalovirus into human fibroblasts. *Antiviral Research*, *51*(2), 141–149.

Bals, R. (2000). Epithelial antimicrobial peptides in host defense against infection. *Respiratory Research*, *1*(3), 141–150.

Belaid, A., Aouni, M., Khelifa, R., Trabelsi, A., Jemmali, M., & Hani, K. (2002). In vitro antiviral activity of dermaseptins against herpes simplex virus type 1. *Journal of Medical Virology*, *66*, 229–234.

Benachir, T., & Lafleur, M. (1995). Study of vesicle leakage induced by melittin. *Biochimica et Biophysica Acta*, *1235*, 452–460.

Boas, L. C. P. V., Campos, M. L., Berlanda, R. L. A., de Carvalho Neves, N., & Franco, O. L. (2019). Antiviral peptides as promising therapeutic drugs. *Cellular and Molecular Life Sciences*, *76*(18), 3525–3542.

Bokesch, H. R., O'Keefe, B. R., McKee, T. C., Pannell, L. K., Patterson, G. M., Gardella, R. S., Sowder, R. C., Turpin, J., Watson, K., Buckheit, R.W., & Boyd, M. R. (2003). A potent novel anti-HIV protein from the cultured cyanobacterium *Scytonema varium*. *Biochemistry*, *42*(9), 2578–2584.

Bokesch, H. R., Pannell, L. K., Cochran, P. K., Sowder, R. C., McKee, T. C., & Boyd, M. R. (2001). A novel anti-HIV macrocyclic peptide from *Palicourea condensata*. *Journal of Natural Products*, *64*(2), 249–250.

Boyd, M. R., Gustafson, K. R., McMahon, J. B., Shoemaker, R. H., O'Keefe, B. R., Mori, T., Gulakowski, R. J., Wu, L., Rivera, M. I., Laurencot, C. M., Currens, M. J., Cardellina 2nd, J. H., Buckheit Jr, R. W., Nara, P. L., Pannell, L. K., Sowder 2nd, R. C., & Henderson, L. E. (1997). Discovery of cyanovirin-N, a novel human immunodeficiency virus-inactivating protein that binds viral surface envelope glycoprotein gp120: Potential applications to microbicide development. *Antimicrobial Agents and Chemotherapy*, *41*, 1521–1530.

Bradford, A. M., Bowie, J. H., Tyler, M. J., & Wallace, J. C. (1996). New antibiotic uperin peptides from the dorsal glands of the Australian toadlet *Uperoleia mjobergii*. *Australian Journal of Chemistry*, *49*(12), 1325–1331.

Buck, C. B., Day, P. M., & Trus, B. L. (2013). The papillomavirus major capsid protein L1. *Virology*, *445*(1–2), 169–174.

Camargo-Filho, I., Cortez, D. A. G., Ueda-Nakamura, T., Nakamura, C. V., & Dias Filho, B. P. (2008). Antiviral activity and mode of action of a peptide isolated from *Sorghum bicolor*. *Phytomedicine*, *15*(3), 202–208.

Castilla, V., Barquero, A. A., Mersich, S. E., & Coto, C. E. (1998). In vitro anti-Junin virus activity of a peptide isolated from *Melia azedarach* L. leaves. *International Journal of Antimicrobial Agents*, *10*(1), 67–75.

Chen, X. S., Garcea, R. L., Goldberg, I., Casini, G., & Harrison, S. C. (2000). Structure of small virus-like particles assembled from the L1 protein of human papillomavirus 16. *Molecular Cell*, *5*(3), 557–567.

Chernysh, S., Kim, S. I., Bekker, G., Pleskach, V. A., Filatova, N. A., Anikin, V. B., Platonov, V. G., & Bulet, P. (2002). Antiviral and antitumor peptides from insects. *Proceedings of the National Academy of Sciences*, *99*(20), 12628–12632.

Chinchar, V. G., Bryan, L., Silphadaung, U., Noga, E., Wade, D., & Rollins-Smith, L. (2004). Inactivation of viruses infecting ectothermic animals by amphibian and piscine antimicrobial peptides. *Virology*, *323*(2), 268–275.

Chiozzi, R. Z., Capriotti, A. L., Cavaliere, C., La Barbera, G., Piovesana, S., Samperi, R., & Laganà, A. (2016). Purification and identification of endogenous antioxidant and ACE-inhibitory peptides from donkey milk by multidimensional liquid chromatography and nanoHPLC-high resolution mass spectrometry. *Analytical and Bioanalytical Chemistry*, *408*(20), 5657–5666.

Choi, K. Y. G., & Mookherjee, N. (2012). Multiple immune-modulatory functions of cathelicidin host defense peptides. *Frontiers in Immunology*, *3*, 149.

Chowdhury, S. M., Talukder, S. A., Khan, A. M., Afrin, N., Ali, M. A., Islam, R., Parves, R., Al Mamun, A., Sufian, M. A., Hossain, M. N., & Hossain, M. A. (2020). Antiviral peptides as promising therapeutics against SARS-CoV-2. *The Journal of Physical Chemistry B*, *124*(44), 9785–9792.

Clarke, N. M., & May, J. T. (2000). Effect of antimicrobial factors in human milk on rhinoviruses and milk-borne cytomegalovirus in vitro. *Journal of Medical Microbiology*, *49*(8), 719–723.

Clifford, G., Smith, J., Plummer, M., Munoz, N., & Franceschi, S. (2003). Human papillomavirus types in invasive cervical cancer worldwide: A meta-analysis. *British Journal of Cancer*, *88*(1), 63.

Dias, A., Bouvier, D., Crepin, T., McCarthy, A. A., Hart, D. J., Baudin, F., Cusack, S., Ruigrok, R. W. H. (2009). The cap-snatching endonuclease of influenza virus polymerase resides in the PA subunit. *Nature*, *458*, 914–918.

Dreier, B., & Pluckthun, A. (2011). Ribosome display: A technology for selecting and evolving proteins from large libraries. *Methods in Molecular Biology*, 687, 283–306.

Ehret-Sabatier, L., Loew, D., Goyffon, M., Fehlbaum, P., Hoffmann, J. A., van Dorsselaer, A., & Bulet, P. (1996). Characterization of novel cysteine-rich antimicrobial peptides from scorpion blood. *Journal of Biological Chemistry*, *271*(47), 29537–29544.

El-Bitar, A. M., Sarhan, M., Abdel-Rahman, M. A., Quintero-Hernandez, V., Aoki-Utsubo, C., Moustafa, M. A., Possani, L. D., & Hotta, H. (2020). Smp76, a scorpine-like peptide isolated from the venom of the scorpion *Scorpio maurus palmatus*, with a potent antiviral activity against hepatitis C virus and dengue virus. *International Journal of Peptide Research and Therapeutics*, *26*(2), 811–821.

Enria, D. A., & Maiztegui, J. I. (1994). Antiviral treatment of Argentine hemorrhagic fever. *Antiviral Research*, 23, 23–31.

Faulkner, D. J. (2000). Marine natural products. *Natural Product Reports*, *17*(1), 7–55.

Fechter, P., Mingay, L., Sharps, J., Chambers, A., Fodor, E., & Brownlee, G. G. (2003). Two aromatic residues in the PB2 subunit of influenza A RNA polymerase are crucial for cap binding. *The Journal of Biological Chemistry*, *278*, 20381–20388.

Férir, G., Hänchen, A., François, K. O., Hoorelbeke, B., Huskens, D., Dettner, F., Süssmuth, R. D., & Schols D. (2012). Feglymycin, a unique natural bacterial antibiotic peptide, inhibits HIV entry by targeting the viral envelope protein gp120. *Virology*, *433*(2), 308–319.

Fukunaga, K., & Taki, M. (2012). Practical tips for construction of custom peptide libraries and affinity selection by using commercially available phage display cloning systems. *Journal of Nucleic Acids*, *2012*, 1–9.

Fusetani, N., & Matsunaga, S. (1993). Bioactive sponge peptides. *Chemical Reviews*, 93(5), 1793–1806.

Gallo, R. L., Kim, K. J., Bernfield, M., Kozak, C. A., Zanetti, M., Merluzzi, L., & Gennaro, R. (1997). Identification of CRAMP, a cathelin-related antimicrobial peptide expressed in the embryonic and adult mouse. *Journal of Biological Chemistry*, *272*(20), 13088–13093.

Gordon-Grossman, M., Gofman, Y., Zimmermann, H., Frydman, V., Shai, Y., Ben-Tal, N., & Goldfarb, D. (2009). A combined pulse EPR and Monte Carlo simulation study provides molecular insight on peptide-membrane interactions. *Journal of Physical Chemistry B*, *113*, 15128.

Gordon-Grossman, M., Zimmermann, H., Wolf, S.G., Shai, Y., & Goldfarb, D. (2012). Investigation of model membrane disruption mechanism by melittin using pulse electron paramagnetic resonance spectroscopy and cryogenic transmission electron microscopy. *Journal of Physical Chemistry B*, *116*, 179–188.

Grover, M., Giouzeppos, O., Schnagl, R. D., & May, J. T. (1997). Effect of human milk prostaglandins and lactoferrin on respiratory syncytial virus and rotavirus. *Acta Paediatrica*, *86*(3), 315–316.

Han, Z., Zhang, Y., Huang, K., Wang, J., Tian, H., Song, Y., Yang, Q., Yan, D., Zhu, S., Yao, M., & Wang, X. (2019). Two Coxsackievirus B3 outbreaks associated with hand, foot, and mouth disease in China and the evolutionary history worldwide. *BMC Infectious Diseases*, *19*(1), 466.

Harder, J., Bartels, J., Christophers, E., & Schröder, J. M. (2001). Isolation and Characterization of human μ-defensin-3, a novel human inducible peptide antibiotic. *Journal of Biological Chemistry*, *276*(8), 5707–5713.

Harmsen, M. C., Swart, P. J., de Be´thune, M. P., Pauwels, R., De Clercq, E., The, T. H., & Meijer, D. K. F. (1995). Antiviral effects of plasma and milk proteins: Lactoferrin shows potent activity against both human immunodeficiency virus and human cytomegalovirus replication in vitro. *Journal of Infectious Diseases*, *172*, 380–388.

Hasegawa, K., Motsuchi, W., Tanaka, S., & Dosako, S. (1994). Inhibition with lactoferrin of in vitro infection with human herpes virus. *Japanese Journal of Medical Science and Biology*, *47*, 73–85.

He, M., Zhang, H., Li, Y., Wang, G., Tang, B., Zhao, J., Huang, Y., & Zheng, J. (2018). Cathelicidin-derived antimicrobial peptides inhibit Zika virus through direct inactivation and interferon pathway. *Frontiers in Immunology*, 9, 722.

Hoffmann, J. A., Kafatos, F. C., Janeway, C. A., & Ezekowitz, R. A. B. (1999). Phylogenetic perspectives in innate immunity. *Science*, *284*(5418), 1313–1318.

Hoffmann, M., Kleine-Weber, H., Schroeder, S., Krüger, N., Herrler, T., Erichsen, S., Schiergens, T. S., Herrler, G., Wu, N. H., Nitsche, A., & Müller, M. A. (2020). SARS-CoV-2 cell entry depends on ACE2 and TMPRSS2 and is blocked by a clinically proven protease inhibitor. *Cell*, *181*(2), 271–280.

Holthausen, D. J., Lee, S. H., Kumar, V. T., Bouvier, N. M., Krammer, F., Ellebedy, A. H., Wrammert, J., Lowen, A. C., George, S., Pillai, M. R., & Jacob, J. (2017). An amphibian host defense peptide is virucidal for human H1 hemagglutinin-bearing influenza viruses. *Immunity*, *46*(4), 587–595.

Huang, X., Lu, Z., Zhao, H., Bie, X., Lü, F., & Yang, S. (2006). Antiviral activity of antimicrobial lipopeptide from *Bacillus subtilis* fmbj against pseudorabies virus, porcine parvovirus, Newcastle Disease virus and infectious bursal disease virus in vitro. *International Journal of Peptide Research and Therapeutics*, *12*(4), 373–377.

Hultmark, D. (2003). Drosophila immunity: Paths and patterns. *Current Opinion in Immunology*, *15*(1), 12–19.

Jenssen, H., Hamill, P., & Hancock, R. E. (2006). Peptide antimicrobial agents. *Clinical Microbiology Reviews 19*, 491–511.

Kirnbauer, R., Booy, F., Cheng, N., Lowy, D., & Schiller, J. (1992). Papillomavirus L1 major capsid protein self-assembles into virus-like particles that are highly immunogenic. *Proceedings of the National Academy of Sciences*, *89*(24), 12180–12184.

Kit, O., & Kit, Y. (2020). Features of the interaction of humans defensins with the SARS-CoV-2 spike protein: An in silico comparative analysis. *Research Gate*.

Kozlov, S. A., Vassilevski, A. A., Feofanov, A. V., Surovoy, A. Y., Karpunin, D. V., & Grishin, E. V. (2006). Latarcins, antimicrobial and cytolytic peptides from the venom of the spider *Lachesana tarabaevi* (Zodariidae) that exemplify biomolecular diversity. *Journal of Biological Chemistry*, *281*(30), 20983–20992.

Kuczer, M., Midak-Siewirska, A., Zahorska, R., Łuczak, M., & Konopińska, D. (2011). Further studies on the antiviral activity of alloferon and its analogues. *Journal of Peptide Science*, *17*(11), 715–719.

Kuhn-Nentwig, L., Müller, J., Schaller, J., Walz, A., Dathe, M., & Nentwig, W. (2002). Cupiennin 1, a new family of highly basic antimicrobial peptides in the venom of the spider *Cupiennius salei* (Ctenidae). *Journal of Biological Chemistry*, *277*(13), 11208–11216.

Ladokhin, A. S., & White, S. H. (2001). 'Detergent-like' permeabilization of anionic lipid vesicles by melittin. *Biochimica et Biophysica Acta*, *1514*, 253–260.

Lamberty, M., Zachary, D., Lanot, R., Bordereau, C., Robert, A., Hoffmann, J. A., & Bulet, P. (2001). Insect immunity: Constitutive expression of a cysteine-rich antifungal and a linear antibacterial peptide in a termite insect. *Journal of Biological Chemistry*, *276*(6), 4085–4092.

Lang, J., Yang, N., Deng, J., Liu, K., Yang, P., Zhang, G., & Jiang, C. (2011). Inhibition of SARS pseudovirus cell entry by lactoferrin binding to heparan sulfate proteoglycans. *PLoS One*, *6*(8), e23710.

Lee, I. H., Zhao, C., Cho, Y., Harwig, S. S., Cooper, E. L., & Lehrer, R. I. (1997). Clavanins, α-helical antimicrobial peptides from tunicate hemocytes. *FEBS Letters*, *400*(2), 158–162.

Li, N., Li L., Fang, J. C., Wong, J. H., Ng, T. B., Jiang, Y., Wang, C. R., Zhang, N. Y., Wen, T. Y., Qu, L. Y., & Lv, P. Y. (2012). Isolation and identification of a novel polysaccharide–peptide complex with antioxidant, anti-proliferative and hypoglycaemic activities from the abalone mushroom. *Bioscience Reports*, *32*(3), 221–228.

Li-Chan, E. C. Y. (2015). Bioactive peptides and protein hydrolysates: Research trends and challenges for application as nutraceuticals and functional food ingredients. *Current Opinion in Food Science*, *1*, 28–37.

Lin, P., & Ng, T. B. (2008). A novel and exploitable antifungal peptide from kale (*Brassica alboglabra*) seeds. *Peptides*, *29*(10), 1664–1671.

Linciano, S., Pluda, S., Bacchin, A., & Angelini, A. (2019). Molecular evolution of peptides by yeast surface display technology. *MedChemComm*, 10, 1569–1580.

Lindenbach, B. D., & Rice, C. M. (2005). Unravelling hepatitis C virus replication from genome to function. *Nature*, *436*(7053), 933–938.

Liu, H. T., Wang, J., Mao, Y., Liu, M., Niu, S. F., Qiao, Y., Su, Y. Q., Wang, C. Z., & Zheng, Z. P. (2015). Identification and expression analysis of a novel stylicin antimicrobial peptide from Kuruma shrimp (*Marsupenaeus japonicus*). *Fish & Shellfish Immunology*, *47*(2), 817–823.

López-Martínez, R., Ramírez-Salinas, G. L., Correa-Basurto, J., & Barrón, B. L. (2013). Inhibition of influenza A virus infection in vitro by peptides designed in silico. *PLoS One*, *8*(10), e76876.

Luo, C., Liu, X., Zhou, X., Guo, J., Truong, J., Wang, X., Zhou, H., Li, X., & Chen, Z. (2015). Unusual biosynthesis and structure of locillomycins from *Bacillus subtilis* 916. *Applied and Environmental Microbiology*, *81*, 6601–6609.

Magliani, W., Conti, S., Ciociola, T., Giovati, L., Zanello, P. P., Pertinhez, T., Spisni, A., & Polonelli, L. (2011). Killer peptide: A novel paradigm of antimicrobial, antiviral and immunomodulatory auto-delivering drugs. *Future Medicinal Chemistry*, *3*(9), 1209–1231.

Mahmoud, A. (2016). New vaccines: Challenges of discovery. *Microbial Biotechnology*, 9(5), 549–552.

Matsubara, T. (2012). Potential of peptides as inhibitors and mimotopes: Selection of carbohydrate-mimetic peptides from phage display libraries. *Journal of Nucleic Acids*, *2012*.

Miyata, T., Tokunaga, F., Yoneya, T., Yoshikawa, K., Iwanaga, S., Niwa, M., Takao, T., & Shimonishi, Y. (1989). Antimicrobial peptides, isolated from horseshoe crab hemocytes, tachyplesin II, and polyphemusins I and II: Chemical structures and biological activity. *The Journal of Biochemistry*, *106*(4), 663–668.

Monie, A., Hung, C.-F., Roden, R., & Wu, T. C. (2008). Cervarix™: A vaccine for the prevention of HPV 16, 18-associated cervical cancer. *Biologics: Targets & Therapy*, 2(1), 107.

Mori, T., O'Keefe, B. R., Sowder II, R. C., Bringans, S., Gardella, R., Berg, S., Cochran, P., Turpin, J. A., Buckheit Jr, R. W., McMahon, J. B., & Boyd, M. R. (2005). Isolation and characterization of griffithsin, a novel HIV-inactivating protein, from the red alga *Griffithsia* sp. *Journal of Biological Chemistry*, *280*(10), 9345–9353.

Mukai, H., Hokari, Y., Seki, T., Takao, T., Kubota, M., Matsuo, Y., Tsukagoshi, H., Kato, M., Kimura, H., Shimonishi, Y., & Kiso, Y. (2008). Discovery of mitocryptide-1, a neutrophil-activating cryptide from healthy porcine heart. *Journal of Biological Chemistry*, *283*(45), 30596–30605.

Mukai, H., Seki, T., Nakano, H., Hokari, Y., Takao, T., Kawanami, M., Tsukagoshi, H., Kimura, H., Kiso, Y., Shimonishi, Y., & Nishi, Y. (2009). Mitocryptide-2: Purification, identification, and characterization of a novel cryptide that activates neutrophils. *The Journal of Immunology*, *182*(8), 5072–5080.

Mulder, K., Lima, L. A., Miranda, V., Dias, S. C., & Franco, O. L. (2013). Current scenario of peptide-based drugs: The key roles of cationic antitumor and antiviral peptides. *Frontiers in Microbiology*, *4*, 321.

Muñoz-Camargo, C., Méndez, M. C., Salazar, V., Moscoso, J., Narváez, D., Torres, M. M., Florez, F. K., Groot, H., & Mitrani, E. (2016). Frog skin cultures secrete anti-yellow fever compounds. *The Journal of Antibiotics*, *69*(11), 783–790.

Nakayama, T., Urano, T., Osano, M., Hayashi, Y., Sekine, S., Ando, T., & Makinom, S. (1989). Outbreak of herpangina associated with Coxsackievirus B3 infection. *The Pediatric Infectious Disease Journal*, *8*, 495–498.

Nevola, L., & Giralt, E. (2015). Modulating protein-protein interactions: The potential of peptides. *Chemical Communications (Cambridge, England)*, *51*, 3302–3315.

Oren, Z., & Shai, Y. (1998). Mode of action of linear amphipathic α-helical antimicrobial peptides. *Biopolymers*, *47*, 451–463.

Orivel, J., Redeker, V., Le Caer, J. P., Krier, F., Revol-Junelles, A. M., Longeon, A., Chaffotte, A., Dejean, A., & Rossier, J. (2001). Ponericins, new antibacterial and insecticidal peptides from the venom of the ant *Pachycondyla goeldii*. *Journal of Biological Chemistry*, *276*(21), 17823–17829.

Pan, C. Y., Chen, J. Y., Cheng, Y. S. E., Chen, C. Y., Ni, I. H., Sheen, J. F., Pan, Y. L., & Kuo, C. M. (2007). Gene expression and localization of the epinecidin-1 antimicrobial peptide in the grouper (*Epinephelus coioides*), and its role in protecting fish against pathogenic infection. *DNA and Cell Biology*, *26*(6), 403–413.

Patching, S. G. (2014). Surface plasmon resonance spectroscopy for characterization of membrane protein–ligand interactions and its potential for drug discovery. *Biochimica et Biophysica Acta*, *1838*, 43–55.

Quintana, V. M., Torres, N. I., Wachsman, M. B., Sinko, P. J., Castilla, V., & Chikindas, M. (2014). Antiherpes simplex virus type 2 activity of the antimicrobial peptide subtilosin. *Journal of Applied Microbiology*, *117*(5), 1253–1259.

Raftery, M. J., Waugh, R. J., Bowie, J. H., Wallace, J. C., & Tyler, M. J. (1996). The structures of the frenatin peptides from the skin secretion of the giant tree frog *Litoria infrafrenata*. *Journal of Peptide Science: An Official Publication of the European Peptide Society*, *2*(2), 117–124.

Raghuraman, H., & Chattopadhyay, A. (2007). Melittin: A membrane-active peptide with diverse functions. *Bioscience Reports*, *27*, 189–223.

Rajendran, L., Knoelker, H.-J., & Simons, K. (2010). Subcellular targeting strategies for drug design and delivery. *Nature Reviews Drug Discovery*, 9, 29–42.

Rashid, M. A., Gustafson, K. R., Cartner, L. K., Shigematsu, N., Pannell, L. K., & Boyd, M. R. (2001). Microspinosamide, a new hiv-inhibitory cyclic depsipeptide from the marine sponge *Sidonops microspinosa*. *Journal of Natural Products*, *64*(1), 117–121.

Reddy, K. V. R., Yedery, R. D., & Aranha, C. (2004). Antimicrobial peptides: Premises and promises. *International Journal of Antimicrobial Agents*, *24*(6), 536–547.

Reed, L., & Muench, H. (1938). A simple method of estimating fifty percent end points. *American Journal of Hygiene*, *27*, 493–497.

Robinson Jr, W.E., McDougall, B., Tran, D., & Selsted, M. E. (1998). Anti⊠HIV⊠1 activity of indolicidin, an antimicrobial peptide from neutrophils. *Journal of Leukocyte Biology*, *63*(1), 94–100.

Roden, R., & Wu, T.-C. (2006). How will HPV vaccines affect cervical cancer? *Nature Reviews Cancer*, *6*(10), 753.

Rodríguez-Valentín, M., López, S., Rivera, M., Ríos-Olivares, E., Cubano, L., & Boukli, N. M. (2018). Naturally derived anti-HIV polysaccharide peptide (PSP) triggers a toll-like receptor 4-dependent antiviral immune response. *Journal of Immunology Research, 2018*.

Rogers, M. S., Cryan, L. M., Habeshian, K. A., Bazinet, L., Caldwell, T. P., Ackroyd, P. C., & Christensen, K. A. (2012). A FRET-based high throughput screening assay to identify inhibitors of anthrax protective antigen binding to capillary morphogenesis gene 2 protein. *PLoS One*, *7*, e39911.

Rothan, H. A., Bahrani, H., Abd Rahman, N., & Yusof, R. (2014). Identification of natural antimicrobial agents to treat dengue infection: In vitro analysis of latarcin peptide activity against dengue virus. *BMC Microbiology*, *14*(1), 1–10.

Ruigrok, R. W. H., Crepin, T., Hart, D. J., & Cusack, S. (2010). Towards an atomic resolution understanding of the influenza virus replication machinery. *Current Opinion in Structural Biology*, *20*, 104–113.

Sala, A., Ardizzoni, A., Ciociola, T., Magliani, W., Conti, S., Blasi, E., & Cermelli, C. (2018). Antiviral activity of synthetic peptides derived from physiological proteins. *Intervirology*, *61*(4), 166–173.

Selsted, M. E., Novotny, M. J., Morris, W. L., Tang, Y. Q., Smith, W., & Cullor, J. S. (1992). Indolicidin, a novel bactericidal tridecapeptide amide from neutrophils. *Journal of Biological Chemistry*, *267*(7), 4292–4295.

Sen, N., Kanitkar, T. R., Roy, A. A., Soni, N., Amritkar, K., Supekar, S., Nair, S., Singh, G., & Madhusudhan, M. S. (2019). Predicting and designing therapeutics against the Nipah virus. *PLoS Neglected Tropical Diseases*, *13*(12), e0007419.

Shah, N. B., & Duncan, T. M. (2014). Bio-layer interferometry for measuring kinetics of protein-protein interactions and allosteric ligand effects. *Journal of Visualized Experiments*, (84), e51383.

Silphaduang, U., & Noga, E. J. (2001). Peptide antibiotics in mast cells of fish. *Nature*, *414*(6861), 268–269.

Sinha, S., Cheshenko, N., Lehrer, R. I., & Herold, B. C. (2003). NP-1, a rabbit α-defensin, prevents the entry and intercellular spread of herpes simplex virus type 2. *Antimicrobial Agents and Chemotherapy*, *47*(2), 494–500.

Skalickova, S., Heger, Z., Krejcova, L., Pekarik, V., Bastl, K., Janda, J., Kostolansky, F., Vareckova, E., Zitka, O., Adam, V., & Kizek, R. (2015). Perspective of use of antiviral peptides against influenza virus. *Viruses*, *7*(10), 5428–5442.

Skerlavaj, B., Benincasa, M., Risso, A., Zanetti, M., & Gennaro, R. (1999). SMAP-29: A potent antibacterial and antifungal peptide from sheep leukocytes. *FEBS Letters*, *463*(1–2), 58–62.

Skerlavaj, B., Gennaro, R., Bagella, L., Merluzzi, L., Risso, A., & Zanetti, M. (1996). Biological characterization of two novel cathelicidin-derived peptides and identification of structural requirements for their antimicrobial and cell lytic activities. *Journal of Biological Chemistry*, *271*(45), 28375–28381.

Swart, P. J., Harmsen, M. C., Kuipers, M. E., Van Dijk, A. A., van der Strate, B. W. A., Van Berkel, P. H. C., Nuijens, J. H., Smit, C., Witvrouw, M., De Clercq, E., de Be´thune, M.-P., Pauwels, R., & Meijer, D. K. F. (1999). Charge modification of plasma and milk proteins results in antiviral active compounds. *Journal of Peptide Science*, *5*(12), 563–576.

Swart, P. J., Kuipers, E. M., Smit, C., Van Der Strate, B. W., Harmsen, M. C., & Meijer, D. K. (1998). Lactoferrin. In *Advances in lactoferrin research* (pp. 205–213). *Springer.*

Tao, J., Zhao, Y. Q., Chi, C. F., & Wang, B. (2018). Bioactive peptides from cartilage protein hydrolysate of spotless smoothhound and their antioxidant activity in vitro. *Marine Drugs*, *16*(4), 100.

Tsai, C. C., Emau, P., Jiang, Y., Agy, M. B., Shattock, R. J., Schmidt, A., Morton, W. R., Gustafson, K. R., & Boyd, M. R. (2004). Cyanovirin-N inhibits AIDS virus infections in vaginal transmission models. *AIDS Research and Human Retroviruses*, *20*(1), 11–18.

Tu, M., Cheng, S., Lu, W., & Du, M. (2018). Advancement and prospects of bioinformatics analysis for studying bioactive peptides from food-derived protein: Sequence, structure, and functions. *TrAC Trends in Analytical Chemistry*, *105*, 7–17.

Turner, R. B. (2001). The treatment of rhinovirus infections: Progress and potential. *Antiviral Research*, *49*(1), 1–14.

Ueki, N., Someya, K., Matsuo, Y., Wakamatsu, K., & Mukai, H. (2007). Cryptides: Functional cryptic peptides hidden in protein structures. *Peptide Science: Original Research on Biomolecules*, *88*(2), 190–198.

Ussery, M. A., Irvin, J. D., & Hardesty, B. (1977). Inhibition of poliovirus replication by a plant antiviral peptide. *Annals of the New York Academy of Sciences*, *284*(1), 431–440.

Valdés, A., Cifuentes, A., & León, C. (2017). Foodomics evaluation of bioactive compounds in foods. *TrAC Trends in Analytical Chemistry*, *96*, 2–13.

Van Compernolle, S. E., Taylor, R. J., Oswald-Richter, K., Jiang, J., Youree, B. E., Bowie, J. H., Tyler, M. J., Conlon, J. M., Wade, D., Aiken, C., & Dermody, T. S. (2005). Antimicrobial peptides from amphibian skin potently inhibit human immunodeficiency virus infection and transfer of virus from dendritic cells to T cells. *Journal of Virology*, *79*(18), 11598–11606.

Van der Strate, B. W. A., Beljaars, L., Molema, G., Harmsen, M. C., & Meijer, D. K. F. (2001). Antiviral activities of lactoferrin. *Antiviral Research*, *52*(3), 225–239.

Villamil, S. M., Alche, L. E., & Coto, C. E. (1995). Inhibition of herpes simplex virus type-1 multiplication by meliacine, a peptide of plant origin. *Antiviral Chemistry and Chemotherapy*, *6*(4), 239–244.

Vorland, L. H. (1999). Lactoferrin: A multifunctional glycoprotein. *APMIS*, *107*(11), 971–981.

Wachsman, M. B., Castilla, V., & Coto, C. E. (1998). Inhibition of foot and mouth disease virus (FMDV) uncoating by a plant-derived peptide isolated from *Melia azedarach* L leaves. *Archives of Virology*, *143*(3), 581–590.

Wachsman, M. B., Farías, M. E., Takeda, E., Sesma, F., de Ruiz Holgado, A. P., de Torres, R. A., & Coto, C. E. (1999). Antiviral activity of enterocin CRL35 against herpesviruses. *International Journal of Antimicrobial Agents*, *12*(4), 293–299.

Walls, A. C., Park, Y. J., Tortorici, M. A., Wall, A., McGuire, A. T., & Veesler, D. (2020). Structure, function, and antigenicity of the SARS-CoV-2 spike glycoprotein. *Cell*, *181*(2), 281–292.

Wan, Y., Shang, J., Graham, R., Baric, R. S., & Li, F. (2020). Receptor recognition by novel coronavirus from Wuhan: An analysis based on decade-long structural studies of SARS. *Journal of Virology*, *94*(7).

Wang, H., & Liu, R. (2011). Advantages of mRNA display selections over other selection techniques for investigation of protein–protein interactions. *Expert Review of Proteomics*, *8*, 335–346.

Wang, W., Owen, S. M., Rudolph, D. L., Cole, A. M., Hong, T., Waring, A. J., Lal, R. B., & Lehrer, R. I. (2004). Activity of α- and θ-defensins against primary isolates of HIV-1. *The Journal of Immunology*, *173*(1), 515–520.

Wang, G., Li, X., & Wang, Z. (2009). APD2: The updated antimicrobial peptide database and its application in peptide design. *Nucleic Acids Research*, *37*, D933–D937.

Wang, G., Li, X., & Wang, Z. (2016). APD3: The antimicrobial peptide database as a tool for research and education. *Nucleic Acids Research*, 44, D1087–D1093.

Wang, G., Watson, K. M., Peterkofsky, A., & Buckheit, R. W. (2010). Identification of novel human immunodeficiency virus type 1-inhibitory peptides based on the antimicrobial peptide database. *Antimicrobial Agents and Chemotherapy*, *54*(3), 1343–1346.

Wang, H., & Ng, T. B. (2000). Ginkbilobin, a novel antifungal protein from *Ginkgo biloba* seeds with sequence similarity to embryo-abundant protein. *Biochemical and Biophysical Research Communications*, *279*(2), 407–411.

Wang, H., & Ng, T. B. (2001). Novel antifungal peptides from Ceylon spinach seeds. *Biochemical and Biophysical Research Communications*, *288*(4), 765–770.

Wang, H., & Ng, T. B. (2002). Ascalin, a new anti-fungal peptide with human immunodeficiency virus type 1 reverse transcriptase-inhibiting activity from shallot bulbs. *Peptides*, *23*(6), 1025–1029.

Wang, H. X., & Ng, T. B. (2005). An antifungal peptide from the coconut. *Peptides*, *26*(12), 2392–2396.

Wang, J., Wang, H. X., & Ng, T. B. (2007). A peptide with HIV-1 reverse transcriptase inhibitory activity from the medicinal mushroom *Russula paludosa*. *Peptides*, *28*(3), 560–565.

Wang, Q., Notay, K., Downey, G. P., & McCulloch, C.A. (2020). The Leucine-rich repeat region of CARMIL1 regulates IL-1-mediated ERK activation, MMP expression, and collagen degradation. *Cell Reports*, *31*(13), 107781.

Wang, Y. D., Kung, C. W., & Chen, J. Y. (2010). Antiviral activity by fish antimicrobial peptides of epinecidin-1 and hepcidin 1–5 against nervous necrosis virus in medaka. *Peptides*, *31*(6), 1026–1033.

Weinberg, A., Quinones-Mateu, M. E., & Lederman, M. M. (2006). Role of human β-defensins in HIV infection. *Advances in Dental Research*, *19*(1), 42–48.

Weissenbacher, M. C., Laguens, R. P., & Coto, C. E. (1987). Argentine hemorrhagic fever. *Current Topics in Microbiology and Immunology*, *134*, 79–116.

Wong, H., Bowie, J. H., & Carver, J. A. (1997). The solution structure and activity of caerin 1.1, an antimicrobial peptide from the Australian green tree frog, *Litoria splendida*. *European Journal of Biochemistry*, *247*(2), 545–557.

Wong, J. H., & Ng, T. B. (2005). Sesquin, a potent defensin-like antimicrobial peptide from ground beans with inhibitory activities toward tumor cells and HIV-1 reverse transcriptase. *Peptides*, *26*(7), 1120–1126.

Yan, R., Zhao, Z., He, Y., Wu, L., Cai, D., Hong, W., Wu, Y., Cao, Z., Zheng, C., & Li, W. (2011). A new natural α-helical peptide from the venom of the scorpion *Heterometrus petersii* kills HCV. *Peptides*, *32*(1), 11–19.

Yan, R., Zhang, Y., Li, Y., Xia, L., Guo, Y., & Zhou, Q. (2020). Structural basis for the recognition of SARS-CoV-2 by full-length human ACE2. *Science*, *367*(6485), 1444–1448.

Yang, Q. Y. (1999). *Advanced research in PSP*. The Hong Kong Association for Health Care, Tsim Sha Tsu, Kowloon.

Yasin, B., Pang, M., Turner, J. S., Cho, Y., Dinh, N. N., Waring, A. J., Lehrer, R. I., & Wagar, E. A. (2000). Evaluation of the inactivation of infectious Herpes simplex virus by host-defense peptides. *European Journal of Clinical Microbiology and Infectious Diseases*, *19*(3), 187–194.

Yazdani, Z., Rafiei, A., Valadan, R., Ashrafi, H., Pasandi, M., & Kardan, M. (2020). Designing a potent L1 protein-based HPV peptide vaccine: A bioinformatics approach. *Computational Biology and Chemistry*, *85*, 107209.

Yeung, J. H., & Or, P. M. (2012). Polysaccharide peptides from *Coriolus versicolor* competitively inhibit model cytochrome P450 enzyme probe substrates metabolism in human liver microsomes. *Phytomedicine*, *19*(5), 457–463.

Yi, M. Y., Kaneko, S., Yu, D. Y., & Murakami, S. (1997). Hepatitis C virus envelope proteins bind lactoferrin. *Journal of Virology*, *71*(8), 5997–6002.

Yuan, H., Estes, P. A., Chen, Y., Newsome, J., Olcese, V. A., Garcea, R. L., & Schlegel, R. (2001). Immunization with a pentameric L1 fusion protein protects against papillomavirus infection. *Journal of Virology*, *75*(17), 7848–7853.

Yuan, L., Zhang, S., Peng, J., Li, Y., & Yang, Q. (2019). Synthetic surfactin analogues have improved anti-PEDV properties. *PLoS One*, *14*, e0215227.

Yuan, P. W., Bartlam, M., Lou, Z. Y., Chen, S. D., Zhou, J., He, X. J., Lv, Z. Y., Ge, R. W., Li, X. M., Deng, T., Fodor, E., Rao, Z., & Liu, Y. (2009). Crystal structure of an avian influenza polymerase PA(n) reveals an endonuclease active site. *Nature*, *458*, 909–913.

Zhan, S., Aweya, J. J., Wang, F., Yao, D., Zhong, M., Chen, J., Li, S., & Zhang, Y. (2019). *Litopenaeus vannamei* attenuates white spot syndrome virus replication by specific antiviral peptides generated from hemocyanin. *Developmental & Comparative Immunology*, *91*, 50–61.

Zhang, G., Pomplun, S., Loftis, A. R., Loas, A., & Pentelute, B. L. (2020). The first-in-class peptide binder to the SARS-CoV-2 spike protein. *bioRxiv preprint*.

Zhang, G., Pomplun, S., Loftis, A. R., Tan, X., Loas, A., & Pentelute, B. L. (2020). Investigation of ACE2 N-terminal fragments binding to SARS-CoV-2 Spike RBD. *BioRxiv*, 2020-03.

Zhao, L., Hao, X., & Wu, Y. (2015). Inhibitory effect of polysaccharide peptide (PSP) against Tobacco mosaic virus (TMV). *International Journal of Biological Macromolecules*, *75*, 474–478.

https://doi.org/10.1142/9789811254796_0009

9 Designing a Multi-epitope Peptide-based Vaccine for Human Influenza A/H1N1 Virus — An Immunoinformatics Approach

Gracy Fathima Selvaraj[†], Kaveri Krishnasamy[*,†], Shanmughavel Piramanayagam[‡] and Velmurugan Devadasan[§]

[†]*Department of Virology, King Institute of Preventive Medicine, Guindy, Chennai 600032, Tamil Nadu, India*
[‡]*Department of Bioinformatics, Bharathiar University, Coimbatore 641046, Tamil Nadu, India*
[§]*Office of the Dean Sponsored Research, Publications and Collaborations, AMET University, Kanathur, ECR Road, Chennai, P.C.-603 112*

Abstract

Influenza A viruses are enveloped and contain eight segments of single-stranded, negative-sense RNA, which encode 11 proteins. The external transmembrane surface glycoproteins, hemagglutinin (HA) and NA are the major antigenic determinants. HA is responsible for binding of virus to the cell that is being infected, which triggers the human immune system to create antibodies to target the virus specifically. So, HA protein is used for vaccine designing. Vaccination is the most effective way to reduce the risk of infection. But the efficacy of the seasonal influenza vaccine is compromised by antigenic changes like antigenic shift, and drift in influenza viruses over time requires annual immunization and

*Corresponding author: e-mail: kaveri_raj1967@yahoo.com

that vaccines are updated frequently. Therefore, it is necessary to develop an effective vaccine that will target a part of the virus that is not affected by these changes, that is, a universal flu vaccine which should only be administered occasionally, rather than every year. Immunoinformatics is a branch of bioinformatics focusing on immunology and vaccinology. This chapter discusses in detail the designing of a multi-epitope peptide-based vaccine for human *Influenza* A/H1N1 virus using B-cell and T-cell epitopes that are more capable of stimulating the immune system, by using immunoinformatics approaches.

1. Introduction

Hemagglutinin (HA) is the main antigenic glycoprotein on the surface of *Influenza* virus recognized by the host immune system and inducing a neutralizing antibody response (Liu *et al.*, 2009). It mediates virus binding to the specific terminal sialic acid on the host cell surface, and hence the HA protein is selected for vaccine designing. Antigenic variation leads to antigenic drift, which results in the selection of new strain frequently for vaccine preparation. The HA protein sequence was explored thoroughly using multiple immunoinformatics-based servers and software, to identify various epitopes for an effective vaccine. Epitope vaccine or an epitope-based subunit vaccine has lesser side effects when compared to the conventional vaccines (Sakib *et al.*, 2014). It is easier to produce and cheaper to manufacture when compared to engineered subunit vaccines. It does not contain any complete component of the pathogens. The peptide vaccine mechanism is the chemical method to synthesize the recognized B-cell and T-cell epitopes that are immunodominant, and it can induce specific immune responses. Peptide-based vaccines do not need *in vitro* culture, making them biologically safe, and their selectivity allows accurate activation of immune responses (Dudek *et al.*, 2010; Purcell *et al.*, 2007).

The concept of a multi-epitope vaccine is to efficiently identify and assemble B- and T-cell epitopes that are more capable of stimulating the immune system and therefore can induce both arms of immune responses. Epitopes of cytotoxic T lymphocyte (CTL), helper T lymphocyte (HTL), and B-cell lymphocytes, the short stretches of amino acid sequences of protein can elicit direct and strong immune response, than the response generated by the whole protein itself (Kao & Hodges, 2009). In this chapter, we predicted the CTL, HTL, and B-cell epitopes and their properties by various bioinformatics tools. The population coverage of these epitopes is also studied worldwide. The interactions between the epitopes and their corresponding alleles were studied. Simultaneously, the multi-epitope vaccine construct (MEVC) was prepared and its biological activity was assessed by bioinformatics tools using the interaction between the vaccine construct and the innate immune system receptors TLR3 and TLR4 and cell-mediated immune receptor HLA*11:01. We strongly believe that the outcome of the present report will provide a potential vaccine candidate against *Influenza* A/H1N1.

2. Materials and Methods

2.1. Sequence Retrieval

The HA protein of vaccine strain (A/Michigan/45/2015(H1N1)) was retrieved from protein sequence database Swissprot (www.expasy.org) (UniprotKB-A0A0X9QTS2_9INFA) to predict the T- and B-cell epitopes and MEVC preparation.

2.2. Prediction of Physiochemical Properties, Antigenicity, Allergenicity and Secondary Structure

The Expasy ProtParam tool was used to evaluate the physical and chemical properties of target protein (Gasteiger *et al.*,

2003). Allergenicity and antigenicity of proteins were checked through AllerTOP v2.0 (https://www.ddg-pharmfac.net/AllerTOP/method.html) (Dimitrov *et al.*, 2013) and VaxiJen v2.0 (http://www.ddg-pharmfac.net/vaxijen/VaxiJen/VaxiJen.html) (Doytchinova & Flower, 2007), respectively. For antigenicity prediction with higher accuracy, Virus model available at the VaxiJen server with a threshold of 0.4 was utilized. The conformational states, for example, helix, sheet, turn and coil were predicted using the online Secondary Structure Analysis Tool (SOPMA) (Geourjon & Deleage, 1995) with default parameters.

2.3. T-cell Epitope Prediction

The T-cell epitopes are important for epitope-based peptide vaccine design. These are typically peptide fragments, which are immunodominant in nature and can promote specific immune responses during infection.

2.3.1. *Cytotoxic T-cell epitope prediction*

The NetCTL 1.2 (http://www.cbs.dtu.dk/services/NetCTL/) server was used for the prediction of CTL epitopes. NetCTL uses NetMHC server's artificial neural networks to predict MHC binding and NetChop-3.0 to predict C-terminal cleavages and a weight matrix to calculate TAP transport efficiency to generate predictions (Larsen *et al.*, 2005, 2007). The NetCTL 1.2 server can predict CD8+ T-cell epitopes for 12 human leukocyte antigens (HLA supertypes such as A1, A2, A3, A24, A26, B7, B8, B27, B39, B44, B58, and B62) taking into account the proteasomal C-terminal cleavage, MHC class I binding, and TAP transport efficiency. Together, these supertypes account for the majority of HLA-A (76.5%) and HLA-B (67.1%) distribution (Rodrigo Dos Santos Francisco *et al.*, 2015). In this chapter, the threshold value for epitope identification was set at 1.25, which has a sensitivity and specificity of 0.54 and 0.993, respectively (Adhikari *et al.*, 2018). The weights on C-terminal cleavage and TAP transport efficiency were used as default parameters. Antigenicity of the predicted epitopes was calculated by VaxiJen v2.0 with a threshold of 0.4, allergenicity was calculated by AllerTOP v2.0, and the toxicity was predicted by ToxinPred (http://crdd.osdd.net/raghava/toxinpred/), a tool which is developed to predict and design toxic/nontoxic peptides based on the machine learning technique and quantitative matrix using different properties of peptides (Gupta *et al.*, 2015). Only the epitopes with VaxiJen score ≥ 0.4 and predicted to be nontoxic and nonallergens, were taken for further screening.

2.3.1.1. Epitope conservancy and immunogenicity prediction

For epitope conservancy and immunogenicity prediction, the conservancy (http://tools.iedb.org/conservancy/) (Bui *et al.*, 2007) and immunogenicity (http://tools.iedb.org/immunogenicity/) (Calis *et al.*, 2013) prediction tools were used. The degree of conservancy of an epitope within a given protein sequence set at different degrees of sequence identity is studied. Immunogenicity prediction can cover the degree of efficiency of the respective epitope to produce an immunogenic response. More immunogenic peptides are superior to the less immunogenic peptides and considered as effective T-cell epitopes.

2.3.1.2. Allele selection

Based on the antigenicity, allergenicity, toxicity, conservancy, and immunogenicity, epitopes are shortlisted from the NetCTL predicted epitopes. To identify frequently and nonfrequently occurring MHC-I-binding alleles, the epitopes were analyzed by the stabilized matrix method (SMM) using the IEDB analysis tool (http://tools.iedb.org/mhci/) (Peters *et al.*, 2005). The amino acid length of peptide 9.0 and the IC_{50} value less than 200 were selected as parameters for the identification of MHC-I-binding alleles. Here, peptides with IC_{50} values <50 nM are considered as high affinity,

<500 nM intermediate affinity, and, <5000 nM low affinity. So the lower IC_{50} value indicates higher affinity (Adhikari *et al.*, 2018).

2.3.1.3. Comparison with IEDB database

The CTL epitopes were compared with the IEDB database to identify their novelty. The Immune Epitope Database and Analysis Resource (IEDB) (https://www.iedb.org/) is a freely available resource and is populated using information captured or curated from peer-reviewed scientific literature and from data submitted by researchers.

2.3.2. *Helper T-cell (HTL) epitope prediction*

HTLs are the key players of the adaptive immune response. To predict HTL epitopes, the IEDB MHC II server (http://tools.iedb.org/mhcii/) was used (Zhang *et al.*, 2008). The SMM-align method was used for the prediction of MHC-II-binding alleles of the best candidate epitope (Nielsen *et al.*, 2007). The server provides the epitope predictions for three human MHC class II isotypes that include HLA-DR, HLA-DP, and HLA-DQ. The percentile rank was given after comparing the peptides score with million 15 mers from the SWISSPROT database. The lower percentile value means a higher binding affinity of MHC II. The epitopes with IC_{50} values up to 1000 nM and with lower percentile rank were in consideration. The predicted HTL epitopes were subjected for further analysis of antigenicity by VaxiJen v2.0, allergenicity by AllerTOP v2.0, and the toxicity was predicted by ToxinPred.

2.4. Population Coverage

The expression and distribution of HLA alleles vary depending on the world's ethnicities and regions, thereby impacting the effective production of an epitope-based vaccine (Adhikari *et al.*, 2018). The population coverage analysis helps in finding the efficacy of epitopes on HLA allele distribution across different populations in the world. Every epitope and its binding HLA alleles are added, and different geographic areas are also selected for this analysis. The population coverage was calculated using the IEDB population coverage tool ((http://tools.iedb.org/population/) and for this purpose selected MHC class I and II epitopes and corresponding HLA-binding alleles were considered.

2.5. Three-dimensional (3D) Structure Design of the Epitope

Based on the above studies, the novel epitope was selected and was submitted for modeling. PEP-FOLD3 peptide structure prediction server (http://bioserv.rpbs.univ-paris-diderot.fr/services/PEP-FOLD3/) (Lamiable *et al.*, 2016; Shen *et al.*, 2014; Thévenet *et al.*, 2012) is a *de novo* approach aimed at predicting peptide structures from amino acid sequences. The best model was selected for analysis of the interaction with MHC-I-binding alleles.

2.6. Molecular Interaction of the MHC and Epitopes

In order to estimate the binding affinities between the epitope and the molecular structure of MHC I and II, *in silico* molecular docking was used. The predicted structure of epitope was subjected to dock with the MHC I (PDB ID: 4NT6:A) and MHC II (4MDI) structures, downloaded from RCSB PDB database (https://www.rcsb.org/) (Berman *et al.*, 2000) by ClusPro v.2 (https://cluspro.bu.edu/) protein–protein docking web server (Kozakov *et al.*, 2017). The server uses three consecutive steps like rigid body docking, clustering of lowest energy structure, and structural refinement by energy minimization (Sayed *et al.*, 2020).

2.7. B-cell Epitope Prediction

2.7.1. *Linear/continuous B-cell epitope prediction*

B-cell epitopes were predicted using the ABCpred server (http://crdd.osdd.net/raghava/abcpred/) (Saha & Raghava, 2006).

This server predicts B-cell epitopes using recurrent neural network algorithm. For higher accuracy, the threshold for the prediction was kept 0.90. The predicted epitopes were checked for their antigenicity using VaxiJen server and toxicity using ToxinPred server. The conservancy was checked by IEDB conservancy tool.

2.7.2. *Structure prediction, refinement and validation*

To identify discontinuous B-cell epitopes, the structure of the selected HA sequence of A/Michigan/45/2015(H1N1) is needed. The secondary structure was predicted by SOPMA (https://npsa-prabi.ibcp.fr/cgi-bin/secpred_sopma.pl) (Geourjon & Deleage, 1995). The tertiary structure of the selected sequence was predicted by SWISS-MODEL (https://swissmodel.expasy.org/) (Waterhouse *et al.*, 2018) and the predicted structures were refined (http://galaxy.seoklab.org/cgi-bin/submit.cgi?-type=REFINE) (Heo *et al.*, 2013). The modeled structure was validated by the Ramachandran plot generated in Procheck (https://servicesn.mbi.ucla.edu/PROCHECK/) (Laskowski *et al.*, 2001) and ProSA (https://prosa.services.came.sbg.ac.at/prosa.php) (Wiederstein& Sippl, 2007).

2.7.3. *Conformational/discontinuous B-cell epitope prediction*

Conformational epitopes are the most prevalent epitopes that are recognized by antibodies. They are present in small segments on linear protein and are brought to proximity while protein folding. All conformational epitope prediction methods require the 3D structures of proteins. Discontinuous epitopes can be predicted using the ElliPro (http://tools.iedb.org/ellipro/) server at IEDB. ElliPro defines PI score of each residue based on the center of mass of residue residing outside the largest possible ellipsoid. The prediction parameters like minimum score and maximum distance (Angstrom) were set as 0.8 and 6, respectively.

2.8. Interferon (IFN)-γ-inducing Epitopes

Since IFN-γ is the signature cytokine of both the innate and adaptive immune systems, epitopes with potency to induce IFN-γ could boost the immunogenic capacity of any vaccine. Thus, IFN-γ-inducing epitopes were predicted for each structural protein by the IFN epitope server (http://crdd.osdd.net/raghava/ifnepitope/index.php) (Dhanda *et al.*, 2013). For IFN-γ-inducing epitopes selection, the Motif/SVM hybrid approach was chosen, and the model was set to be IFN-γ versus non-IFN-γ.

2.9. Designing of MEVC

The main strategy in the present chapter was to design and construct a novel multi-epitope vaccine from HA of A/Michigan/45/2015(H1N1) based on *in silico* methods to elicit humoral and cellular immune responses. To construct a multi-epitope vaccine, the selected best HTL, CTL, and B-cell epitopes were linked by using GPGPG, AAY, EAAAK, and KK linkers, respectively. Five adjuvants, namely, β-defensin, universal memory T-cell helper peptide (TpD), PADRE (Pan HLA-DR reactive epitope), RS09 TLR4 agonist, and an M-cell ligand were also linked by linkers into the vaccine construct. To enhance the immunogenicity, β-defensin was added to the N-terminal, whereas in the C-terminal, M-cell ligand was added which was followed by adding of HHHHHH for easy purification of vaccine. For the construction of a multi-epitope vaccine against *Influenza* A/H1N1, we followed Chauhan *et al*. (2019): (i) they should be promiscuous, (ii) should have overlapping CTL and HTL epitopes, (iii) immunogenicity, (iv) population coverage, (v) high affinity toward HLA alleles, and (vi) should not overlap with any human gene.

The antigenicity of the MEVC was determined using the VaxiJen server (http://www.ddg-pharmfac.net/vaxijen/VaxiJen/VaxiJen.html), the allergenicity was checked using AllerTOP v2.0 (http://www.ddg-pharmfac. net/AllerTOP/), and the physiochemical characteristics were determined using the ProtParam tool of the ExPASy database server (http://web. expasy.org/protparam/).

2.10. Structure Prediction, Validation and Docking with the Receptor

The secondary structure of the MEVC was predicted using PSIPred 4.0 Protein Sequence Analysis Workbench (http://bioinf.cs.ucl.ac.uk/psipred/), while the tertiary structure was predicted by GalaxyWeb server (http://galaxy.seoklab.org/tbm) (Shin *et al.*, 2014). The best-modeled structure was refined using the Galaxy Refine server (http://galaxy.seoklab.org/cgi-bin/submit.cgi?-type=REFINE) (Heo *et al.*, 2013). Galaxy refined the model by molecular dynamics simulation. PROCHECK v.3.5 (https://servicesn.mbi.ucla.edu/PROCHECK/) and ProSA (https://prosa.services.came.sbg.ac.at/prosa.php) web servers validated the model of the MEVC with the best TMscore. The biological activity of the engineered fusion protein was assessed by bioinformatics tools using the interaction between the vaccine candidate and the innate immune system receptors (TLR3 and TLR4) and cellular immune system receptor (HLA-A*11:01). Vaccine-receptor docking was performed by the ClusPro v.2 (https://cluspro.bu.edu/) protein–protein docking web server (Kozakov *et al.*, 2017) to determine the binding affinity of the vaccine with the TLR3 (PDB ID: 2A0Z), TLR4 receptor (PDB ID: 3FXI), and HLA-A*11:01) (PDB ID-6JP3). Based on the lowest energy weight score and members, the final vaccine-TLR3 and TLR4 complex and vaccine-HLA-A11:01 models were selected.

2.11. Population Coverage of MEVC

To check the population coverage of the vaccine construct, population coverage tool available at IEDB (http://tools.iedb.org/population/) server was utilized. The HLA class I and II alleles in the final construct were entered in the tool, and the population coverage of the alleles was calculated for the top 27 countries and across the world. Those epitopes exhibiting 50% or more population coverage were scrutinized and to reduce the probability of autoimmunity, all the selected epitopes were subjected to BlastP search analysis against the Human proteome. Epitopes showing similarity to any human protein were excluded from the further analysis.

2.12. Immune Simulations of Vaccine Construct

To characterize the real-life immunogenic profiles and immune response of the multi-epitope vaccine, C-ImmSim server (Rapin *et al.*, 2010) was utilized. Position-specific scoring matrix and machine learning are the two methods, based on which C-ImmSim predicts immune epitopes and immune interactions. It simultaneously simulates three different anatomical regions of mammals, that is, bone marrow, thymus, and tertiary lymphatic organs. The parameters like Random seed, simulation volume, and simulation step and the host HLA selection parameter for MHC class I were set on HLA-A*10:10, HLA-A*11:01, and HLA-B*07:02 and for DR MHC class II was set on DBR1*01:01 alleles were kept as default values and based on literatures the time step to injection parameter was set to administer three injections at time steps 1, 84, and 168, corresponding to time 0, 4, and 8 weeks with a total of 1,050 simulation steps. The immune system simulation server mentioned here provides an opportunity to study the overall immunogenicity of the generic protein sequence in the context of its amino acid sequence (Rapin *et al.*, 2011). The total simulation is focused on three events: (i) B-cell epitopes binding, (ii) HLA class I and II epitopes binding, and (iii) TCR binding in which HLA–peptide complex interaction should be present. Such processes are independently conducted by cells described by agents and occupy a specified simulated biological amount.

3. Results and Discussion

The advancement of newer immunoinformatics tools has made a broader way in developing vaccine or vaccine candidates through the satisfactory understanding of the immune response of the human body against an organism within a short time (De Groot & Rappuoli, 2004).

3.1. Sequence Retrieval and Prediction of Physiochemical Properties

The surface glycoprotein HA of vaccine strain A/Michigan/45/2015(H1N1) sequence was retrieved from protein sequence database Swissprot to predict various B-cell and T-cell epitopes against *Influenza* A/H1N1. The predicted physiochemical characteristics are as follows. The protein has 566 amino acids, and a molecular weight of 63,376.70 Da. The total number of positively charged residues (Arg+Lys) and negatively charged residues (Asp+Glu) were 60 and 59, respectively. The theoretical isoelectric point (PI) was calculated at 7.51. Instability index (II) is one of the key parameters that is significantly considered, as it helps in discarding the unstable protein candidates. A protein whose II is smaller than 40 is predicted as stable, and a value above 40 predicts that the protein may be unstable. Here, the II was 29.36, which classifies the protein as stable. The aliphatic index of HA protein was calculated to be 80.42, which indicates that this protein has stability at several temperatures. Its grand average of hydropathicity (GRAVY) is −0.384 (**Table 1**).

3.2. Antigenicity and Allergenicity

Prediction of the antigenicity represents a numerical criterion for the capability of the protein to bind to the B- and T-cell receptors and increase the immune response in the host cell. VaxiJen v2.0 was used to predict the antigenicity of the selected protein

Table 1 Physiochemical properties of A/Michigan/45/2015 (H1N1) HA sequence.

Features	Value
Number of amino acids	566
Molecular weight	63,376.7
Theoretical pI	7.51
Total number of negatively charged residues (Asp+Glu)	59
Total number of positively charged residues (Arg+Lys)	60
Total number of atoms	8,840
Instability index	29.36
Aliphatic index	80.42
Grand average of hydropathicity (GRAVY)	−0.384

and the results showed potent antigenicity of 0.5269 with a 0.4% threshold. The score suggested that the HA protein is the most potent antigenic protein to generate immune response. Allergen proteins induce an IgE antibody response (Dimitrov *et al.*, 2013). The allergenicity of the sequence was predicted as non-allergen using the AllerTOP tool.

3.3. T cell Prediction

T-cell epitopes reside on the antigen-presenting cell surface, where they bind to major histocompatibility molecules (MHC) to induce the immune response (Madden, 1995). T-cell epitope prediction comprises identification of MHC I and II binding epitopes, in order to activate both CTL- and HTL-mediated immune response.

3.3.1. *Cytotoxic T-cell epitope prediction*

CTL epitopes are essential for inducing MHC-I cellular immune response by neutralizing virus-infected cells and damaged cells via releasing cytotoxic proteins like granzymes, perforins, and so on. The CTL epitopes were predicted for all selected proteins using the NetCTL 1.2 server. The combined score was considered for the epitope selection. In this chapter, we unraveled 47 epitopes in total, which achieved the selected threshold value of 1.25. The predicted T-cell epitopes were further evaluated by the VaxiJen server, IEDB immunogenicity prediction tool, and conservancy analysis tool. Herein, among 47 primarily selected T-cell epitopes, 24 epitopes were below the threshold value 0.4 of VaxiJen server, whereas 20 epitopes contained the immunogenicity value less than 0.00. Two of them showed 75% conservancy. The results thus revealed that all epitopes with the highest combined score could not be the best epitopes. Among 47 epitopes, we selected 11 epitopes which have positive antigenicity and immunogenicity scores and with 100% conservancy, so that these highly antigenic epitopes can interact with the MHC alleles with high affinity and can create an effective immune response.

Based on the allergenicity and toxicity analysis, we finally identified eight epitopes (**Table 2**), which contained 100% conservancy, higher immunogenicity and antigenicity, that are non-allergen and non-toxic in nature. The conservancy score is an important issue during the development of an effective vaccine. Epitope conservancy among different strains of the selected protein can provide immunization effectively. Antigenicity score plays an important role in the selection of epitopes. Here, in the selected eight epitopes, six of them showed VaxiJen score more than 1 and two epitopes showed 0.9827 and 0.5187, respectively, which explained that all epitopes are highly antigenic in nature. The immunogenicity score of the epitope can be a good criterion for the selection of the best epitope. The higher score designates a greater probability of eliciting an effective immune response.

3.3.1.1. Allele selection

The selected eight T-cell epitopes were found to be recognized by the significant MHC class I molecule such as HLA-A, HLA-B, and

Table 2 **CTL epitopes with combined score, antigenicity, immunogenicity, conservancy, allergenicity, and toxicity. The high scores indicate the best epitopes.**

S. No.	Epitope	Combined Score	Antigenicity	Immunogenicity	Conservancy (%)	Position	Allergenicity	Toxicity
1	NADTLCIGY	2.2541	1.1988	0.11683	100.00	16–24	NA	No
2	RMNYYWTLV	1.294	1.4842	0.22537	100.00	243–251	NA	No
3	YVFVGTSRY	1.8925	0.9827	0.0397	100.00	215–223	NA	No
4	FIEGGWTGM	1.2905	1.1543	0.36067	100.00	353–361	NA	No
5	LPFQNIHPI	1.3495	1.7205	0.06124	100.00	307–315	NA	No
6	YNAELLVLL	1.6	0.5187	0.12057	100.00	438–446	NA	No
7	VSLGAISFW	1.6567	1.337	0.12266	100.00	545–553	NA	No
8	VVSLGAISF	1.3748	1.7163	0.02063	100.00	544–552	NA	No

HLA-C according to IEDB MHC class I-binding analysis resource. We selected humans as MHC source species and the SMM method for the prediction of a distinct set of MHC HLA alleles for the humans. This tool gives an output result for HLA-binding affinity of the epitopes in IC_{50} nM unit. A lower IC_{50} value indicates higher binding affinity of the epitopes with the MHC class I molecule. So, in this chapter, we chose IC_{50} values less than 200 nM (IC_{50} <200) for ensuring higher affinity (**Table 3**). The epitopes showed affinity to different number of HLA alleles with lower IC_{50} values. In addition to that, all the epitopes showed the highest affinity with the allele HLA-C*12:03 with various IC_{50} values. For MHC I processing, the analysis tool of the IEDB generates an overall score for each epitope's intrinsic potential of being a T-cell epitope based on proteasomal processing, TAP transport, and MHC-I-binding efficiency. Effective immune response depends not only on the successful recognition of epitopes by HLA molecules with significant affinity but also on the antigenicity and immunogenicity scores.

3.3.1.2. Comparison with IEDB database

IEDB database contains collection of experimental data of immune epitopes. The comparison of the predicted eight CTL epitopes with IEDB database showed that RMNYYWTLV epitope is a novel one and it is suggested to be used for subunit vaccine preparation due to its higher antigenicity, non-allergenic, non-toxic, and high conservancy. Epitope-based vaccines offer a viable alternative since they can elicit potent immune responses by selectively stimulating antigen specific B- and T-cells without causing undesirable allergic reactions.

3.3.2. *HTL epitope prediction*

HTLs act as the central mediators of immune response and coordinate with B lymphocytes, TC cells, and macrophages via signaling

Table 3 Allele selection for CTL epitopes. The alleles for the epitopes with lower IC_{50} value, which show higher binding affinity, were selected.

No.	Epitope	MHC I Alleles (IC_{50}, nM)
1	NADTLCIGY	HLA-C*12:03 (2.41)
		HLA-C*05:01 (4.71)
		HLA-B*35:01 (84.64)
		HLA-A*01:01 (145.73)
		HLA-B*15:02 (170.70)
2	RMNYYWTLV	HLA-A*02:01 (28.78)
		HLA-A*02:06 (31.96)
		HLA-C*12:03 (42.38)
		HLA-A*31:01 (118.43)
		HLA-C*05:01 (143.44)
3	YVFVGTSRY	HLA-A*29:02 (11.66)
		HLA-C*12:03 (14.07)
		HLA-B*35:01 (23.80)
		HLA-B*15:02 (36.08)
		HLA-C*07:01 (58.50)
		HLA-B*15:01 (91.41)
		HLA-A*25:01 (122.20)
		HLA-A*68:01 (159.77)
		HLA-C*03:03 (174.02)
		HLA-C*06:02 (174.51)
		HLA-A*26:01 (175.23)
		HLA-A*30:02 (186.84)
4	FIEGGWTGM	HLA-C*03:03 (14.61)
		HLA-C*12:03 (26.68)
		HLA-C*05:01 (34.33)
		HLA-B*15:02 (50.03)
		HLA-A*02:06 (126.93)

(*Continued*)

Table 3 (***Continued***)

No.	Epitope	MHC I Alleles (IC_{50}, nM)
5	LPFQNIHPI	HLA-C*12:03 (15.68)
		HLA-C*03:03 (42.33)
		HLA-B*35:01 (141.44)
		HLA-B*07:02 (169.00)
6	YNAELLVLL	HLA-B*15:02 (51.43)
		HLA-C*03:03 (97.86)
		HLA-C*12:03 (136.84)
7	VSLGAISFW	HLA-B*58:01 (12.6)
		HLA-C*03:03 (18.52)
		HLA-B*57:01 (34.90)
		HLA-C*12:03 (43.17)
8	VVSLGAISF	HLA-C*03:03 (43.32)
		HLA-C*12:03 (82.64)
		HLA-C*14:02 (169.68)

through interleukins and cytokines synthesis. HTLs recognize the epitopes presented on MHC-II-binding cleft. The eight MHC II server-predicted epitopes were selected based on the percentile rank and IC_{50} value. Here, the selected epitopes had percentile rank ≤1 (**Table 4**) and the IC_{50} is also less, which indicated that these epitopes have higher binding affinity. The resultant epitopes were checked for their antigenicity, allergenicity, and toxicity.

Based on this, among eight predicted HTL epitopes, seven were selected and subjected for their corresponding allele selection, which showed highest affinity (**Table 5**). The epitope RMNYYWTLV was subjected for the prediction of MHC II alleles. Six epitopes which contained this RMNYYWTLV as core peptide were selected based on the IC_{50} value less than 1,000 with lower percentile rank. The corresponding alleles for the epitopes were also identified (**Table 6**).

Table 4 Helper T-cell epitopes with percentile rank ≤1 and the lower IC_{50} value were selected and their antigenicity, allergenicity, and toxicity were studied.

S. No.	Epitope	Core Peptide	Percentile Rank	Position	IC_{50}	Antigenicity	Allergenicity	Toxicity
1	ILAIYSTVASSLVLV	YSTVASSLV	0.02	530–544	5	0.4789	NA	NT
2	INTSLPFQNIHPITI	INTSLPFQN	0.12	303–317	8	1.1509	NA	NT
3	NQSYINDKGKEVLVL	YINDKGKEV	0.31	179–193	53	0.6324	NA	NT
4	VVLLYTFTTANADTL	LYTFTTANA	0.38	6–20	58	0.0977	A	NT
5	NHLEKRIENLNKKVD	RIENLNKKV	0.69	415–429	48	0.5135	NA	NT
6	NGKLCKLRGVAPLHL	NGKLCKLRG	0.76	55–69	18	0.5453	NA	NT
7	GKCPKYVKSTKLRLA	PKYVKSTKL	0.88	318–332	19	0.5574	NA	NT
8	AELLVLLENERTLDY	LVLLENERT	0.98	440–454	30	0.8295	NA	NT

Table 5 Alleles selection for HTL epitopes based on percentile rank ≤1 and the lower IC_{50}, which show higher affinity.

S. No.	Epitope	Allele
1	ILAIYSTVASSLVLV	HLA-DRB1*07:01
		HLA-DRB1*09:01
		HLA-DRB1*01:01
		HLA-DRB1*04:01
2	INTSLPFQNIHPITI	HLA-DRB1*07:01
		HLA-DRB1*13:02
3	NQSYINDKGKEVLVL	HLA-DRB3*01:01
4	NHLEKRIENLNKKVD	HLA-DRB1*13:02
5	NGKLCKLRGVAPLHL	HLA-DRB1*07:01
		HLA-DRB1*01:01
6	GKCPKYVKSTKLRLA	HLA-DRB1*07:01
		HLA-DRB1*11:01
7	AELLVLLENERTLDY	HLA-DRB1*04:04
		HLA-DRB1*04:05

Table 6 Allele selection for RMNYYWTLV epitope based on lower IC_{50} to get higher affinity.

Epitope Sequence	MHC II Alleles	Position	Peptide	IC_{50}
RMNYYWTLV	HLA-DPA1*03:01(4P4R)/DPB1*04:02	240–254	QEGRMNYYWTLVEPG	509
	HLA-DRB1*04:05	238–252	RDQEGRMNYYWTLVE	614
	HLA-DPA1*01/DPB1*04:01	240–254	QEGRMNYYWTLVEPG	634
	HLA-DRB1*15:01	238–252	RDQEGRMNYYWTLVE	645
	HLA-DPA1*02:01/DPB1*01:01	239–253	DQEGRMNYYWTLVEP	766
	HLA-DRB1*04:04	238–252	RDQEGRMNYYWTLVE	919

3.4. Population Coverage of RMNYYWTLV Epitope

MHC HLA allele distribution differs among diverse geographic regions and ethnic groups around the world. Therefore, population coverage must be taken into consideration during the design of an effective vaccine. To study the population coverage of RMNYY-WTLV epitope, MHC-I- and II-binding alleles were considered. A significant population coverage was found for the selected epitope in different geographic regions of the world. This epitope and its HLA-alleles cover 90.07% of the world population. The highest population coverage was found in Mexico (99.24%) which was closely followed by Liberia, Ecuador, Ireland, Uganda, Venezuela, Nigeria, France, Finland, Brazil, Argentina, Cameroon, England, Sweden, Germany, and Saudi Arabia, with a population coverage of 98.73%, 97.59%, 97.4%, 97.33%, 96.73%, 96.5%, 96.4%, 96.35%, 96.31%, 96.29%, 95.93%, 95.53%, 95.47%, 95.34%, and 94.5%, respectively. The lowest population coverage was found in Rwanda (2.97%). The first case of A/H1N1 pdm09 was reported in Mexico in 2009. The population coverage of Mexico was 99.24%. Most of the countries in East Asia, South Asia, Southwest Asia, many Europe counties, East, West and Central African countries, North, Central and South American countries showed more than 90% of population coverage. Thus, the RMNYYWTLV epitope showed high population coverage.

3.5. 3D Structure Design of the RMNYYWTLV Epitope and its Molecular Interaction with MHC I and II

MHC class I and II alleles have a specific binding groove where the peptide binds and were presented on the cell surface for immune system activation. The RMNYYWTLV epitope structure was modeled using Pepfold-3. To check the molecular interaction of our selected epitope with their respective HLA alleles, protein–protein docking was performed using ClusPro. HLA alleles were taken as receptors and epitopes as ligands. ClusPro v.2 predicted five models for MHC I–epitope complex and three models for

Table 7 Docking results of MHC I. The ClusPro docking clusters and scores of RMNYYWTLV epitope and MHC I were tabulated.

Cluster	Members	Representative	Weighted Score
0	486	Center	–684.9
		Lowest energy	–809.9
1	203	Center	–682.0
		Lowest energy	–809.4
2	168	Center	–686.9
		Lowest energy	–769.4
3	134	Center	–679.4
		Lowest energy	–778.5
4	3	Center	–688.0
		Lowest energy	–700.5

Table 8 Docking results of MHC II. The ClusPro docking clusters and scores of RMNYYWTLV epitope and MHC II were tabulated.

Cluster	Members	Representative	Weighted Score
0	535	Center	–830.2
		Lowest energy	–947.5
1	254	Center	–830.2
		Lowest energy	–936.1
2	211	Center	–824.2
		Lowest energy	–907.1

MHC II–epitope complex with their corresponding cluster scores (**Tables 7 and 8**). Among these models, the model number 0 in both MHC I–epitope and MHC II–epitope complex were selected as a best docked complex with the lowest energy score of –809.9 with 486 members (MHC I) and lowest energy score of –947.5 with 535 members (MHC II). The ligplot of the interaction showed the hydrogen bonding and hydrophobic interactions between MHC molecules and the epitope. This signifies potential

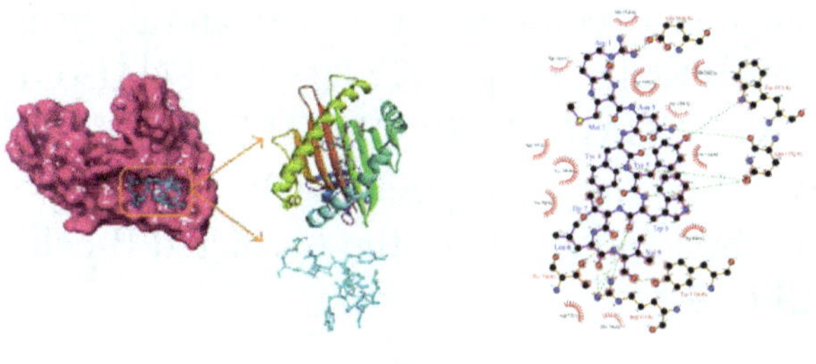

(a) (b)

Fig. 1 Docking results of MHC I: The interactions between the RMNYYWTLV epitope and MHC II showed in both (a) 3D and (b) 2D view.

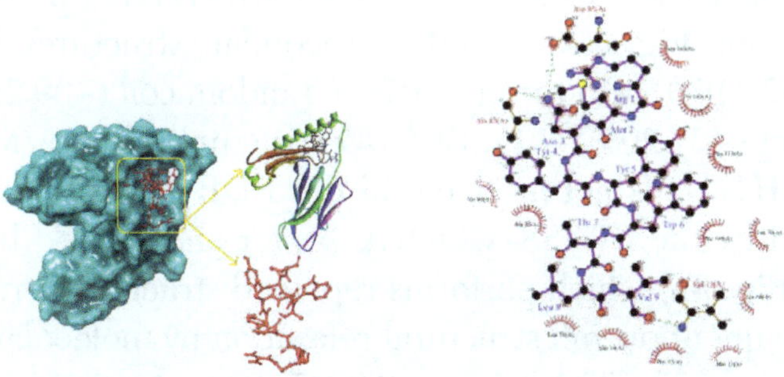

Fig. 2 Docking results of MHC II: The interactions between the RMNYYWTLV epitope and MHC II showed in both 2D and 3D view.

molecular interaction between RMNYYWTLV epitope with MHC I and MHC II proteins (**Figs. 1 and 2**). The protein-peptide docking of the HLA alleles and the epitope RMNYYWTLV showed efficient binding with high score.

3.6. Linear/continuous B-cell Epitope Prediction

B-cell epitope is a precise portion of an antigen recognized by either a specific B-cell receptor or the elicited antibody in a humoral response (Peters *et al.*, 2005; Sun *et al.*, 2013). The B-cell epitopes are divided into two main categories: continuous or linear epitope and discontinuous or conformational epitope. Linear epitopes were predicted by the web server ABC pred with a cutoff value of 0.90. A total of seven epitopes were predicted. The analysis of antigenicity, conservancy, toxicity, and allergenicity of B-cell epitopes revealed that the epitopes VPSIQSRGLFGAIAGF, LVEPGDKITFEATGNL, EGAINTSLPFQNIHPI, and ERTLDYHDSNVKNLYE could be the most potential B-cell epitope candidates. The exact position and length of the predicted B-cell epitopes are shown in **Table 9**.

3.7. Secondary and Tertiary Structure Prediction, Refinement and Validation

The 2D structures of A/Michigan/45/2015(H1N1) predicted by SOPMA tool (**Fig. 3a**) showed the secondary structures like alpha helix (~32.51%), beta turn (~7.07%), random coil (~39.22%), and beta sheet (~21.20%) (**Fig. 3b**). 3D structure of the A/Michigan/45/2015(H1N1) is not available in the PDB database. So, it was predicted by the SWISS-MODEL server and refined by Galaxy Refine (**Fig. 4a**) which performs repeated structure perturbation and subsequent overall structural relaxation by molecular dynamics simulation. The TM score is −0.9947, RMSD is 0.256, and MolProbity is 1.787 for the selected best model. Here, PROCHECK was used to check the stereochemical quality of the structure by considering residue geometry and overall structural geometry. The results showed that among the amino acid residues, 93.5% in most favored regions, 5.9% in the additional allowed region, 0.2% in the generously allowed region, and 0.4% in the disallowed region in the Ramachandran plot statistics (**Fig. 4b**). To check the potential errors of the protein 3D model, ProSA was used, and it predicts the negative Z-score of −9.17, which ensures the good quality of the model (**Fig. 4c**). All the results showed that the predicted model is good in quality.

3.8. Conformational/discontinuous B-cell Epitope Prediction

It has been found that most of the B-cell epitopes are conformational epitopes, and the amount of this epitope is more than 90%. In this chapter, a total of seven discontinuous or conformational

Table 9 Linear or continuous B-cell epitopes. The epitopes with score of more than 0.9 were selected, their antigenicity, allergenicity, toxicity, and conservancy were calculated, and the high-score epitopes were selected.

No.	Epitope	Score	Start Position	Antigenicity	Toxicity	Allergenicity	Conservancy
1	GSGIIISDTPVHDCNT	0.97	279	−0.0968	NT	NA	0.99
2	VPSIQSRGLFGAIAGF	0.95	338	0.5652	NT	NA	1
3	LVEPGDKITFEATGNL	0.93	250	0.5479	NT	NA	1
4	EGAINTSLPFQNIHPI	0.92	300	0.8671	NT	NA	1
5	GWTGMVDGWYGYHHQN	0.91	357	0.509	NT	A	1
6	ERTLDYHDSNVKNLYE	0.9	449	0.6597	NT	NA	1
7	AGFIEGGWTGMVDGWY	0.9	351	0.1004	NT	A	1

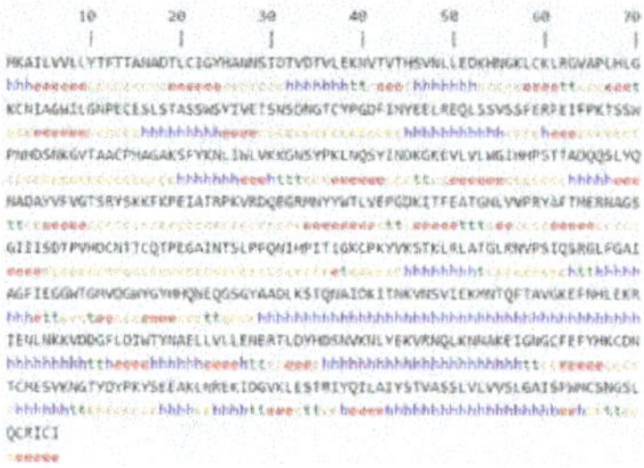

(a)

```
SOPMA :
 Alpha helix         (Hh) :   184 is  32.51%
 3₁₀ helix           (Gg) :     0 is   0.00%
 Pi helix            (Ii) :     0 is   0.00%
 Beta bridge         (Bb) :     0 is   0.00%
 Extended strand     (Ee) :   120 is  21.20%
 Beta turn           (Tt) :    40 is   7.07%
 Bend region         (Ss) :     0 is   0.00%
 Random coil         (Cc) :   222 is  39.22%
 Ambiguous states (?)     :     0 is   0.00%
 Other states             :     0 is   0.00%
```

(b)

Fig. 3 Secondary structure prediction for HA sequence of A/Michigan/45/2015(H1N1). (a) The secondary structures were mentioned in sequence. (b) The percentage of alpha helix, beta turn, random coil, and beta sheet are shown.

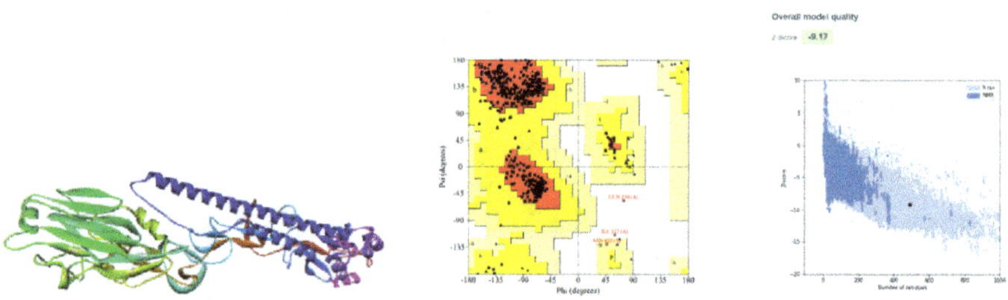

(a) (b) (c)

Fig. 4 Tertiary structure prediction for HA sequence of A/Michigan/45/2015(H1N1). (a) The 3D structure of HA protein. (b) Ramachandran plot explained the amino acids in the favored, allowed, and disallowed regions. (c) ProSA showed the quality of the model.

B-cell epitopes were predicted using the ElliPro tool of IEDB. The epitopes with a protrusion index (PI) score of above 0.8 were taken into consideration. The PI value of the seven predicted epitopes ranged from 0.813 to 0.884. The residues with higher scores indicate better solvent accessibility. The predicted model was submitted for conformational epitope prediction. Conformational epitopes and their individual residues, residue position, length, and the scores are shown in **Table 10**, whereas the positions of epitopes on 3D structures are exhibited in **Fig. 5a–g**.

Table 10 Conformational/discontinuous B-cell epitope prediction. The epitopes with PI score above 0.8 were listed along with the number of residues in each epitope.

Predicted Discontinuous Epitope(s):

No.	Residues	Number of residues	Score
1	A:Y501, A:D502, A:Y503, A:P504, A:K505, A:S507, A:E509, A:A510, A:N513, A:R514, A:K516	11	0 884
2	A:R420, A:N423, A:L424, A:K427	4	0 871
3	A:M1, A:K2, A:A3, A:14, A:L5, A:V6, A:V7, A:L8, A:L9, A:Y10, A:AT11, A:N372, A:E373, A:Q374, A:G375, A:I517, A:D518, A:G519, A:V520, A:E523, A:S524, A:T525, A:R526, A:Y534, A:T536, A:V537, A:A538, A:S540, A:L541, A:V542, A:L543, A:V544, A:V545, A:S546, A:F552, A:M554, A:C555, A:S556, A:N557, A:G558, A:S559, A:L560, A:Q561, A:C562, A:R562, A:R563, A:I564, A:C565, A:I566	49	0.87
4	A:1133, A:N179, A:Q180, A:S181, A:182, A:I183, A:N184, A:D185, A:K186, A:G187, A:K188, A:E189, A:G219, A:T220, A:S221, A:R222, A:Y223, A:E252, A:P253, A:G254, A:D255, A:K256, A:T258	23	0.851
5	A:Y108, A:P109, A:P199, A:S200, A:T201, A:T202, A:A203, A:E230, A:I231, A:A232, A:T233, A:R234, A:P235, A:K236, A:V237, A:R238, A:D239, A:Q240, A:E241, A:G242	20	0.832
6	A:F134, A:P135, A:T137, A:S138	4	0.822
7	A:V149, A:T150, A:A151, A:A152, A:C153, A:P154, A:H155, A:A156, A:G157, A:A158, A:K159, A:S160	12	0.813

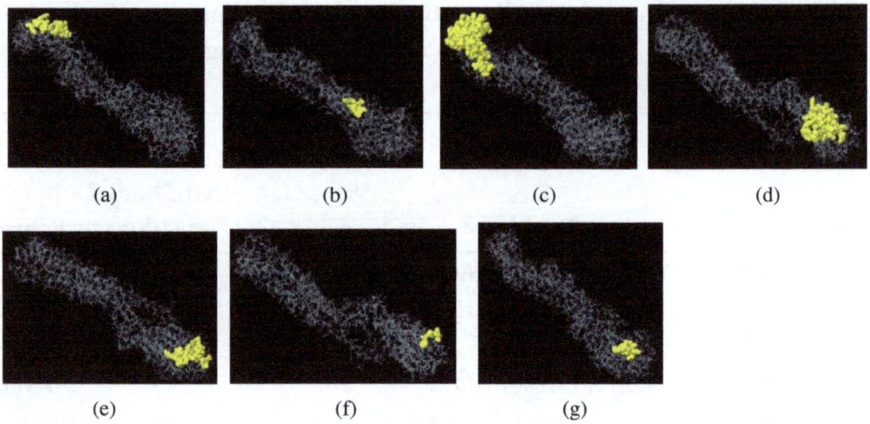

Fig. 5 (a–g) Positions of conformational epitopes in the protein structure. Each epitope was present at different positions with different number of residues.

3.9. IFN-γ-inducing Epitopes

The ability of the predicted linear B-cell and T-cell epitopes to mount IFN-γ response was assessed using the IFN epitope. The server IFN epitope predicted seven CTL epitopes, five HTL epitopes, and three B-cell epitopes (**Table 11**) as IFN-γ-inducing epitopes. These epitopes have the capability to induce Th1 type immune response accompanied by IFN-γ production. These epitopes are equally effective in immune regulatory, antiviral, and antitumor activities.

3.10. Designing of MEVC

The antigenic seven HTL and eight CTL epitopes having highest affinity for the respective HLA alleles and four B-cell epitopes that are non-allergenic, non-toxic, and can generate a potential immune response were selected for incorporation into the MEVC (**Fig. 6a**). The adjuvant β-defensin was coupled at the N-terminal by EAAAK linker with HTL epitope and subsequently, AAY (Schubert & Kohlbacher, 2016) linker was used to couple HTL epitopes and GPGPG (Nezafat *et al.*, 2014) linker was used to

Table 11 IFN-γ-inducing property of the predicted CTL, HTL, and B-cell epitopes was predicted using different algorithms. Based on the results, most of the epitopes are capable to induce IFN-γ.

Epitope	Score	Status
CTL		
NADTLCIGY	-0.24641244	Negative
RMNYYWTLV	0.026202802	Positive
YVFVGTSRY	0.26427831	Positive
FIEGGWTGM	0.26595345	Positive
LPFQNIHPI	0.77151794	Positive
YNAELLVLL	0.15240811	Positive
VSLGAISFW	0.20798546	Positive
VVSLGAISF	0.11495552	Positive
HTL		
ILAIYSTVASSLVLV	0.83953483	Positive
INTSLPFQNIHPITI	0.40168795	Positive
NQSYINDKGKEVLVL	-0.35179566	Negative
NHLEKRIENLNKKVD	-0.2887081	Negative
NGKLCKLRGVAPLHL	0.038186701	Positive
GKCPKYVKSTKLRLA	6	Positive
AELLVLLENERTLDY	0.90173735	Positive
B cell		
VPSIQSRGLFGAIAGF	0.57242885	Positive
LVEPGDKITFEATGNL	-0.14942908	Negative
EGAINTSLPFQNIHPI	0.47403865	Positive
ERTLDYHDSNVKNLYE	1	Positive

couple CTL epitopes. KK (Nezafat *et al.*, 2017) linker was used to couple B-cell epitopes. Adjuvants are the small peptides that when added along with the antigenic vaccine enhances the specific immunogenic response by influence its onset, strength, and longevity to antigens and induce protection against infection (Lee

GIINTLQKYYCRVRGGRCAVLSCLPKEEQIGKCSTRGRKCCRRKKEAAAKILAIYST
VASSLVLVAAYINTSLPFQNIHPITIAAYNQSYINDKGKEVLVLAAYNHLEKRIENLN
KKVDAAYNGKLCKLRGVAPLHLAAYGKCPKYVKSTKLRLAAAYAELLVLLENERT
LDYEAAAKILMQYIKANSKFIGIPMGLPQSIALSSMVAQEAAAKNADTLCIGYGPGP
GRMNYYWTLVGPGPGYVFVGTSRYGPGPGFIEGGWTGMGPGPGLPFQNIHPIGPG
PGYNAELLVLLGPGPGVSLGAISFWGPGPGVVSLGAISFEAAAKAKFVAAWTLKAA
AEAAAKVPSIQSRGLFGAIAGFKKLVEPGDKITFEATGNLKKEGAINTSLPFQNIHPI
KKERTLDYHDSNVKNLYEEAAAKCTGKSCHHHHHH

(a)

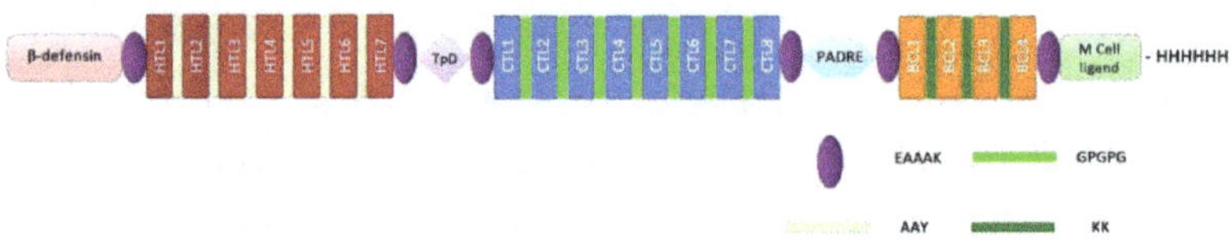

(b)

Fig. 6 Multi-epitope vaccine construct. (a) The multi-epitope vaccine construct sequence. (b) Graphical representation of multi-epitope vaccine construct contained epitopes, adjuvants, and linker molecules represented by various colors and shapes.

& Nguyen, 2015; Schijns & Lavelle, 2011). Adjuvants like universal memory T-cell helper peptide (TpD), PADRE (Pan HLA-DR reactive epitope), RS09 TLR4 agonist, and an M-cell ligand were coupled by using EAAAK linkers into the vaccine construct (**Fig. 6b**). HHHHHH was coupled at C-terminal by EAAAK linker for the easy purification of the vaccine. Both T- and B-cell epitopes in the construct will play roles in the generation of humoral and cellular-mediated memory immunity, which will lead to fast and long-lasting immune response during viral infection. The final MEVC was composed of 431 amino acid residues, which was then validated for antigenicity, allergenicity, and physiochemical properties.

3.10.1. *Physiochemical properties, antigenicity and allergenicity of MEVC*

Analysis of the physiochemical properties of a multi-subunit vaccine helps in analyzing the optimal immune response of the vaccine and its stability inside the host. The physiochemical properties were calculated by ProtParam tool (**Table 12**).

Table 12 Physiochemical properties of multi-epitope vaccine construct.

Features	Value
Number of amino acids	431
Molecular weight	46,165.7
Theoretical pI	9.5
Total number of negatively charged residues (Asp+Glu)	28
Total number of positively charged residues (Arg+Lys)	51
Total number of atoms	6,557
Instability index	27.09
Aliphatic index	90.21
Grand average of Hydropathicity (GRAVY)	-0.062

A vaccine construct must possess both immunogenicity and antigenicity to elicit the humoral and cell-mediated immune response. Upon analyzing the antigenicity of vaccine construct, the score was 0.6100 which signifies that the vaccine construct may have the potential to evoke the immune response inside the host. On allergenicity analysis, the tool AllerTOP supported the non-allergenic nature of the vaccine construct while toxicity analysis revealed the non-toxic behavior of the construct. In summary, the constructed epitope was observed to be stable, soluble, antigenic, nonallergenic, and nontoxic.

3.10.2. *Secondary and tertiary structure prediction and validation*

Secondary and tertiary structure helps in the functional annotation of the multi-epitope vaccines. It also helps in analyzing the interaction of this vaccine construct with the immunological receptors like TLRs. Secondary structure of the protein was analyzed by using SOPMA server (**Fig. 7a**) that revealed the presence of ~38.98% alpha helix, ~17.40% β-sheet, ~36.43% coils, and ~7.19% beta turns (**Fig. 7b**) in the vaccine construct.

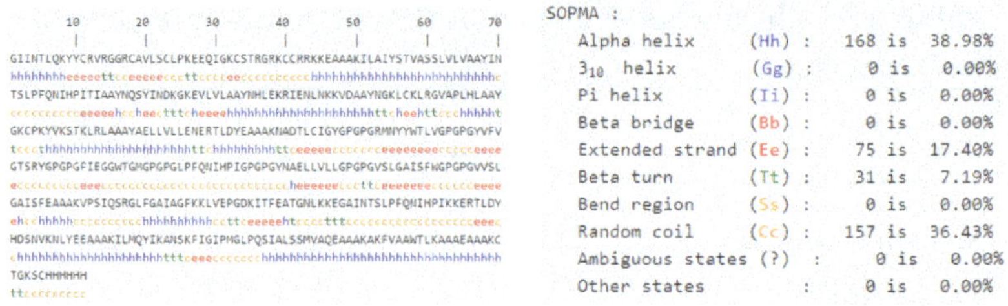

(a) (b)

Fig. 7 Secondary structure prediction of multi-epitope vaccine construct. (a) The secondary structures were mentioned in the sequence. (b) The percentage of alpha helix, beta turn, random coil, and beta sheet are shown.

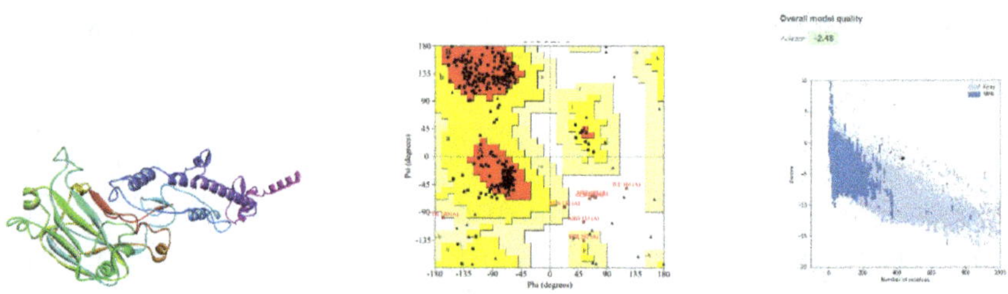

(a) (b) (c)

Fig. 8 Tertiary structure prediction of multi-epitope vaccine construct. (a) The 3D structure of HA protein. (b) Ramachandran plot explained the amino acids in the favored, allowed, and disallowed regions. (c) ProSA showed the quality of the model.

Tertiary structure of the MEVC (**Fig. 8a**) was predicted by Galaxy WEB server and refined by Galaxy Refine, which performs repeated structure perturbation and subsequent overall structural relaxation by molecular dynamics simulation. The TM score is −0.9948, RMSD is 0.245, and MolProbity is 2.196 for the selected best model. Here, PROCHECK was used to check the stereochemical quality of the structure by considering residue geometry and overall structural geometry. Ramachandran plot analysis of the modeled structure revealed the presence of 90.6% residues in the most favored regions and 8.1% in the additionally allowed regions (**Fig. 8b**). To check the potential errors of the protein 3D model, ProSA was used, and it predicts the negative Z-score of -2.48, which ensures the good quality of the model (**Fig. 8c**). All the results showed that the predicted model is good in quality.

3.10.3. *Docking of MEVC with receptors*

The 3D structures of human TLR3 and TLR4 were retrieved from protein data bank (PDB ID: 2A0Z and 3FXI). Molecular docking was performed using the ClusPro v.2 protein–protein docking server to analyze the interaction pattern of vaccine with TLR3 and TLR4. The server provides cluster scores based on rigid docking by sampling billions of conformation, pairwise RMSD energy minimization. ClusPro v.2 predicted 30 models each of vaccine receptor TLR3 complex, TLR4 complex, and HLA-A*11:01 complex with their corresponding cluster. Among these models, the model number 1 in TLR3 complex, model number 2 in TLR4 complex, and model number in HLA-A*11:01 were selected as a best docked complex with the lowest energy score of -1268.9 with 33 members, -1254.1 with 42 members, -1139.9 with 53 members for TLR3, TLR4, and HLA-A*11:01, respectively. This signifies potential molecular interaction between predicted vaccine construct with TLR3, TLR4, and HLA-A*11:01 (**Fig. 9a–c**) receptors. The molecular interaction of vaccine with TLR3, TLR4, and HLA-A*11:01 through docking analysis suggested that the constructed vaccine has a significant affinity toward the toll-like receptors to recognize molecular patterns of pathogen to initiate immune response. The significant affinity toward HLA-A*11:01

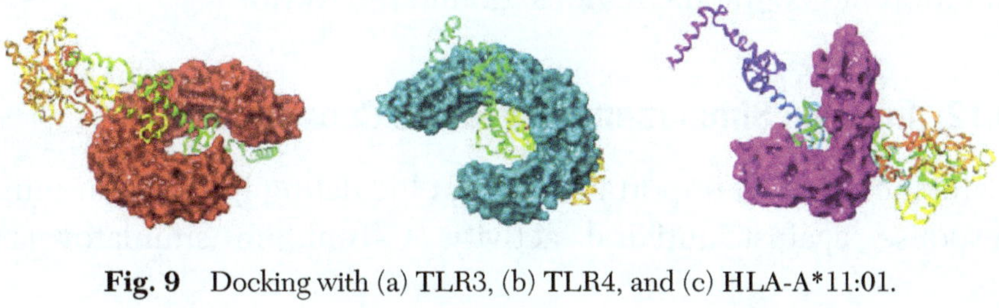

Fig. 9 Docking with (a) TLR3, (b) TLR4, and (c) HLA-A*11:01.

indicated the cell-mediated immune response. Thus, the vaccine TLR complex is capable of generating an effective innate and cell-mediated immune response against *Influenza* A/H1N1.

3.11. Population Coverage of MEVC

Population coverage gives information about the efficiency of epitopes to generate immune response in different population groups located in geographical locations across the world. This analysis is based on the distribution of HLA alleles among different population groups throughout the world (Bui *et al.*, 2006). As our vaccine construct harbors HTL epitopes for seven MHC class II and CTL epitopes for eight MHC class I alleles, the occurrence of these HLA alleles depicted the population coverage of 96.69% throughout the world. Five countries showed ≥99% population coverage, while ≥95% of population was covered in 16 countries whereas ≥90% was covered by 13 countries. The predicted epitopes can bind to MHC alleles, which show distribution throughout the world. The vaccine designed using these epitopes can provide immunity to all the population groups in the world. For determining the homology of these epitopes with human proteins BLAST analysis was done. None of the epitopes shared identity with human protein sequences eliminating the chances of these being recognized as self-epitopes. MHC I and II HLA allele specificity of T-cell epitopes should be considered as the initial criteria to induce extensive immune responses in diverse ethnic human populations (Maenaka & Jones, 1999; Stern & Wiley, 1994). The results revealed that the selected epitopes and their alleles have ideal population coverage in different geographic regions around the world.

3.12. Immune Simulations of Vaccine Construct

Cytokines play an important role in elucidating humoral immune response against antiviral activity. C-ImmSim simulator was used to analyze the immune response produced by the final vaccine construct. The tool utilizes the Celada–Seiden model for describing both humoral and cellular profiles of a mammalian immune system against designed vaccine. The tool generated the immune response simulations that match the response of a real immune system (**Fig. 10a–j**). The cumulative results of immune responses after three times antigen exposure revealed that the primary immune response against the antigenic fragments was elevated and it was indicated by gradual increase of IgM level after each antigen exposure. Similarly, the secondary response was characterized by increased with adequate generation of IgM+IgG more than IgM. An increased level of IgG1+IgG2 and IgG1 (**Fig. 10a**) was also observed. On the subsequent exposure of vaccine, a decrease in the level of antigens was observed, indicating the development of immunogenic response in the form of immune memory. The elevated level of all circulating immunoglobulins indicates the accuracy of relevant clonal proliferation of B-cell and T-cell population. Furthermore, an increase in the B-cell population (**Fig. 10b and c**) was characterized by an increase in the expression of immunoglobulins, which resulted in a decrease in the concentration of the antigen. In addition, there is a consistent rise in Th (helper) and Tc (cytotoxic) cell population with memory development (**Fig. 10d–f**). Total NK cells, dendritic cells, and macrophages were also increased (**Figure 10g–i**). It was also observed that the production of IFN-γ was stimulated after immunization (**Fig. 10j**). These results signified that the vaccine proposed in this chapter has generated a strong immune response and immunity increases even on subsequent repeated exposure. So, the analysis clearly revealed that the immunoinformatics or *in silico* approaches could make a great contribution in vaccine lead identification for experimental study and/or the design of an effective vaccine. With all these immunoinformatics approaches, the vaccine designed against *Influenza* A/H1N1 showed promising results in inducing immune response.

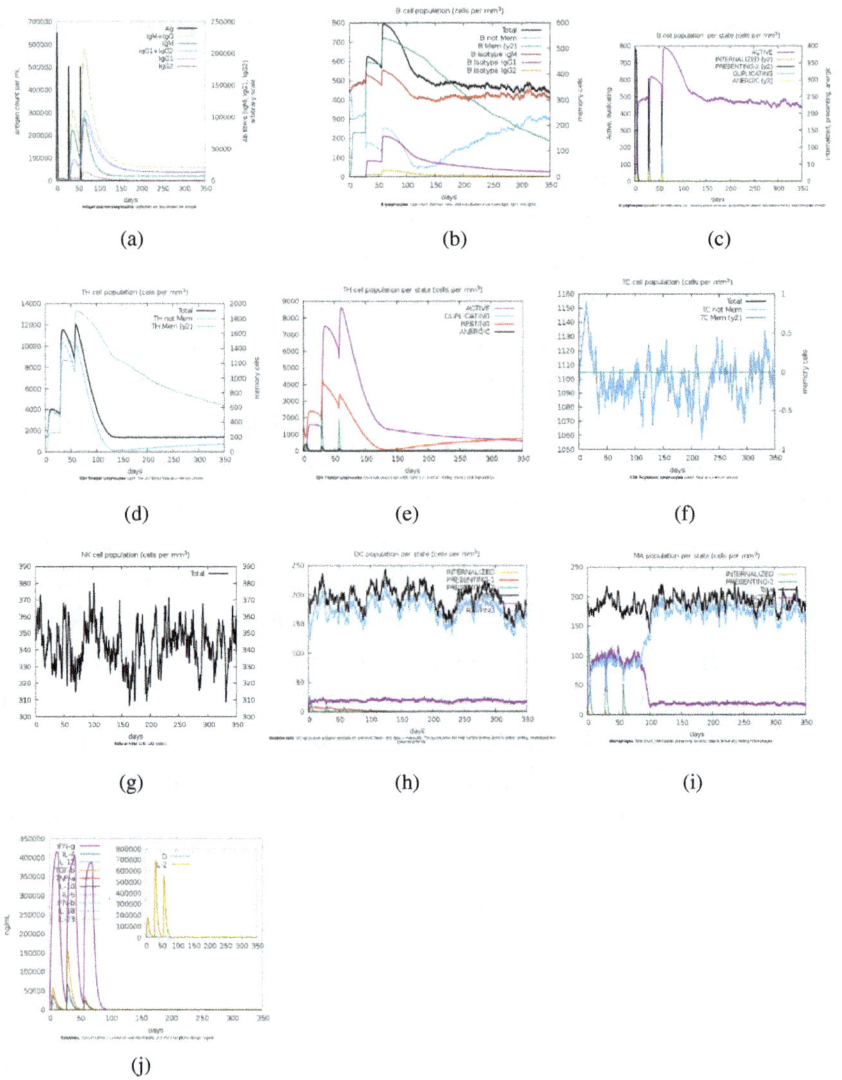

Fig. 10 (a–j) Immune simulations of vaccine construct.

4. Conclusion

Vaccine development and its application could play a key role in eliminating the virus from the human population. However, an effective vaccine progression and production are costly and can take years to be completed. So, the researchers have to try for many years to minimize the cost and time for the development of vaccines. Antigenic variation is another big challenge, which made researchers to select new strains frequently. The epitope prediction for subunit vaccine and the construction of peptide based multi-epitope vaccine are the fewer ways to address the problems. Currently, immunoinformatics tools play hence a major role in the development of vaccine by understanding the immune response of the human body against an organism within a short time. The epitope ^{243}RMNYYWTLV^{251} showed higher antigenicity, non-allergenic, non-toxic, and high conservancy. In addition to that, the detailed interaction between the generated ^{243}RMNYYWTLV^{251} epitope and the MHC II alleles and I allows a hypothetical analysis of potential therapeutic strategy for *Influenza* A/H1N1 infections. So, this epitope can be suggested for subunit vaccine preparation. In the similar way, the detailed interaction of constructed multi-epitope-based vaccine with the innate immune system receptors (TLR3 and TLR4) and cellular immune system receptor (HLA-A*11:01) also provides the idea of efficacy of the vaccine construct. The identified epitope and the vaccine construct also require proper experimental validation for a vaccine against *Influenza* A/H1N1 virus.

Acknowledgment

Gracy Fathima would like to thank Dr Siva Subramanian, Scientist, Department of Virology, King Institute of Preventive Medicine, for his guidance and support.

References

Adhikari, U. K., Tayebi, M., & Rahman, M. M. (2018). Immunoinformatics approach for epitope-based peptide vaccine design and active site prediction against polyprotein of emerging Oropouche virus. *Journal of Immunology Research*, *2018*, 20, Article ID 6718083.

Berman, H. M., Westbrook, J., Feng, Z., Gilliland, G., Bhat, T. N., Weissig, H., Shindyalov, I. N., & Bourne, P. E. (2000). The protein data bank. *Nucleic Acids Research*, *28*, 235–242.

Bui, H.-H., Sidney, J., Li, W., Fusseder, N., & Sette, A. (2007). Development of an epitope conservancy analysis tool to facilitate the design of epitope-based diagnostics and vaccines. *BMC Bioinformatics*, *8*, 361.

Calis, J. J. A., Maybeno, M., Greenbaum, J. A., *et al.* (2013). Properties of MHC class I presented peptides that enhance immunogenicity. *PLoS Computational Biology*, *9*(10), e1003266.

De Groot, A. S., & Rappuoli, R. (2004). Genome-derived vaccines. *Expert Review of Vaccines*, *3*(1), 59–76.

Dhanda, S. K., Vir, P., & Raghava, G. P. (2013). Designing of interferon-gamma inducing MHC 536 class-II binders. *Biology Direct*, *8*, 30.

Dimitrov, I., Flower, D. R., & Doytchinova, I. (2013). AllerTOP—A server for in silico prediction of allergens. *BMC bioinformatics*, *14*, S4.

Doytchinova, I. A., & Flower, D. R. (2007). VaxiJen: A server for prediction of protective antigens, tumour antigens and subunit vaccines. *BMC Bioinformatics*, *8*, 4.

Dudek, N. L., Perlmutter, P., Aguilar, M. I., Croft, N. P., & Purcell, A. W. (2010). Epitope discovery and their use in peptide based vaccines. *Current Pharmaceutical Design*, *16*(28), 3149–3157.

Gasteiger, E., Gattiker, A., Hoogland, C., Ivanyi, I., Appel, R. D., & Bairoch, A. (2003). ExPASy: The proteomics server for in-depth protein knowledge and analysis. *Nucleic Acids Research*, *31*, 3784–3788.

Geourjon, C., & Deleage, G. (1995). SOPMA: Significant improvement in protein secondary structure prediction by consensus prediction from multiple alignments. *CABIOS*, *11*, 681–684.

Gupta, S., Kapoor, P., Chaudhary, K., Gautam, A., Kumar, R., & Raghava, G. P. (2015). Peptide toxicity prediction. In *Computational peptidology* (143–157). Springer.

Heo, L., Park, H., & Seok, C. (2013). GalaxyRefine: Protein structure refinement driven by side-chain repacking. *Nucleic Acids Research*, *41*, W384–W388.

Kao, D. J., & Hodges, R. S. (2009). Advantages of a synthetic peptide immunogen over a protein immunogen in the development of an anti-pilus vaccine for *Pseudomonas aeruginosa*. *Chemical Biology & Drug Design*, *74*, 33–42.

Kozakov, D., Hall, D. R., Xia, B., Porter, K. A., Padhorny, D., Yueh, C., Beglov, D., & Vajda, S. (2017). The ClusPro web server for protein-protein docking. *Nature Protocols*, *12*(2), 255–278.

Larsen, M. V., Lundegaard, C., Lamberth, K., Buus, S., Lund, O., & Nielsen, M. (2007). Large-scale validation of methods for cytotoxic T-lymphocyte epitope prediction. *BMC Bioinformatics*, *8*(1), 424.

Larsen, M. V., Lundegaard, C., Lamberth, *et al.* (2005). An integrative approach to CTL epitope prediction: A combined algorithm integrating MHC class I binding, TAP transport efficiency, and proteasomal cleavage predictions. *European Journal of Immunology*, *35*(8), 2295–2303.

Lamiable, A., Thévenet, P., Rey, J., Vavrusa, M., Derreumaux, P., & Tufféry, P. (2016 July). PEP-FOLD3: Faster de novo structure prediction for linear peptides in solution and in complex. *Nucleic Acids Research*, *44*(W1), W449–W454.

Laskowski, R.A., MacArthur, M.W., & Thornton, J. M. (2001). PROCHECK: Validation of protein structure coordinates. In M. G. Rossmann & E. Arnold (Eds.), *International tables of crystallography, Volume F. Crystallography of biological macromolecules* (pp. 722–725). Dordrecht, The Netherlands: Kluwer Academic Publishers.

Lee, S., & Nguyen, M. T. (2015). Recent advances of vaccine adjuvants for infectious diseases. *Immune Network*, *15*(2), 51–57.

Liu, N., Wang, G., Lee, K. C., Guan, Y., Chen, H., & Cai, Z. (2009). Mutations in influenza virus replication and transcription: Detection of amino acid substitutions in hemagglutinin of an avian influenza virus (H1N1). *FASEB Journal*, *23*, 3377–3382.

Madden, D. R. (1995). The three-dimensional structure of peptide-MHC complexes. *Annual Review of Immunology*, *13*, 587–622.

Maenaka, K., & Jones, E. Y. (1999). MHC superfamily structure and the immune system. *Current Opinion in Structural Biology*, *9*(6), 745–753.

Nezafat, N., Eslami, M., Negahdaripour, M., Rahbar, M. R., & Ghasemi, Y. (2017). Designing an efficient multi-epitope oral vaccine against *Helicobacter pylori* using immunoinformatics and structural vaccinology approaches. *Molecular BioSystems*, *13*(4), 699–713.

Nezafat, N., Ghasemi, Y., Javadi, G., Khoshnoud, M. J., & Omidinia, E. (2014). A novel multi-epitope peptide vaccine against cancer: An insilico approach. *Journal of Theoretical Biology*, *349*, 121–134.

Nielsen, M., Lundegaard, C., & Lund, O. (2007). Prediction of MHC class II binding affinity using SMM-align, a novel stabilization matrix alignment method. *BMC Bioinformatics*, *8*(1), 238.

Peters, B., Sidney, J., Bourne, P., *et al.* (2005). The design and implementation of the immune epitope database and analysis resource. *Immunogenetics*, *57*(5), 326–336.

Purcell, A. W., McCluskey, J., & Rossjohn, J. (2007). More than one reason to rethink the use of peptides in vaccine design. *Nature Reviews Drug Discovery*, *6*(5), 404–414.

Rapin, N., Lund, O., Bernaschi, M., & Castiglione, F. (2010). Computational immunology meets bioinformatics: The use of prediction tools for molecular binding in the simulation of the immune system. *PLoS One*, 5, e9862.

Rapin, N., Lund, O., & Castiglione, F. (2011). Immune system simulation online. *Bioinformatics*, *27*, 2013–2014.

Rodrigo Dos Santos Francisco, R., Buhler, S., Nunes, J. M., *et al.* (2015). HLA supertype variation across populations: New insights into the role of natural selection in the evolution of HLA⊠A and HLA⊠B polymorphisms. *Immunogenetics*, *67*, 651–663.

Saha, S., & Raghava, G. P. (2006). Prediction of continuous B-cell epitopes in an antigen using recurrent neural network. *Proteins*, *65*(1), 40–48.

Sakib, M. S., Islam, M. R., Hasan, A. K. M. M., & Nabi, A. H. M. N. (2014). Prediction of epitope based peptides for the utility of vaccine development from fusion and glycoprotein of Nipah virus using in silico approach. *Advances in Bioinformatics*, *2014*, 1–17.

Sayed, S. B., Nain, Z., Khan, M. S. A., Abdulla, F., Tasmin, R., & Adhikari, U. K. (2020). Exploring Lassa virus proteome to design a multi-epitope vaccine through immunoinformatics and immune simulation analyses. *International Journal of Peptide Research and Therapeutics*, *26*, 2089–2107.

Schijns, V. E. J. C., & Lavelle, E. C. (2011). Trends in vaccine adjuvant. *Expert Review of Vaccines*, *10*(4), 539–550.

Schubert, B., & Kohlbacher, O. (2016). Designing string of beads vaccines with optimal spacers. *Genome Medicine*, *8*, 9.

Shen, Y., Maupetit, J., Derreumaux, P., & Tufféry, P. (2014). Improved PEP-FOLD approach for peptide and miniprotein structure prediction. *Journal of Chemical Theory and Computation*, *10*(10), 4745–4758.

Shin, W.-H., Lee, G. R., Heo, L., Lee, H., & Seok, C. (2014). Prediction of protein structure and interaction by GALAXY protein modeling programs. *Bio Design*, *2*, 1–11.

Stern, L. J., & Wiley, D. C. (1994). Antigenic peptide binding by class I and class II histocompatibility proteins. *Structure*, *2*(4), 245–251.

Sun, P., Ju, H., Liu, Z., *et al.* (2013). Bioinformatics resources and tools for conformational B-cell epitope prediction. *Computational and Mathematical Methods in Medicine*, *2013*, article ID 943636.

Thévenet, P., Shen, Y., Maupetit, J., Guyon, F., Derreumaux, P., & Tufféry P. (2012). PEP-FOLD: An updated de novo structure prediction server for both linear and disulfide bonded cyclic peptides. *Nucleic Acids Research*, *40*(W1), W288–W293.

Waterhouse, A., Bertoni, M., Bienert, S., Studer, G., Tauriello, G., Gumienny. R., Heer, F. T., de Beer, T. A. P., Rampfer, C., Bordoli, L., Lepore, R., & Schwede, T. (2018). SWISS-MODEL: Homology modelling of protein structures and complexes. *Nucleic Acids Research*, *46*(W1), W296–W303.

Wiederstein, M., & Sippl, M. J. (2007). ProSA-web: Interactive web service for the recognition of errors in three-dimensional structures of proteins. *Nucleic Acids Research*, *35*(Suppl. 2), W407–W410.

Zhang, Q., *et al.* (2008). Immune epitope database analysis resource (IEDB-AR). *Nucleic Acids Research*, *36*(Web Server issue), W513–W518. doi: 10.1093/nar/gkn254

https://doi.org/10.1142/9789811254796_0010

10 Identification of Potent Inhibitors from Some Medicinally Important Plants for the Treatment Against Various Types of Cancers

R. Pachaiappan[†], Vinduja Vasudevan[†],
Atanu Bhattacharjee[‡] and D. Velmurugan*[,§]

[†]*Department of Biotechnology, School of Bioengineering, SRM Institute of Science and Technology, Kattankulathur Campus, Chennai 603203, Tamil Nadu, India*
[‡]*Department of Biotechnology and Bioinformatics, North Eastern Hill University, Shillong 793022, Meghalaya, India*
[§]*Office of the Dean Sponsored Research, Publications and Collaborations, AMET University, Kanathur, ECR Road, Chennai, P.C.-603 112*

Abstract

Although there is a rapid progress in the discovery of synthetic drugs in treating various types of cancers, the impact and demand of medicinally important plants/herbs as an alternative or complementary medicine also grow globally. In earlier times cancers were given importance in developed countries alone. But at present the number of cancer patients and associated deaths is increasing in the developing countries as well. It is well known that immediate effects regarding the cure of cancer are not possible with the use of herbs. Even then these medicinally important

*Corresponding author: e-mail: shirai2011@gmail.com

plants are still being used in the developing countries due to their less cost and less side effects. This chapter deals in detail with the phyto-constituents from certain medicinally important plants being used for treating various types of cancer in India by certain herbalists. In order to explain the principles behind the control of cancers with these plants, molecular docking analysis has been performed for some of their phyto-constituents with various cancer-related targets, and the results have also been compared with the standard synthetic drug complexes for which the structures are available from the Protein Data Bank.

1. Introduction

Cancer has been known as a human malady for thousands of years, but only in the last century medical science had acknowledged what cancer is and how it spreads. It is a serious illness that has become a significant issue in both developed and developing nations. The demand for new ways to avoid the illness is rising. Various treatments for curing this disease are available, like chemotherapy and radiation. But inspite of their harmful side effects they are still being utilized due to lack of targeted, less harmful therapeutics. Plants have often served as a backbone for traditional systems of medicine, and they have supplied humankind with continuous treatments for centuries. There has lately been a surge in scientific interest in the analysis of plant-derived compounds as anticancer substances. Also, nanoparticles are now becoming progressively relevant in modern cancer treatment due to their precise targeting capabilities and improved efficacy. This review highlights various phytochemicals against cancer and the role of nanoparticles in targeted drug delivery.

Cancer is a generic term which refers to a wide range of diseases which could affect any part of the body. In all forms of cancer some of the body's cells start to multiply uncontrollably as well as spread into adjacent tissues. It is regarded as one of the leading causes of illness and death in millions around the world, and because of its severity, there is unquestionably an unfulfilled necessity to develop new anticancer drugs (Rayan *et al.*, 2017).

Cancer is the second leading cause of death globally, and despite the advances in drug development, developing new plant-based medicines is still needed. In 2018, the World Health Organization recorded 9.6 million deaths worldwide (WHO, 2018). Mummies from ancient Egypt were found with bone cancer around 1600 BC and breast cancer around 1500 BC. Between 1950 and 1980, on an average, two new drugs were approved for their anticancer activities per year. In the years between 2011 and 2019, an average of 10 novel oncologic drugs hit the market (Kinch, 2014). The reason behind the low numbers is that it takes nearly 13–15 years for the validation of drugs in the preclinical and clinical phases. Out of the latest drug approved by the Food and Drug Administration (FDA), USA, in the last decade, nearly 89% of the drugs in the last three decades for the cancer treatment are either natural products or their derivatives. In the last decade more than 50 small molecules that have antitumor agents have been approved by the FDA (Sharifi-Rad *et al.*, 2019). Traditional plant species have been used in East Asia to cure a variety of illnesses including cancer, since earlier times. Due to their various anti-proliferative and pro-apoptotic features, natural antioxidants as well as several phytochemicals have lately been proposed as anticancer adjuvant therapies (Chikara *et al.*, 2018).

Biochemical and pharmacological mechanisms involved in the plant compounds are mostly lacking due to which the plant-based medicine to treat cancer was underestimated. There are several plant-derived anticancer compounds like vinblastine, taxol, camptothecin, elliptimaum, homoharringtonine, and so on which have been successfully used as anticancer drugs in various clinical studies. National Cancer Institute has approximately screened 35,000 plant species for their potential anticancer activities and 3000 plant species among them have shown reproducible anticancer activity (Desai *et al.*, 2008; Roy *et al.*, 2017).

One of the main strategies is to build drug delivery mechanisms which are more targeted toward cancer cells, in addition to producing novel therapeutics with a higher safety profile and lower toxic effects. The primary goal of choosing natural products to fight cancer depends on an effective drug carrier. Luckily, the introduction of nanotechnology for targeted drug delivery has accelerated this field in recent times (Ashraf, 2020). Nanotechnology provides a unique chance to establish new diagnosis and therapeutic techniques that can improve the cancer patient's longevity (Zhu & Liao, 2015). Nanoparticles or nanomedicines aim to enhance the anticancer activities of plant-derived drugs by controlling the release of the compounds. The review presented here deals with the impact of naturally derived compounds from medicinal plants which bind at the active sites of cancer related macromolecular targets.

2. Types of Cancer

Based on the tissue or origin, cancers are mainly categorized into five different types: carcinoma, sarcoma, leukemia, lymphoma, and myeloma. Leukemia is a form of cancer that affects the bone marrow that is responsible for the production of blood cells. Lymphoma and myeloma are immune system cancers.

2.1. Carcinoma

Carcinoma is a form of cancer which originates in the skin or the tissues that surround other organs. Carcinoma is of various types including basal cell carcinoma (BCC), squamous cell carcinoma (SCC), renal cell carcinoma (RCC), ductal carcinoma in situ (DCIS), and adenocarcinoma.

BCC is a malignant epidermal skin tumor that grows slowly and is locally invasive (Braun *et al.*, 2005; Cigna *et al.*, 2011). Metastasis is highly unusual. However morbidity is caused by local tissue invasion as well as destruction, especially on the face, head, and neck (Ting *et al.*, 2005). Sun exposure is the most dangerous risk factor as UVB radiation induces direct disruption of DNA and RNA by triggering formation of cyclopyrimidine dimers (TT) as well as pyrimidine–pyrimidine adducts (Kyrgidis *et al.*, 2010). A mutation in the repair protein genes is implicated in a number of disorders defined by the proliferation of BCC. One of these syndromes is Gorlin–Goltz syndrome, which is caused by a mutation in the patched gene (PTCH) resulting in the loss of heterozygosity (Hooper & Scott, 2005; Lear *et al.*, 2000).

SCC is an epithelial cancer that develops in organs that are usually lined by squamous epithelium that comprises the urinary tract, skin, lungs, mouth, esophagus, lips, prostate, vagina, and cervix. Non-melanoma skin cancer, head and neck cancer, esophageal cancer, and non-small cell lung cancer are the four anatomic sites that constitute the majority of SCC occurrences. Tobacco use as well as HPV infection also considered to be carcinogenic factors for these four subtypes (Yan *et al.*, 2011). Genetic alterations are usually oncogene activation, consisting of recessive oncogenes as well as loss of heterozygosity, tumor suppressor gene inactivation via mutations, deletions, and mechanisms like methylation and gene expression by miRNA modulation (Fearon & Vogelstein, 1990; Minna *et al.*, 2002).

RCC is a form of cancer that develops from renal epithelium. While somatic VHL mutations were known for some time, latest cancer genome studies have observed mutations in epigenetic regulatory genes and revealed significant intra-tumor heterogeneity, which may have prognostic, predictive, and therapeutic implications (Hsieh *et al.*, 2017).

DCIS corresponds to cancerous breast epithelial cells which remain in their natural location in the ducts and lobules. DCIS is a non-lethal form of cancer since it remains in its natural location. DCIS, on the other hand, is critical because it is the immediate precursor to invasive breast cancers that could be fatal (Allred, 2010). BRCA1 and BRCA2 mutation carriers acquire DCIS more often and even at a younger age than the general population

(Hwang *et al.*, 2007; Mazzola *et al.*, 2013), and are considerably more prone to have occult DCIS in preventative mastectomies than age-matched non-carriers in autopsy studies (Gorringe & Fox, 2017; Kauff *et al.*, 2003).

Adenocarcinomas are malignant tumors that develop from glandular structures in epithelial tissue. It is most often found in the breast, lung, prostate, and gastrointestinal tract, including the colon, rectum, pancreas, stomach, and esophagus (Mullangi & Lekkala, 2020). The risk factors of lung adenocarcinoma include radiation exposure, environmental pollutants such as arsenic, chromium, and nickel, and genetic factors (Alberg & Samet, 2003; Hubbard *et al.*, 2000). Breast adenocarcinoma risk is increased by genetic factors such as mutations in the BRCA1/2, PTEN, p53, PALB2, and others, as well as family history (Lu *et al.*, 2019). Age is the most significant risk factor for prostate adenocarcinoma. Patients suffering with prostate cancer before the age of 40 are extremely rare (Delongchamps *et al.*, 2006). Cigarette smoking, a family medical history of prostate cancer, and germline mutations such as BRCA2/1 and ATM are also risk factors (Nicolosi *et al.*, 2019). Colorectal adenocarcinoma risk is increased by environmental and genetic factors. Many familial colorectal cancer syndromes, such as familial adenomatous polyposis and Lynch syndrome, as well as non-Lynch syndromes such as biallelic MUTYH, PALB2, BRCA1/2, CDKN2A, FAP and TP53, raise the risk of colorectal cancer (Burt *et al.*, 1995; Yurgelun *et al.*, 2017).

2.2. Sarcoma

Sarcoma is a form of cancer that affects connective tissues including bones, muscles, cartilage, and blood vessels. Although the majority of sarcomas develop on their own, several risk factors have been reported. Ionizing radiation exposure raises the risk of sarcomas for more than 7–10 years following exposure, most often in patients receiving radiation therapy for breast and cervical cancers, and also lymphoma. Patients who received ionizing radiation for cancer developed osteosarcoma as well as STS, including angiosarcoma.

Other risks include chronic lymphedema, that raises the occurrence of STS, soft tissue sarcoma, (particularly angiosarcoma), and exposure to chemicals (e.g., vinyl chloride, which raises the likelihood of hepatic angiosarcoma). Sarcoma emergence is also linked to certain genetic syndromes. Neurofibromatosis type 1 (NF1) is an autosomal dominant disorder resulting from mutations in the NF1 gene, which encode for protein neurofibromin. Patients with NF1 have a higher prevalence of benign schwannomas and neurofibromas, and also a higher likelihood of acquiring malignant neurofibrosarcomas and schwannomas. A number of other genetic disorders have been linked to an increased risk of sarcomas, like Li–Fraumeni syndrome that occurs when mutations in the TP53 gene intervenes its tumor suppressor role (Skubitz & D'Adamo, 2007).

2.3. Leukemia

Leukemia is characterized by the clonal multiplication of hematopoietic stem cells in the bone marrow. Acute lymphoblastic, acute myelogenous, chronic lymphocytic, and chronic myelogenous are the four diverse subtypes most often observed by general practitioners. Several genetic disorders, like Down syndrome and neurofibromatosis, are linked to an elevated risk of childhood acute lymphoblastic and acute myelogenous leukemia. People who have been exposed to ionizing radiation, as well as cancer patients who are undergoing radiation therapy, are at a higher risk of acquiring acute lymphoblastic leukemia (ALL), acute myelogenous leukemia, and chronic myelogenous leukemia. Pesticide exposure at home, during pregnancy, and the first three years of life has been linked to a higher threat of childhood ALL (Davis *et al.*, 2014).

2.4. Lymphoma

Lymphomas are a diverse class of tumors that grow in the reticulo-endothelial as well as lymphatic systems. Hodgkin lymphoma and non-Hodgkin lymphoma are the two most common forms.

Among the most common lymphomas is Hodgkin lymphoma (HL), a B cell–derived cancer. In Hodgkin and Reed–Sternberg (HL), tumor cells — Hodgkin and Reed–Sternberg (HRS) cells — are generally quite rare in the tissue. While HRS cells are formed from mature B cells, they lack much of their B cell phenotype and exhibit very abnormal co-expression of markers from different hematopoietic cell types. The induction of several signaling pathways as well as transcription factors in HRS cells is dysregulated. These pathways and factors are activated in part by associations of HRS cells with various other types of cells in the micro-environment, as well as by genetic lesions. Although the transformative processes underlying the pathogenesis of HL are only partially known, mutations impacting the NF-B and JAK/STAT pathways are common. HRS cells' reliance on micro-environmental interactions and deregulated signaling pathways can open up new avenues for targeted treatments (Küppers *et al.*, 2012).

Non-Hodgkin lymphomas are a diverse type of cancer, with B lymphocytes accounting for 85%–90% of cases and T or NK lymphocytes accounting for the rest. This broad array of malignancies typically develops in lymph nodes, but can also arise almost in any tissue, and varies from follicular lymphoma to the aggressive diffuse large B-cell and also Burkitt's lymphomas. Non-Hodgkin lymphomas lacking IgV (variable immunoglobulin) mutations are non-Hodgkin lymphomas derived from the pre-germinal core (e.g., most cases of mantle cell lymphoma). Follicular lymphoma, Burkitt's lymphoma, mucosa-associated lymphoid tissue lymphoma, lymphoplasmacytic lymphoma, and diffuse massive B-cell lymphoma are all non-Hodgkin lymphomas with IgV mutations which originate from germinal center or post germinal-center B cells (Küppers & Rajewsky, 2010; Shankland *et al.*, 2012).

2.5. Myeloma

Multiple myeloma is described by unrestricted multiplication of monoclonal plasma cells in bone marrow, which results in the formation of nonfunctional unchanged immunoglobulins or immunoglobulin chains. Obesity and chronic illness, along with ionizing radiation, pesticides, as well as benzol, have been reported as risk factors for multiple myeloma. A detailed history and physical examination, as well as numerous lab examinations, such as study of a 24-hour urine sample, a bone-marrow biopsy, and skeletal radiography, are used to diagnose multiple myeloma. After organ damage has been diagnosed systemic therapy should be used (Gerecke *et al.*, 2016).

3. Role of Nanoparticles Against Cancer

Nanoparticles are smaller than 100 nm in at least one dimension. They can be anywhere between 1 and 100 nm in size. This size spectrum of nanoparticles has been engineered for drug development as well as delivery (Edis *et al.*, 2021; Mattheolabakis *et al.*, 2012; Zhu & Liao, 2015). In 1995, the FDA certified the first nano-drug, liposomal doxorubicin (Doxil), for the therapy of AIDS-related Kaposi's sarcoma in AIDS patients whose disease had advanced on past combination chemotherapy or in patients who were resistant to such treatment. Doxil has a long drug circulation period and a stable and high doxorubicin loading. Doxil is introduced to cancer by passive targeting, and doxorubicin is delivered and made accessible to tumor cells through unknown mechanisms. Following bortezomib, it is also now approved for ovarian cancer and also multiple myeloma (Barenholz, 2012; Prescott, 1995). Myocet is a non-pegylated liposomal doxorubicin that is used in conjunction with cyclophosphamide to combat metastatic breast cancer in Canada and Europe. Its design principles are close to that of Doxil. Since the myocet liposome does not provide a polyethylene glycol layer like Doxil, it doesn't cause Hand Foot Syndrome, which is a rate-limiting toxicity for other doxorubicin liposomal formulations (Batist, 2001). The FDA licensed DaunoXome®, a non-pegylated liposomal daunorubicin, for the first-line management of advanced AIDS-related Kaposi's sarcoma (Rivera, 2003).

In 2012, the FDA approved Marqibo (vincristine sulfate liposome injection) for the treatment of Philadelphia chromosome negative (Ph^-) ALL (Bedikian *et al.*, 2011). When nanoparticles adhere to unique receptors and enter the cell, they are normally enveloped by endosomes through receptor-mediated endocytosis, circumventing P-glycoprotein recognition, which is one of the most common drug resistance pathways (Cho *et al.*, 2008).

For anticancer medicines to be successful in cancer treatment, they must first be capable of penetrating barriers within body and enter the target tumor tissues with limited loss of volume or function in blood circulation following administration. Then, with a regulated release process of the active form, drugs should be able to exclusively destroy tumor cells without harming normal cells once they enter the tumor tissue. By increasing the intracellular dosage of drugs while subsequently lowering dose-limiting toxicities, these two essential techniques have been correlated to significant improvement in patient survival as well as quality of life. Nanoparticles are rapidly emerging to have the ability to meet each of these criteria for successful drug delivery systems (Cho *et al.*, 2008).

4. Anticancer Compounds from Plants

Actein is the main compound of the plant *Actaea racemosa* belonging to the family Ranunculaceae. This compound shows the inhibition of human — HepG2 — liver cancer cell growth (Einbond *et al.*, 2009). Compounds ardisiacrispin A, B from *Ardisia crenata* belonging to Myrsinaceae family are reported to inhibit the uncontrolled proliferation of liver cancer cell line (Li *et al.*, 2008). Stigmasterol extracted from *Bacopa monnieri* has been discovered to have anticancer properties by stimulating apoptosis via the activation protein phosphatase 2A (Ghosh *et al.*, 2011; Roy *et al.*, 2017). Vinblastine and vincristine, which are extracted from the Apocynaceae family's *Catharanthus roseus*, have been used to cure a variety of cancers, including leukemias, lymphomas, advanced testicular cancer, breast cancer, and lung cancer (Ashraf, 2020; Buyel, 2018; Chando *et al.*, 2019; Cragg & Newman 2005).

The medicinal plants like Citrus, *Cynodon dactylon*, *galangal*, *Piper longum*, *Picrorhiza kurroa*, *Plumbago zeylanica*, *Punica granatum*, *Tinospora cordifolia*, *Thymus vulgaris*, and *Zanthoxylum nitidum* are reported for treatment against various types of cancers (Roy *et al.*, 2017). Anticancer activity of novel plant extracts and compounds from *Adenosma bracteosum* in human lung and liver cancer cells have been elaborately discussed by Nguyen *et al.* (2020). The detailed anticancer activities of certain medicinal plants such as *Aloe barbadensis*, *Azadirachta indica*, *Glycericia glabra*, *Curcuma longa*, *Hypericum perforatum*, *Acacia nilotica*, *Vachellia nilotica*, *Acacia catechue*, *Senegalia catechue*, *Camellia sinensis*, and *Vitis vinifera* were reported by Padmaharish and Lakshmi (2017). Berberin, the main constituent of *Coptis chinensis* has been used in the treatment of oral cancer cells (Lin *et al.*, 1999).

There are many traditional herbalists throughout the North Eastern Region of India as the allopathy medicine practitioners are less in number, mostly in villages. Suhitha *et al.* (2015) eviewed some herbs and their phyto-constituents that are being used by some herbalists for curing various ailments. In the state of Meghalaya in India there are two well-known herbalists, and their speciality is in treating cancer patients. One herbalist uses two types of formulations from a mixture of herbs and the other one uses a rhizome locally called as Jabung (*Stephania hernandifolia*). The two formulations have been thoroughly analyzed using tools like GC-MS, HPLC and LC-MS/MS. Cell line studies and *in silico* molecular modeling studies have also been carried out by this group (Mohan *et al.*, 2018a). Two major compounds, namely, ethyl-p-methoxycinnamate and pinostrobin chalcone, have been identified from the two formulations. IC50 (μg/mL) values of these two compounds for HCT-116 cell line are 30 and 33 and that for MCF-7 cell lines are 43 and 46, respectively. Literature study showed that these compounds interfere in the TNF-alpha

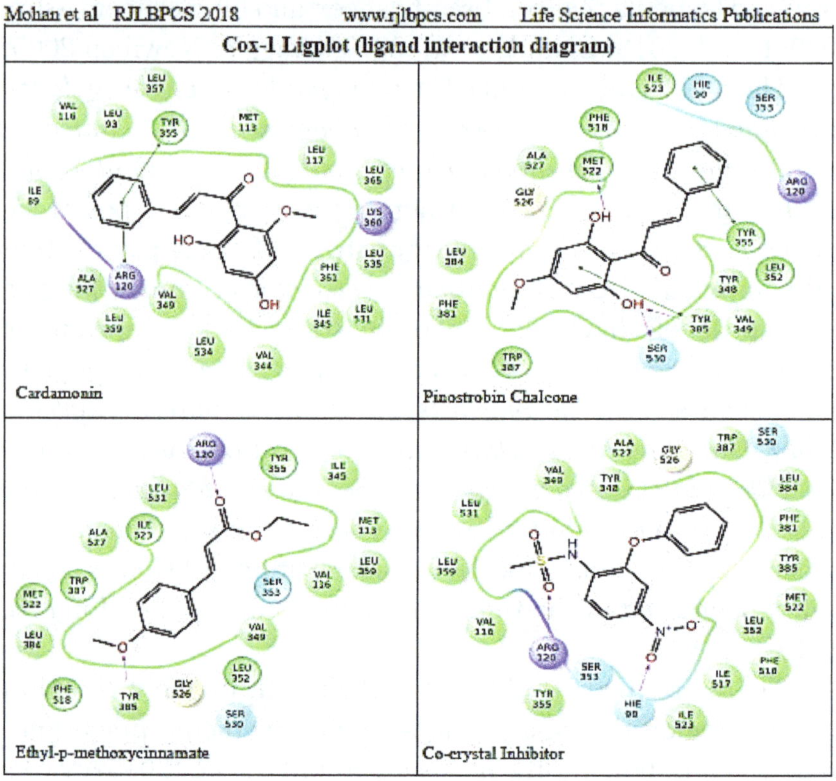

Fig. 1 The ligand interaction diagram of COX-1 (PDB ID: 3N8X) with plant secondary metabolite(s) by ligplot.

and NF-κB pathways, respectively. Modeling studies have been carried out for these compounds with COX-1 and COX-2 as the targets, and the corresponding ligplots are shown in Figs. 1 and 2, and the results are displayed in Table 1. Mohan *et al.* (2018b) discovered a novel anticancer compound isolated from the rhizome Jabung. The three-dimensional molecular structure of the compound dl-tetrahydropalmatine (THP) has been determined by single crystal X-ray diffraction method (Suhitha *et al.*, 2015). Cell line studies of THP showed anticancer activities against colorectal, lung, and breast cancers. Its hydroxyl analog, Stepholidine was reported for its anticancer activity (Mohan *et al.*, 2018c). The

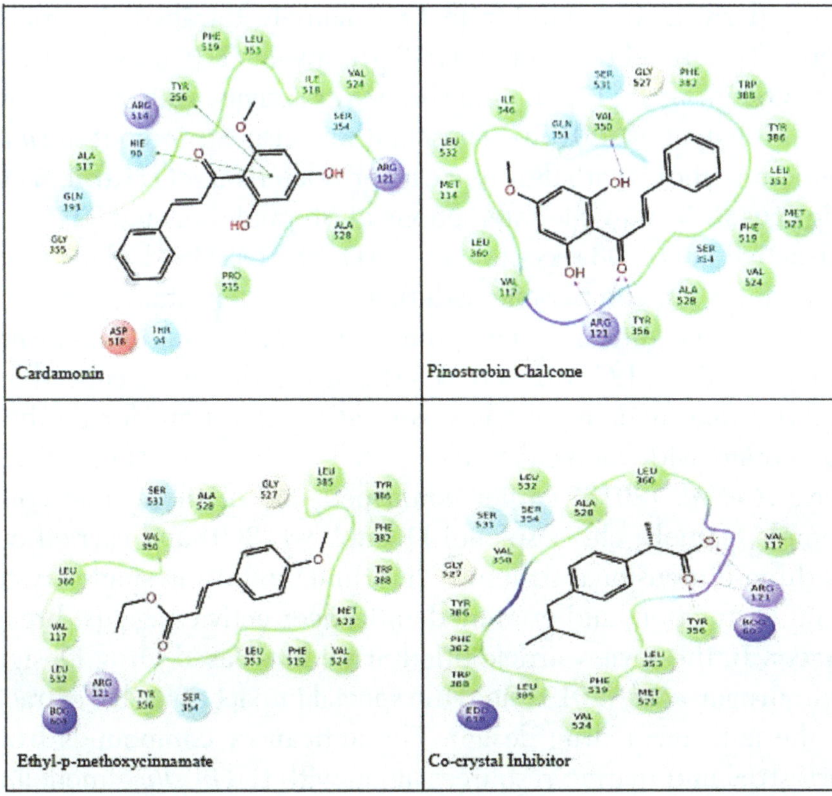

Fig. 2 The ligand interaction diagram of COX-2 (PDB ID: 4PH9) with plant secondary metabolite (s) by ligplot.

Table 1 ***In silico*** **modelling study with COX-1 and COX-2 targets.**

	COX-1 (PDB ID: 3N8X)		COX-2 (PDB ID: 4PH9)	
Sample Description	**Docking Score (kcal/mole)**	**Glide Energy (kcal/mole)**	**Docking Score (kcal/mole)**	**Glide Energy (kcal/mole)**
Cardamonin	-9	-41.01	-7.41	-43.32
Pinostrobin chalcone	-10.48	-44.75	-10.01	-47.03
Ethyl-p-methoxy cinnamate	-6.98	-37.04	-7.74	-36.61
Co-crystal	-7.68	-37.04	-8.63	-36.35

newly derived compound from THP, namely, tetrahydroprotoberberine (where all the four –OCH3 groups in THP are substituted for –OH groups) (THPB) showed better activity against lung cancer (Mohan *et al.*, 2018b). These authors also carried out *in silico* modeling studies with different cancer-related targets (**Table 2–4**). **Figures 3–5** show the interactions of Stepholidine and THPB at the active site of D3 receptor (PDB ID: 3PBL). The docking score and energy are comparable with that of the co-crystal.

The nine anticancer compounds from *Sphaeranthus amaranthoides*. HPLC, LC-MS, and LC-MS/MS studies were carried out and *in silico* modeling studies were also carried out for the best compound with molecular mass 516 Da (Mohan *et al.*, 2018c). Gayatri *et al.* (2016) earlier confirmed one of these nine compounds, namely, chrysosplenol D (mol. wt. 360) and carried out its three-dimensional structure determination using single crystal X-ray diffraction, and examined anticancer activity against breast cancer. In the review article titled Structure-Based Drug Design, Velmurugan *et al.* (2019) cited the special impact of herbal extracts in the anticancer drug design. The anticancer compounds from terrestrial and marine resources along with the *in silico* modeling studies carried out by Velmurugan *et al.* (2020). The anticancer properties and enhancement of therapeutic potential of cisplatin by the leaf extract of *Zanthoxylum armatum* DC (ZALE) reported by Singh *et al.* (2015). In prostrate, cervical, as well as osteosarcoma cancer cell lines, ZALE had a synergistic interaction with cisplatin. The GC-MS and *in silico* modeling studies of compounds isolated from *Scoparia dulcis* (Linn) extract confirmed the binding affinity of some of its compounds with Estrogen alpha and beta which occur in the cancer pathways (Wangsa *et al.*, 2020). The chromatic fractionation and *in silico* validation of bioactive compounds from *Cynoglossum zeylanicum* (Lehm) for binding affinity with human estrogen and progesterone that are the targets in the cancer pathways (Gowala *et al.*, 2020).

Table 2 Results of induced fit docking studies of ligand interaction of selected plant secondary metabolite(s) with the breast cancer target protein (PDB ID: 5NZP).

Ligand	Docking Score (kcal/mole)	Glide Energy (kcal/mole)	Interaction	Distance (Å)	Hydrophobic Interaction
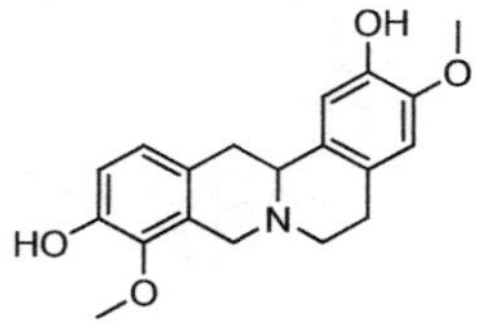 Stepholidine	−6.724	−38.241	—	—	Leu151, Tyr174, Pro176, Leu193, Trp197, Pro208, Leu210, and Leu216
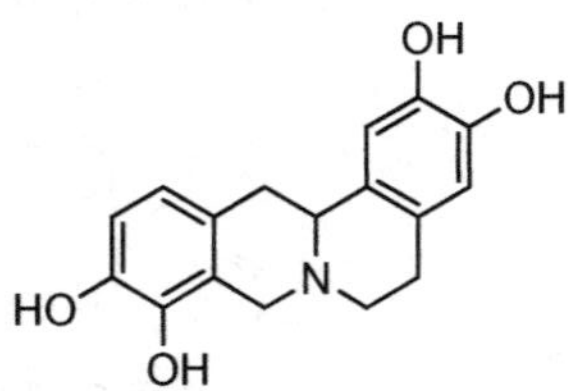 Tetrahydroprotoberberine (MW: 299 Da)	−6.824	−41.946	(O–H…O)Asp175 Ser212(O–H…O) (O–H…O)Ser212	3.06 2.94 2.98	Leu151, Leu153, Tyr174, Pro176, Ile177, Leu193, Pro208, Leu210, and Leu216
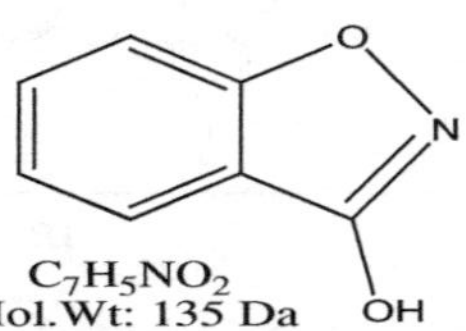 $C_7H_5NO_2$ Mol.Wt: 135 Da benzo[*d*]isoxazol-3-ol Native	−6.256	−26.262	Asp175(O–H…O)	3.15	Leu151, Leu153, Tyr174, Pro176, Ile177, Pro208, Leu210, and Leu216

Table 3 Results of induced fit docking studies of ligand interaction of selected plant secondary metabolite(s) with the σ1 receptor (PDB ID: 6DK0).

Ligand	Docking Score (kcal/mole)	Glide Energy (kcal/mole)	Interaction	Distance (Å)	Hydrophobic Interaction
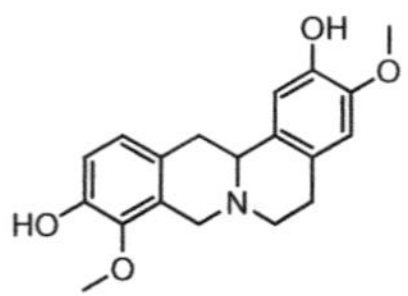 Stepholidine	−8.811	−54.819	(O–H…O) Tyr120 (O–H…O) Gln135	3.04 3.18	Val84, Trp89, Met93, Leu105, Phe107, Tyr120, Ile124, Phe133, Val152, Val153, Val162, Trp164, Met170, Phe184, and Ala185
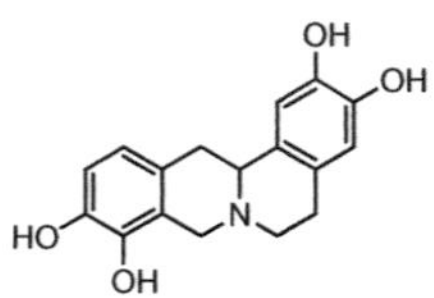 Tetrahydroprotoberberine (MW: 299 Da)	−7.069	−49.288	(O–H…O) Asp126 (O–H…O) Thr181	3.04 2.94	Val84, Trp89, Tyr103, Phe107, Tyr120, Ile124, Phe133, Val152, Val162, Trp164, Met170, Leu182, and Ala185
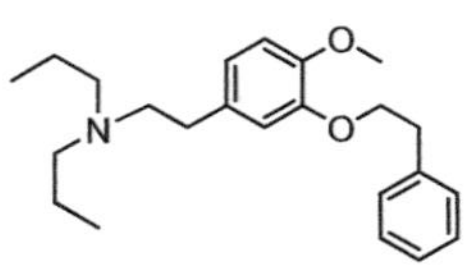 N-(4-methoxy-3-(phenethyloxy) phenethyl)-N-propylpropan-1-amine Native	−7.834	−55.524	Tyr89(O–H…O) Tyr120(O–H…O)	3.05 3.01	Val84, Ala86, Trp89, Met93, Leu95, Tyr103, Leu105, Phe107, Ile124, Ile128, Phe133, Val152, Val153, Val162, Trp164, Met170, Leu182, Phe184, and Ala185

Table 4 Results of induced fit docking studies of ligand interaction of selected plant secondary metabolite(s) with D3 receptor (PDB ID: 3PBL).

Ligand	Docking Score (kcal/mole)	Glide Energy (kcal/mole)	Interaction	Distance (Å)	Hydrophobic Interaction
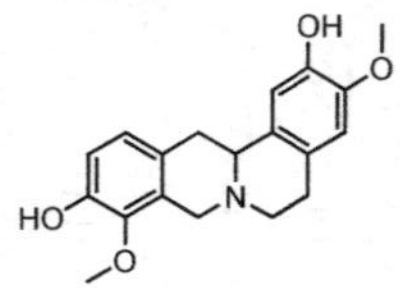 Stepholidine	−7.436	−49.094	Tyr36(O–H...O) (O–H...O)Glu90 (O–H...O) Asp110	3.05 2.89 3.12	Val86, Leu89, Phe106, Val107, Val111, Cys181, Ile183, Phe345, Tyr365, and Tyr373
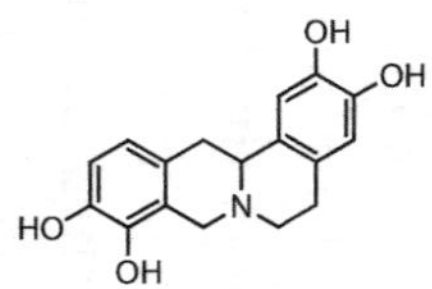 Tetrahydroprotoberberine (MW: 299 Da)	−8.636	−52.840	(O–H...O)Cys181 (O–H...O)Ser192 (O–H...O)Ser192 (O–H...O)Tyr365	3.02 2.94 2.98 3.18	Leu89, Phe106, Val107, Val111, Ile183, Phe188, Val189, Phe345, Phe346, and Val350
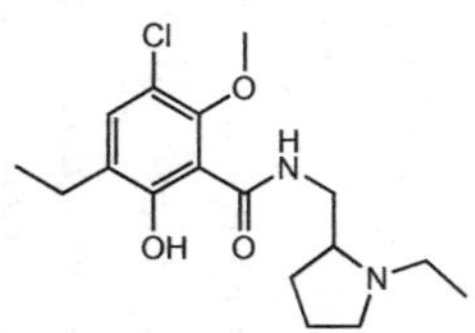 3-Chloro-5-ethyl-N-((1-ethylpyrrolidin-2-yl)methyl)-6-hydroxy-2-methoxybenzamide Native	−7.876	−51.950	(O–H...O) Asp110 (N–H...O) Asp110 His349(O–H...O)	3.15 3.06 2.97	Leu89, Phe106, Val107, Val111, Cys114, Cys181, Ile183, Phe188, Val189, Trp342, Phe345, Phe346, Tyr365, and Tyr373

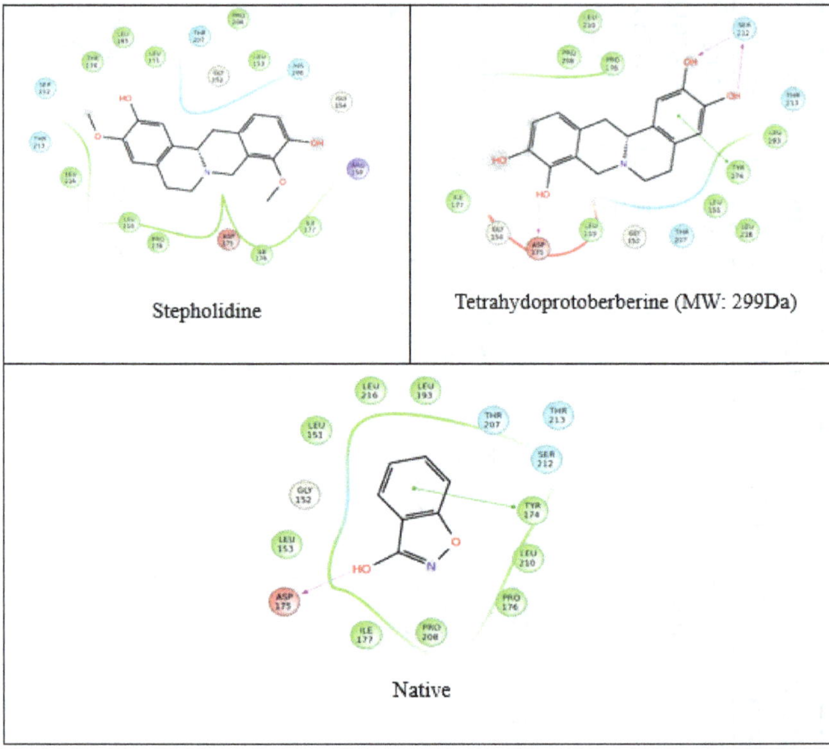

Fig. 3 Induced fit docking studies of ligand interaction of the selected plant secondary metabolite(s) with the breast cancer target protein (PDB ID: 5NZP) by ligplot.

The role of the compound Paclitaxel (Taxol) from *Taxus brevifolia* is well known. It disrupts microtubules, impedes mitosis, as well as induces apoptosis. Microtubules are polymerized and stabilized by paclitaxel. This compound is used to treat non-small lung cancer, breast cancer, ovarian cancer, and Kaposi sarcoma (Che *et al*., 2015; Cragg & Newman, 2005; Jordan & Wilson, 2004). Epipodophyllotoxin from *Podophyllum peltatum* species is used for treating lymphomas and testicular cancer (Solowey *et al*., 2014). Etoposide and teniposide, the two semi-synthetic derivatives of epipodophyllotoxin from *P. peltatum*, were used in the treatment of lymphomas, bronchial and testicular cancers (Cragg & Newman, 2005). Epigallocatechin-3-gallate from green tea

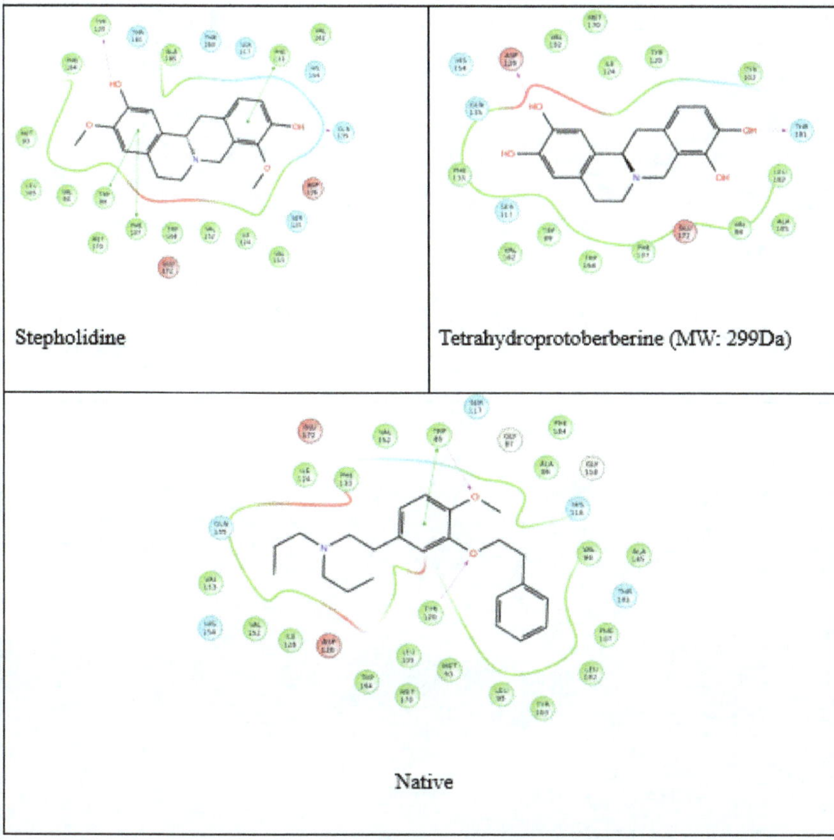

Fig. 4 Induced fit docking studies of ligand interaction of the selected plant secondary metabolite(s) with the σ1 receptor (PDB ID: 6DK0) by ligplot.

has been in clinical trials in prostate cancer treatment (Raza & John, 2005). For treating lymphomas and leukemias, flavopiridol from *Dysoxylum binectariferum* was reported to be very effective (Newcomb *et al.*, 2004). Camptothecin isolated from the Chinese ornamental tree *Camptotheca acuminate* was advanced to clinical trials by National Cancer Institute in 1970s itself but it was dropped due to its severe bladder toxicity. Later, topotecan and irinotecan, the semi-synthetic derivatives were used for the treatment of ovarian and small cell lung cancers, respectively (Creemers *et al.*, 1996). Homoharringtonine isolated from the Chinese

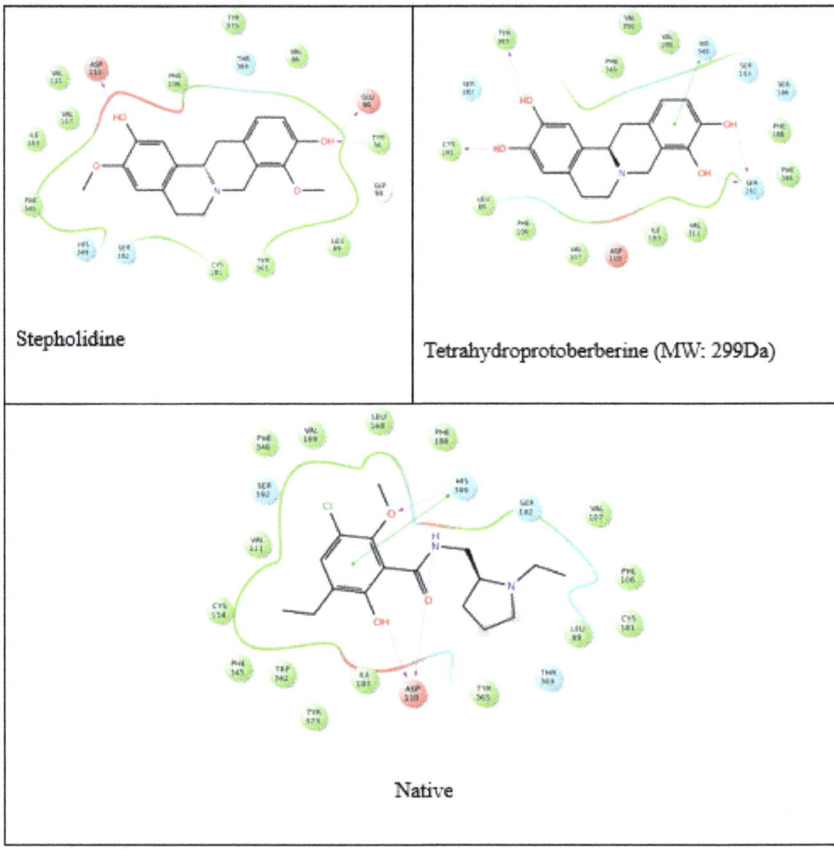

Fig. 5 Induced fit docking studies of ligand interaction to the selected plant secondary metabolite(s) with D3 receptor (PDB ID: 3PBL) by ligplot.

tree, *Cephalotaxus harringtonia* and a racemic mixture of it and harringtonine are clinically used for treatment of acute and also chronic myelogenous leukemia. The elliptinium, a derivative of ellipticine, isolated from a Fijian medicinal plant *Bleekeria vitiensis* for the treatment of breast cancer (Cragg & Newman, 2005). Betulinic acid displayed selective cytotoxicity against human melanoma cell lines (Balunas & Kinghorn, 2005). Betulinic acid is a common secondary metabolite (a pentacyclic triterpene) of plants (*Betula* sp. and *Ziziphus* sp.). Sylvestrol was first isolated from the fruits of *Aglaila sylvestre*, and it was shown to exhibit cytotoxicity against lung and breast cancer cells (Cragg & Newman, 2005).

Essential oils from *Artemisia capillaris* had an anticancer effect related to the induction of apoptosis and activation the mitogen-activated protein kinase (MAPK) signaling pathway (Cha *et al.*, 2009). The limonoids azadirachtin and nimbolide of *A. indica* exhibited apoptosis on the Hamster buccal pouch carcinogenesis model (Kumar *et al.*, 2010). *In vitro* studies of the compounds ganoderma (Liang *et al.*, 2014), aloe-emodin (Cheng & Dong 2018), triterpenes (Thyagarajan *et al.*, 2010), genistein (Luo *et al.*, 2014), stictic acid (Pejin *et al.*, 2017), apigenin (Lefort & Blay, 2011), quercetin (Psahoulia *et al.*, 2007), lycopene (Cha *et al.*, 2017), and the extract of *Ginkgo biloba* (Chen *et al.*, 2011) showed anticancer effects on gastrointestinal cancer cell lines.

4.1. Phytochemical Compounds Against Breast Cancer

Cardamonin from *Alpiniae katsumadai* during the *in vitro* experiments with MDA-MB-231 cells proved inhibition of the HIF 1α pathway and modulator cancer cell metabolism (Jin *et al.*, 2019). Neobractatin from *Garcinia bracteata* had shown the prevention of metastasis cell line experiments with MDA-MB-231 and MCF-7 (Zhang *et al.*, 2019). In vivo experiments in MDA-231 and MDA-435S cells with Sanguinarine from *Sanguinaria canadensis* changed the expression levels with various apoptotic proteins (Kim *et al.*, 2008). Piperin from *Piper nigrum* has shown the induction of apoptosis of FT1 cells and suppression of primary tumor growth FT1 during the *in vitro* and *in vivo* experiments (Lai *et al.*, 2012). Curcumin and carvacrol from *Curcuma longa* in the in vivo and *in vitro* experiments with MDA-MB-231 had shown induction of apoptosis cells and inhibition of tumor regression (Arunasree, 2010; Somasundaram *et al.*, 2002). Essential oils from *Boswellia sacra*, *Boswellia carterii*, *Nigella sativa*, and *Thymus cecphylum* in the *in vitro* experiments with MCF-7 cells showed cytotoxic effect and induction of apoptosis in cancer cells (Hussain *et al.*, 2013; Periasamy *et al.*, 2016; Suhail *et al.*, 2011).

4.2. Phytochemical Compounds Against Pancreatic Cancer — *In vitro* Cell Line Studies

In vitro studies for plumbagin from *Plumbago zylanica* have been carried out by Hafeez *et al.* (2013), targeting EGFR, STAT3, and NF-κB signaling pathways. Nimosine and epigallocatechin-3-gallate from *Moringa oleifera* have been proved to inhibit the cell growth and induced apoptosis (Berkovich *et al.*, 2013). Terpenoids and a flavonoids glycoside from *Acacia pennata* leaves (Rifai *et al.*, 2010) and extract from *Amoora rohituka* and Chittagonga (Chan *et al.*, 2011) have been shown to have cytotoxic activity against pancreatic cancer cell line. Triptolide (Zhou *et al.*, 2008) and luteolin (Li *et al.*, 2018) from *Tripterygium wilfordii* inhibit apoptosis in pancreatic cell lines.

4.3. Phytochemical Compounds Against Brain Cancer

In vitro studies of carvone and β-elemene from *Juliferous phoenicea* showed the inhibition of growth of brain tumors and brain carcinomas (Okokon *et al.*, 2013; Wu *et al.*, 2009). Isoflavones, retinoids, and epigallocatechin gallate from *Angelica sinensis* have been shown to induce apoptosis with activation of caspase 8 (Das *et al.*, 2008; Zhang *et al.*, 2016).

4.4. Phytochemical Compounds Against Skin Cancer

4-Nerolidylcatechol from *Piper umbellatum* exhibited inhibition of matrix metalloproteinase (MMPs) — MMP2 and MMP9 — activities (Brohem *et al.*, 2009). Fucoidans from *Ficus evanescens* inhibited colony formation and cell proliferation in SK-MEL-28 and SK-MEL-5 cell lines (Anastyuk *et al.*, 2012). Elangin from

Alpinia affecinarum has been shown to reduce the mitochondrial membrane potential during the *in vitro* studies with B16F10 murine melanoma cell (Zhang *et al*., 2013). Linalool from *Sature jathymvra* has been shown to inhibit tumor cell growth during the *in vitro* studies on amelanotic melanoma C32 cell line (Loizzo *et al*., 2007). Resveratrol from *V. vinifera* has been shown to arrest cell cycle at G1 phase and downregulation of the protein expression of cyclin D1, D2, & E and also CDK2, CDK4, and CDK6 during the *in vitro* studies on melanoma cell lines A-375, A-431, and SK-MEL-28 (Aggarwal *et al*., 2004; Niles *et al*., 2003). *In vitro* studies of silybin from *Silybum marianum* showed downregulation of the expression of NF-κB and STAT3. It also inhibits the phosphorylation of ERK1/2 and RSK2 and also inhibits the activity of MEK 1 and 2. The tested cell lines were human melanoma SK-MEL-5 and SK-MEL-28 (Lee *et al*., 2013). *In vitro* experiments with silymarin from *S. marianum* on human malignance melanoma A375-S2 cells proved the activation and cleavage of procaspase-8 causing cell death by apoptosis (Ramasamy & Agarwal, 2008). Thermoquinone from *Nigella sativa* showed cytotoxicity against skin cancer (Kuppusamy *et al*., 2013). Apigenin from *Lycopodium clavatum* have been shown to inhibit the formation of ROS, interfering with NF-κB and p38 MAPK signaling pathways (Das *et al*., 2013).

4.5 Anticancer Compounds from Marine Plants

The marine environment represents nearly 70% of the earth surface, and there is the huge biodiversity. This great diversity of secondary metabolites from algae offers an abundant source of drugs which could be the potential candidates for treating various diseases including cancer. There is a great chemical diversity in marine plants, including marine algae and mangroves. Many products isolated from these plants have been proven to be anticancer drugs. A review on the anticancer activity of marine herbs was presented by Vignesh *et al.* (2011). An interesting field of marine drugs is marine blue, green algae termed as cyanobacteria which is an effective agent in killing cancer cells by enhancing the apoptotic death. Lophocladine A and B from the red algae *Lophocladia* have been found to be active against various cancer cell lines (Gross *et al.*, 2006). Marine algae or seaweeds demonstrate metabolic plasticity and produce several compounds useful for drug development (Romano *et al.*, 2017). *Chlorella* species contains diverse carotenoids such as lutein, beta-carotene, zeaxanthin, and astaxanthin. Fucoxanthin from brown seaweeds and some microalgae was isolated by Satomi (2017) and Peng *et al.* (2011). Fucoxanthin inhibits proliferation in colorectal cancer. Anticancer effects of fucoxanthin and fucoxanthinol have been demonstrated by Takahashi *et al.* (2015). Fucoxanthinol, the D acetylated derivative of fucoxanthin, reduces the cell viability of breast cancer cells via modulation of NF-κB pathway. Fucoxanthinol is more potent in inducing apoptosis compared to fucoxanthin (Tamura *et al.*, 2019). An extract of the brown seaweed *Sargassum thunbergii* displayed antitumor activity against sarcoma 180 and Ehrlich solid carcinoma in the in vivo study (Zhuang *et al.*, 1995). The anticancer and anti-proliferative effects of caulerpenyne from *Caulerpa* sp. algae was demonstrated by Barbier *et al.* (2001). The brown algae *Ecklonia cava* and isolated sulfated polysaccharide had cytotoxic effect against murine colon carcinoma and human leukemic monocyte lymphoma cell lines (Athukorala *et al.*, 2006). Dolastatin 10 and curacin A are the two cyanobacteria-derived antimicrotubule agents. They have been clinically evaluated for cancer treatment and served as lead structures for the synthesis of a number of synthetic derivatives (Tan, 2007). The anticancer potent activity of Calothrixins A & B against human HeLa cancer cells has been reported by Rickards *et al.* (1999). These pentacyclic metabolites were isolated from *Calothrix* cyanobacteria. The cyanobacteria *Prochloran* species and *Lissoclinum patella* were found to contain ulithiacyclamide and petellamide, exhibiting potent cytotoxic activity (Williams *et al.*, 1989). The cynobacterial compound aprotoxins inhibit a variety of cancer cell lines at nano molar dose levels. Cynobacteria also produces a family of antitumor agents known as cryptophycins, interfering with tubulin assemblage (Bhatnagar & Kim, 2010). Polysaccharides are present in large amounts in marine algae and some of them exert anticancer effect. Alginic acid, fucoidan, from brown seaweed was found to possess anticancer activity (Senthilkumar *et al.*, 2013). Carrageenans, isolated from the red seaweed *Kappaphycus*, have been proven to suppress the growth of breast, colon, liver, and osteosarcoma cell lines (Suganya *et al.*, 2016). Fucoidan suppresses cell proliferation, apoptosis, and migration in colon cancers; the brown seaweeds *Cladosiphon okamuranus* and *F. evanescens* and the fucoidan from brown seaweeds consist of fucose, galactose, mannose, and xylose and administration of fucoidan for four weeks inhibited tumor growth and angiogenesis (Rui *et al.*, 2017).

5. Targets for Anticancer Drug Design

The need for less harmful, more selective, and more reliable cancer treatments has become more pressing. Inhibiting angiogenesis is still one of the most active areas of cancer drug research today. Observations into tumor angiogenesis biology also led to the discovery of many molecules that are essential for the continuation of these processes.

A group of growth factors, namely fibroblast growth factor, platelet-derived growth factor, and vascular endothelial growth factor, is of specific importance. These growth factors and their receptor tyrosine kinases (RTKs) have emerged as key targets for inhibiting the multiplication of endothelial cells, the prime constituent of blood vessels. Anti-angiogenic strategies that are being investigated are endothelial cell proliferation inhibition; restriction or neutralization of angiogenic factors or receptors such as endothelial cell growth factor receptors (bFGF, vascular endothelial growth factor [VEGF]); and suppression of extracellular matrix proteinases, especially MMPs (Nam & Parang, 2003).

RTKs are a group of cell surface receptors that are responsible for the regulation cell growth, motility, differentiation, and survival (Butti *et al.*, 2018). RTKs have correlation with the abnormalities in the downstream signaling pathways such as MAPK, phosphoinositide-3-kinase/protein kinase B (PI3K/AKT) and Janus kinase/signal transducers, and activators of transcription (JAK/STAT) pathways, which may finally result in cancer development and uncontrolled proliferation of cells (Du & Lovly, 2018). The 2019 FDA-approved drug erdafitinib is a fibroblast growth factor receptor, a kinase inhibitor utilized for treating patients suffering from advanced urothelial carcinoma. Overproduction of several VEGF receptors is associated with abnormal tumor growth and metastasis by stimulating the formation of new blood vessels from existing vasculature (Kelly & Rixe, 2009).

Aside from growth factor RTKs, a plethora of other protein kinases associated with cancer is defined, like non-receptor kinases such as Bcl-Abl and Src kinases. Furthermore, cell cycle regulators (cyclin-dependent kinases, p21 gene) and cell death modulators (Bcl-2 oncoprotein, p53 tumor suppressor gene, survivin protein, and so on) have spurred growing focus as promising anticancer drug candidates. Other molecular targets comprise protein farnesyltransferase (FTase), histone deacetylase, and telomerase, all of which play important roles in cellular signal transduction and cell longevity (telomerase) (Nam & Parang, 2003).

DNA is the molecular target for several cancer therapeutic drugs and is regarded as a non-specific target of cytotoxic agents. Alkylating agents usually associate with DNA in a non-specific manner; the more powerful ones appear to crosslink DNA. Antitumor antibiotics have a higher degree of specificity in their interactions with DNA, and they are often correlated with low sequence selectivity and also the targeting of protein–DNA complexes. Secondary DNA structures, like G-quadruplex structures, bring a promising type of molecular targets for DNA-interactive molecules that may be beneficial for telomere targeting as well as transcriptional regulation. DNA-targeted drugs like cisplatin, mitomycin, melphalan, cyclophosphamide, and so on crosslink the DNA interstrands. Bleomycin is a radiomimetic drug that causes double-stranded breaks in DNA. Actinomycin D impedes DNA-directed synthesis of RNA. Antibodies could be used to target drugs as well: SGN-15 is an antibody conjugate made up of doxorubicin and a monoclonal antibody. This could be directed at a tumor-specific antigen on cancer cell, resulting in tumor specificity (Hurley, 2002; Smith, 2001).

In a number of pathophysiological processes, the two isoforms cyclooxygenase-1 and -2 catalyze the first step in the formation of prostaglandins. They appear to affect apoptosis, angiogenesis, as well as invasion, and also play a role in carcinogen production. Cancer cells usually have a high degree of COX-2 activity. However, low COX-2 expression has been found in certain cancers, such as prostate and breast cancers. Numerous preliminary studies show positive results when chemotherapy or radiotherapy is combined with COX inhibitors. Reports have shown that by combining a COX inhibitor with drugs like cisplatin and cyclophosphamide slowed tumor development and reduced the amount of lung neoplasms (Teicher *et al.*, 1994). Also, selective COX-2 inhibitors have been shown to improve the impact of radiation on cancers that express COX-2 but not on cancers that do not express COX-2 (Pyo *et al.*, 2001). Preclinical trials with the combined use of epidermal growth factor receptor inhibitors and COX-2 inhibitors have also yielded positive results. Targeting the COX-2 pathway is an effective option for solid tumor treatment and prevention (Méric *et al.*, 2006).

Recent research has rekindled interest in direct RAS inhibition, including strategies that aim RAS dimerization or drugs that covalently attach G12C mutant RAS, preventing it from being activated by guanosine diphosphate (Moore *et al.*, 2020). Targeting oncogene amplification has proved difficult. MYC and MYCN transcription factors, for example, are often amplified or translocated in a variety of cancers, and the MYC network is disrupted in a large proportion of cancer types (Dang, 2012; Schaub *et al.*, 2018). Owing to the absence of enzyme and drug-binding sites, clinical targeting of MYC has been difficult. Indirect targeting of MYC through BRD4 inhibition, MYC stability regulators, and inhibition of downstream interacting kinases are all valuable areas of research (Hahn *et al.*, 2021). mTOR, mechanistic target of rapamycin, is often up-regulated in cancer, like hepatocellular carcinoma (HCC), and has been linked to a grim prognosis, poorly differentiated tumors, and earlier relapse. Obstructing mTOR with rapamycin as well as first-generation mTOR inhibitors known as rapalogs has demonstrated impressive outcomes in preclinical models of HCC tumor development. Rapamycin/rapalogs are presently being studied in multiple clinical trials for the therapy of advanced HCC, as well as adjuvant therapy in HCC patients following liver transplant as well as TACE (Matter *et al.*, 2014).

Notch, Hedgehog, and Wnt signaling pathways, for example, have emerged as major targets for novel anticancer drugs. Although Notch and Hedgehog inhibitors are currently in clinical studies, Wnt inhibitors are only in preclinical testing, and only a few compounds have progressed to phase-I clinical trials, as this pathway was only recently identified as having a critical role in tumor growth. Multiple studies have given evidence that specific targeting of molecules in this pathway can partially or completely turn off canonical as well as non-canonical Wnt signaling, resulting in significant antitumor activity. As a result, pharmaceutical and biotechnology firms are continuously working on Wnt signaling inhibitors (Pez *et al.*, 2013).

It is now practical to define and validate a broad array of cancer targets. Furthermore, subsequent work will be required to establish reliable methods for testing possible combinations (Carneiro & El-Deiry, 2020; Hahn *et al.*, 2021).

6. Conclusion

Cancer is a disease that impacts human population worldwide. New treatments to cure and mitigate this life-threatening disease are still in progress. Natural-derived compounds are attracting academic and medical attention because they are thought to have less adverse side effects than conventional therapies. From the publications of clinical, animal, and *in vitro* studies, we can foresee that some of the herbal medicines along with nanoparticle formulations hold great promise in treating cancer with minimum side effects.

References

Aggarwal, B. B., Bhardwaj, A., Aggarwal, R. S., Seeram, N. P., Shishodia, S., & Takada, Y. (2004). Role of resveratrol in prevention and therapy of cancer: Preclinical and clinical studies. *Anticancer Research 24*(5A), 2783–2840.

Alberg, A. J., & Samet, J. M. (2003). Epidemiology of lung cancer. *Chest*, *123*(1 Suppl), 21S–49S.

Allred, D. C. (2010). Ductal carcinoma in situ: Terminology, classification, and natural history. *Journal of the National Cancer Institute Monographs*, *2010*(41), 134–138.

Anastyuk, S. D., Shevchenko, N. M., Ermakova, S. P., Vishchuk, O. S., Nazarenko, E. L., Dmitrenok, P. S., & Zvyagintseva, T. N. (2012). Anticancer activity in vitro of a fucoidan from the brown alga *Fucus evanescens* and its low-molecular fragments, structurally characterized by tandem mass-spectrometry. *Carbohydrate Polymers*, *87*(1), 186–194.

Arunasree, K. M. (2010). Anti-proliferative effects of carvacrol on a human metastatic breast cancer cell line, MDA-MB 231. *Phytomedicine*, *17*(8–9), 581–588.

Ashraf, M. A. (2020). Phytochemicals as potential anticancer drugs: Time to ponder nature's bounty. *BioMed Research International*, *2020*, 8602879.

Athukorala, Y., Kim, K.-N., & Jeon, Y.-J. (2006). Antiproliferative and antioxidant properties of an enzymatic hydrolysate from brown alga, *Ecklonia cava*. *Food and Chemical Toxicology*, *44*(7), 1065–1074.

Balunas, M. J., & Kinghorn, A. D. (2005) Drug discovery from medicinal plants. *Life Science*, *78*(5), 431–441.

Barbier, P., Guise, S., Huitorel, P., Amade, P., Pesando, D., Briand, C., & Peyrot, V. (2001). Caulerpenyne from *Caulerpa taxifolia* has an anti-proliferative activity on tumor cell line SK-N-SH and modifies the microtubule network. *Life Science*, *70*(4), 415–429.

Barenholz, Y. C. (2012). Doxil®—The First FDA-approved nano-drug: Lessons learned. *Journal of Controlled Release*, *160*(2), 117–134.

Batist, G., Ramakrishnan, G., Rao, C. S., Chandrasekharan, A., Gutheil, J., Guthrie, T., Shah, P., Khojasteh, A., Nair, M. K., Hoelzer, K., Tkaczuk, K., Park, Y. C., & Lee, L. W. (2001). Reduced cardiotoxicity and preserved antitumor efficacy of liposome-encapsulated doxorubicin and cyclophosphamide compared with conventional doxorubicin and cyclophosphamide in a randomized, multicenter trial of metastatic breast cancer. *Journal of Clinical Oncology*, *19*(5), 1444–1454.

Bedikian, A. Y., Silverman, J. A., Papadopoulos, N. E., Kim, K. B., Hagey, A. E., Vardeleon, A., Hwu, W.-J., Homsi, J., Davies, M., & Hwu, P. (2011). Pharmacokinetics and safety of Marqibo (vincristine sulfate liposomes injection) in cancer patients with impaired liver function. *Journal of Clinical Pharmacology*, *51*(8), 1205–1212.

Berkovich, L., Earon, G., Ron, I., Rimmon, A., Vexler, A., & Lev-Ari, S. (2013). *Moringa oleifera* aqueous leaf extract down-regulates nuclear factor-kappa B and increases cytotoxic effect of chemotherapy in pancreatic cancer cells. *BMC Complementary and Alternative Medicine*, *13*(1).

Bhatnagar, I., & Kim, S.-K. (2010). Immense essence of excellence: Marine microbial bioactive compounds. *Marine Drugs*, *8*(10), 2673–2701.

Braun, R. P., Klumb, F., Bondon, D., Salomon, D., Skaria, A., Adatto, M., French, L. E., Saurat, J.-H., & Vallée, J.-P. (2005). Three-dimensional reconstruction of basal cell carcinomas. *Dermatologic Surgery*, *31*(5), 562–569.

Brohem, C. A., Sawada, T. C. H., Massaro, R. R., Almeida, R. L., Rivelli, D. P., Ropke, C. D., da Silva, V. V., de Lima, T. M., Curi, R., Barros, S. B. M., & Maria-Engler, S. S. (2009). Apoptosis induction by 4-nerolidylcatechol in melanoma cell lines. *Toxicology In Vitro*, *23*(1), 111–119.

Burt, R. W., DiSario, J. A., & Cannon-Albright, L. (1995). Genetics of colon cancer: Impact of inheritance on colon cancer risk. *Annual Review of Medicine*, *46*(1), 371–379.

Butti, R., Das, S., Gunasekaran, V. P., Yadav, A. S., Kumar, D., & Kundu, G. C. (2018). Receptor Tyrosine Kinases (RTKs) in breast cancer: Signaling, therapeutic implications and challenges. *Molecular Cancer*, *17*(1).

Buyel, J. F. (2018). Plants as sources of natural and recombinant anti-cancer agents. *Biotechnology Advances*, *36*(2), 506–520.

Carneiro, B. A., & El-Deiry, W. S. T. (2020). Targeting apoptosis in cancer therapy. *Nature Reviews Clinical Oncology*, *17*(7), 395–417.

Cha, J. D., Moon, S. E., Kim, H. Y., Lee, J. C., & Lee, K. Y. (2009). The essential oil isolated from *Artemisia capillaris* prevents LPS-induced production of NO and PGE2 by inhibiting MAPK-mediated pathways in Raw 264.7 macrophages. *Immunological Investigations*, *38*(6), 483–497.

Cha, J. H., Kim, W. K., Ha, A. W., Kim, M. H., & Chang, M. J. (2017). Anti-inflammatory effect of lycopene in SW480 human colorectal cancer cells. *Nutrition Research and Practice*, *11*(2), 90–96.

Chan, L. L., George, S., Ahmad, I., Gosangari, S. L., Abbasi, A., Cunningham, B. T., & Watkin, K. L. (2011). Cytotoxicity effects of *Amoora rohituka* and Chittagonga on breast and pancreatic cancer cells. *Evidence-Based Complementary and Alternative Medicine*, *2011*, 860605.

Chando, R. K., Hussain, N., Rana, M. I., Sayed, S., Alam, S., Fakir, T. A., Ashraf, M. A., K., R., Hussain, N., Rana, M. I., Sayed, S., Alam, S., Fakir, T. A., & Ashraf, M. A. (2019). CDK4 as a phytochemical based anticancer drug target. *bioRxiv*.

Che, E., Gao, Y., Wan, L., Zhang, Y., Han, N., Bai, J., Li, J., Sha, Z., & Wang, S. (2015). Paclitaxel/gelatin coated magnetic mesoporous silica nanoparticles: Preparation and antitumor efficacy in vivo. *Microporous and Mesoporous Materials*, *204*, 226–234.

Cheng, C., & Dong, W. (2018). Aloe-emodin induces endoplasmic reticulum stress-dependent apoptosis in colorectal cancer cells. *Medical Science Monitor*, *24*, 6331–6339.

Chikara, S., Nagaprashantha, L. D., Singhal, J., Horne, D., Awasthi, S., & Singhal, S. S. (2018). Oxidative stress and dietary phytochemicals: Role in cancer chemoprevention and treatment. *Cancer Letters*, *413*, 122–134.

Cho, K., Wang, X., Nie, S., Chen, Z. G., & Shin, D. M. (2008). Therapeutic nanoparticles for drug delivery in cancer. *Clinical Cancer Research*, *14*(5), 1310–1316.

Cigna, E., Tarallo, M., Maruccia, M., Sorvillo, V., Pollastrini, A., & Scuderi, N. (2011). Basal cell carcinoma: 10 years of experience. *Journal of Skin Cancer*, *2011*, 476362.

Cragg, G. M., & Newman, D. J. (2005). Plants as a source of anti-cancer agents. *Journal of Ethnopharmacology*, *100*(1–2), 72–79.

Creemers, G. J., Bolis, G., Gore, M., Scarfone, G., Lacave, A. J., Guastalla, J. P., Despax, R., Favalli, G., Kreinberg, R., Van Belle, S., Hudson, I., Verweij, J., & Ten Bokkel Huinink, W. W. (1996). Topotecan, an active drug in the second-line treatment of epithelial ovarian cancer: Results of a large European phase II study. *Journal of Clinical Oncology*, *14*(12), 3056–3061.

Dang, C. V. (2012). MYC on the path to cancer. *Cell*, *149*(1), 22–35.

Das, A., Banik, N. L., & Ray, S. K. (2008). N-(4-Hydroxyphenyl) retinamide induced both differentiation and apoptosis in human glioblastoma T98G and U87MG cells. *Brain Research*, *1227*, 207–215.

Das, S., Das, J., Paul, A., Samadder, A., & Khuda-Bukhsh, A. R. (2013). Apigenin, a bioactive flavonoid from *Lycopodium clavatum*, stimulates nucleotide excision repair genes to protect skin keratinocytes from ultraviolet B-induced reactive oxygen species and DNA damage. *Journal of Acupuncture and Meridian Studies*, *6*(5), 252–262.

Davis, A. S., Viera, A. J., & Mead, M. D. (2014). Leukemia: An overview for primary care. *American Family Physician*, *89*(9), 731–738.

Delongchamps, N. B., Singh, A., & Haas, G. P. (2006). The role of prevalence in the diagnosis of prostate cancer. *Cancer Control*, *13*(3), 158–168.

Desai, A. G., Qazi, G. N., Ganju, R. K., El-Tamer, M., Singh, J., Saxena, A. K., Bedi, Y. S., Taneja, S. C., & Bhat, H. K. (2008). Medicinal plants and cancer chemoprevention. *Current Drug Metabolism*, *9*(7), 581–591.

Devadass, V., Raman, P., & Gayathri, D. (2020). Anti-cancer compounds from terrestrial and marine resources – In silico and experimental studies. *Current Computer-Aided Drug Design*, *16*.

Du, Z., & Lovly, C. M. (2018). Mechanisms of receptor tyrosine kinase activation in cancer. *Molecular Cancer*, *17*(1), 1–13.

Edis, Z., Wang, J., Waqas, M. K., Ijaz, M., & Ijaz, M. (2021). Nanocarriers-mediated drug delivery systems for anticancer agents: An overview and perspectives. *International Journal of Nanomedicine*, *16*, 1313–1330.

Einbond, L. S., Soffritti, M., Esposti, D. D., Park, T., Cruz, E., Su, T., & Vladimirova, A. (2009). Actein activates stress-and statin-associated responses and is bioavailable in Sprague-Dawley rats. *Fundamental & Clinical Pharmacology*, *23*(3), 311–321.

Fearon, E. R., & Vogelstein, B. A. (1990). Genetic model for colorectal tumorigenesis. *Cell*, *61*(5), 759–767.

Gayatri, S., Suresh, R., Reddy, C. U. M., & Chitra, K. (2016). Isolation and characterization of chemopreventive agent from *Sphaeranthus amaranthoides* Burm F. *Pharmacognosy Research*, *8*(1), 61–65.

Gerecke, C., Fuhrmann, S., Strifler, S., Schmidt-Hieber, M., Einsele, H., & Knop, S. (2016). The diagnosis and treatment of multiple myeloma. *Deutsches Ärzteblatt International*, *113*(27–28), 470–476.

Ghosh, T., Maity, T. K., & Singh, J. (2011). Evaluation of antitumor activity of stigmasterol, a constituent isolated from *Bacopa monnieri* Linn aerial parts against Ehrlich ascites carcinoma in mice. *Oriental Pharmacy and Experimental Medicine*, *11*(1), 41–49.

Gorringe, K. L., & Fox, S. B. (2017). Ductal carcinoma in situ biology, biomarkers, and diagnosis. *Frontiers in Oncology*, *7*, 248.

Gowala, U., Ananthakrishnan, D., Velmurugan, D., Saikia, A., & Sarma, H. N. (2020). Chromatographic fractionation and in silico validation of bioactive compounds from *Cynoglossum Zeylanicum* (Lehm) for binding affinity with human ER & PR. *Journal of Biologically Active Products from Nature*, *10*(2), 122–140.

Gross, H., Goeger, D. E., Hills, P., Mooberry, S. L., Ballantine, D. L., Murray, T. F., Valeriote, F. A., & Gerwick, W. H. (2006). Lophocladines, bioactive alkaloids from the red alga *Lophocladia* sp. *Journal of Natural Products*, *69*(4), 640–644.

Hafeez, B. B., Zhong, W., Fischer, J. W., Mustafa, A., Shi, X., Meske, L., & Verma, A. K. (2013). Plumbagin, a medicinal plant (*Plumbago zeylanica*)-derived 1,4-naphthoquinone, inhibits growth and metastasis of human prostate cancer PC-3M-luciferase cells in an orthotopic xenograft mouse model. *Molecular oncology*, *7*(3), 428–439.

Hahn, W. C., Bader, J. S., Braun, T. P., Califano, A., Clemons, P. A., Druker, B. J., Ewald, A. J., Fu, H., Jagu, S., Kemp, C. J., Kim, W., Kuo, C. J., McManus, M., B Mills, G., Mo, X., Sahni, N., Schreiber, S. L., Talamas, J. A., Tamayo, P., … Gerhard, D. S. (2021). Cancer target discovery and development network. An expanded universe of cancer targets. *Cell*, *184*(5), 1142–1155.

Hooper, J. E., & Scott, M. P. (2005). Communicating with hedgehogs. *Nature Reviews Molecular Cell Biology*, *6*(4), 306–317.

Hsieh, J. J., Purdue, M. P., Signoretti, S., Swanton, C., Albiges, L., Schmidinger, M., Heng, D. Y., Larkin, J., & Ficarra, V. (2017). Renal cell carcinoma. *Nature Reviews Disease Primers*, *3*(1).

Hubbard, R., Venn, A., Lewis, S., & Britton, J. (2000). Lung cancer and cryptogenic fibro sing alveolitis. A population-based cohort study. *American Journal of Respiratory and Critical Care Medicine*, *161*(1), 5–8.

Hurley, L. H. (2002). DNA and its associated processes as targets for cancer therapy. *Nature Reviews Cancer*, *2*(3), 188–200.

Hussain, H., Al-Harrasi, A., Al-Rawahi, A., & Hussain, J. (2013). Chemistry and biology of essential oils of genus *Boswellia*. *Evidence-Based Complementary and Alternative Medicine*, *2013*, 140509.

Hwang, E. S., McLennan, J. L., Moore, D. H., Crawford, B. B., Esserman, L. J., & Ziegler, J. L. (2007). Ductal carcinoma in situ in BRCA mutation carriers. *Journal of Clinical Oncology*, *25*(6), 642–647.

Jin, J., Qiu, S., Wang, P., Liang, X., Huang, F., Wu, H., Zhang, B., Zhang, W., Tian, X., Xu, R., Shi, H., & Wu, X. (2019). Cardamonin inhibits breast cancer growth by repressing HIF-1α-dependent metabolic reprogramming. *Journal of Experimental & Clinical Cancer Research*, *38*(1), 377.

Jordan, M. A., & Wilson, L. (2004). Microtubules as a target for anticancer drugs. *Nature Reviews Cancer*, *4*(4), 253–265.

Kauff, N. D., Brogi, E., Scheuer, L., Pathak, D. R., Borgen, P. I., Hudis, C. A., Offit, K., & Robson, M. E. (2003). Epithelial lesions in prophylactic mastectomy specimens from women with BRCA mutations. *Cancer*, *97*(7), 1601–1608.

Kelly, R. J., & Rixe, O. (2009). Axitinib—A selective inhibitor of the Vascular Endothelial Growth Factor (VEGF) receptor. *Targeted Oncology*, *4*(4), 297–305.

Kim, S., Lee, T.-J., Leem, J., Choi, K. S., Park, J.-W., & Kwon, T. K. (2008). Sanguinarine-induced apoptosis: generation of ROS, down-regulation of Bcl-2, c-FLIP, and synergy with TRAIL. *Journal of Cellular Biochemistry*, *104*(3), 895–907.

Kinch, M. S. (2014). An analysis of FDA-approved drugs for oncology. *Drug Discovery Today*, *19*(12), 1831–1835.

Kumar, G. H., Priyadarsini, R. V., Vinothini, G., Letchoumy, P. V., & Nagini, S. (2010). The neem limonoids azadirachtin and nimbolide inhibit cell proliferation and induce apoptosis in an animal model of oral oncogenesis. *Investigational New Drugs*, *28*(4), 392–401.

Küppers, R., Engert, A., & Hansmann, M.-L. (2012). Hodgkin lymphoma. *Journal of Clinical Investigation*, *122*(10), 3439–3447.

Küppers, R., & Rajewsky, K. (2010). *Developmental and functional biology of B lymphocytes* (pp. 26–40). Philadelphia, PA: Wolters Kluwer and Lippincott Williams & Wilkins.

Kuppusamy, P., Yusoff, M. M., Maniam, G. P., & Govindan, N. (2013). A case study – Regulation and functional mechanisms of cancer cells and control its activity using plants and their derivatives. *Journal of Pharmacy Research*, *6*(8), 884–892.

Kyrgidis, A., Vahtsevanos, K., Tzellos, T. G., Xirou, P., Kitikidou, K., Antoniades, K., Zouboulis, C. C., & Triaridis, S. (2010). Clinical, histological and demographic predictors for recurrence and second primary tumours of head and neck basal cell carcinoma. A 1062 patient-cohort study from a tertiary cancer referral hospital. *European Journal of Dermatology*, *20*(3), 276–282.

Lai, L.-H., Fu, Q.-H., Liu, Y., Jiang, K., Guo, Q.-M., Chen, Q.-Y., Yan, B., Wang, Q.-Q., & Shen, J.-G. (2012). Piperine suppresses tumor growth and metastasis in vitro and in vivo in a 4T1 murine breast cancer model. *Acta Pharmacologica Sinica*, *33*(4), 523–530.

Lear, J. T., Smith, A. G., Strange, R. C., & Fryer, A. A. (2000). Detoxifying enzyme genotypes and susceptibility to cutaneous malignancy: Detoxifying enzymes and skin cancer. *British Journal of Dermatology*, *142*(1), 8–15.

Lee, M.-H., Huang, Z., Kim, D. J., Kim, S.-H., Kim, M. O., Lee, S.-Y., Xie, H., Park, S. J., Kim, J. Y., Kundu, J. K., Bode, A. M., Surh, Y.-J., & Dong, Z. (2013). Direct targeting of MEK1/2 and RSK2 by silybin induces cell-cycle arrest and inhibits melanoma cell growth. *Cancer Prevention Research*, *6*(5), 455–465.

Lefort, E. C., & Blay, J. (2011). The dietary flavonoid apigenin enhances the activities of the anti-metastatic protein CD26 on human colon carcinoma cells. *Clinical & Experimental Metastasis*, *28*(4), 337–349.

Li, M., Wei, S. Y., Xu, B., Guo, W., Liu, D. L., Cui, J. R., & Yao, X. S. (2008). Pro-apoptotic and microtubule-disassembly effects of ardisiacrispin (A+B), triterpenoid saponins from *Ardisia crenata* on human hepatoma Bel-7402 cells. *Journal of Asian Natural Products Research*, *10*(8), 729–736.

Li, Z., Zhang, Y., Chen, L., & Li, H. (2018). The dietary compound luteolin inhibits pancreatic cancer growth by targeting BCL-2. *Food & Function*, *9*(5), 3018–3027.

Liang, Z., Guo, Y.-T., Yi, Y.-J., Wang, R.-C., Hu, Q.-L., & Xiong, X.-Y. (2014). *Ganoderma lucidum* polysaccharides target a Fas/Caspase dependent pathway to induce apoptosis in human colon cancer cells. *Asian Pacific Journal of Cancer Prevention*, *15*(9), 3981–3986.

Lin, H. L., Liu, T. Y., Lui, W. Y., & Chi, C. W. (1999). Up-regulation of multidrug resistance transporter expression by berberine in human and murine hepatoma cells. *Cancer: Interdisciplinary International Journal of the American Cancer Society*, *85*(9), 1937–1942.

Loizzo, M. R., Tundis, R., Menichini, F., Saab, A. M., Statti, G. A., & Menichini, F. (2007). Cytotoxic activity of essential oils from Labiatae and Lauraceae families against in vitro human tumor models. *Anticancer Research*, *27*(5A), 3293–3299.

Lu, H.-M., Li, S., Black, M. H., Lee, S., Hoiness, R., Wu, S., Mu, W., Huether, R., Chen, J., Sridhar, S., Tian, Y., McFarland, R., Dolinsky, J., Tippin Davis, B., Mexal, S., Dunlop, C., & Elliott, A. (2019). Association of breast and ovarian cancers with predisposition genes identified by large-scale sequencing. *JAMA Oncology*, *5*(1), 51–57.

Luo, Y., Wang, S.-X., Zhou, Z.-Q., Wang, Z., Zhang, Y.-G., Zhang, Y., & Zhao, P. (2014). Apoptotic effect of genistein on human colon cancer cells via inhibiting the Nuclear Factor-Kappa B (NF-*K*B) pathway. *Tumour Biology*, *35*(11), 11483–11488.

Matter, M. S., Decaens, T., Andersen, J. B., & Thorgeirsson, S. S. (2014). Targeting the MTOR pathway in hepatocellular carcinoma: Current state and future trends. *Journal of Hepatology*, *60*(4), 855–865.

Mattheolabakis, G., Rigas, B., & Constantinides, P. P. (2012). Nanodelivery strategies in cancer chemotherapy: Biological rationale and pharmaceutical perspectives. *Nanomedicine (London, England)*, *7*(10), 1577–1590.

Mazzola, E., Cheng, S.-C., & Parmigiani, G. (2013). The penetrance of ductal carcinoma in situ among BRCA1 and BRCA2 mutation carriers. *Breast Cancer Research and Treatment*, *137*(1), 315–318.

Méric, J.-B., Rottey, S., Olaussen, K., Soria, J.-C., Khayat, D., Rixe, O., & Spano, J.-P. (2006). Cyclooxygenase-2 as a target for anticancer drug development. *Critical Reviews in Oncology Hematology*, *59*(1), 51–64.

Minna, J. D., Roth, J. A., & Gazdar, A. F. (2002). Focus on lung cancer. *Cancer Cell*, *1*(1), 49–52.

Mohan, K., Marthong, B., Atanu, B., Wadhwani, A., Gayathri, D., & Velmurugan, D. (2018). Identification and in-silico analysis of anti-cancer compounds from herbal mix of north-east India. *RJLBPCS Journal*, *4*(5), 40.

Mohan, K., Pakyntein, H. C., Bhattacharjee, A., Viswanathan, V., & Velmurugan, D. (2018). Discovery of novel-anti-cancer compound from the identified phytoconstituent of "Jabung". *RJLBPCS Journal*, *4*(6), 47.

Mohan, K., Rangasamy, K. S., Viswanathan, V., & Velmurugan, D. (2018). Identification of potential anti-cancer leads from sivakaranthai-*Sphaeranthus amaranthoides* using tandem mass and their in-silico studies. *RJLBPCS Journal*, *4*(6), 26.

Moore, A. R., Rosenberg, S. C., McCormick, F., & Malek, S. (2020). RAS-targeted therapies: Is the undruggable drugged? *Nature Reviews Drug Discovery*, *19*(8), 533–552.

Mullangi, S., & Lekkala, M. R. (2021). *Adenocarcinoma*. StatPearls Publishing.

Nam, N.-H., & Parang, K. (2003). Current targets for anticancer drug discovery. *Current Drug Targets*, *4*(2), 159–179.

Newcomb, E. W., Tamasdan, C., Entzminger, Y., Arena, E., Schnee, T., Kim, M., Crisan, D., Lukyanov, Y., Miller, D. C., & Zagzag, D. (2004). Flavopiridol inhibits the growth of GL261 Gliomas in vivo: implications for malignant glioma therapy. *Cell Cycle*, *3*(2), 230–234.

Nguyen, N. H., Ta, Q. T. H., Pham, Q. T., Luong, T. N. H., Phung, V. T., Duong, T.-H., & Vo, V. G. (2020). Anticancer activity of novel plant extracts and compounds from *Adenosma bracteosum* (Bonati) in human lung and liver cancer cells. *Molecules*, *25*(12), 2912.

Nicolosi, P., Ledet, E., Yang, S., Michalski, S., Freschi, B., O'Leary, E., Esplin, E. D., Nussbaum, R. L., & Sartor, O. (2019). Prevalence of germline variants in prostate cancer and implications for current genetic testing guidelines. *JAMA Oncology*, *5*(4), 523–528.

Niles, R. M., McFarland, M., Weimer, M. B., Redkar, A., Fu, Y. M., & Meadows, G. G. (2003). Resveratrol is a potent inducer of apoptosis in human melanoma cells. *Cancer Letters*, *190*(2), 157–163.

Okokon, J. E., Dar, A., & Choudhary, M. I. (2013). Immunomodulatory, cytotoxic and antileishmanial activity of phytoconstituents of *Croton zambesicus*. *Phytopharmacology Journal*, *4*(1), 31–40.

Padmaharish, V., & Lakshmi, T. (2017). Anticancer activities of medicinal plants – An update. *Journal of Pharmaceutical Sciences and Research*, 9(4), 432.

Pejin, B., Iodice, C., Bogdanović, G., Kojić, V., & Tešević, V. (2017). Stictic acid inhibits cell growth of human colon adenocarcinoma HT-29 cells. *Arabian Journal of. Chemistry*, *10*, S1240–S1242.

Peng, J., Yuan, J.-P., Wu, C.-F., & Wang, J.-H. (2011). Fucoxanthin, a marine carotenoid present in brown seaweeds and diatoms: Metabolism and bioactivities relevant to human health. *Marine Drugs*, *9*(10), 1806–1828.

Periasamy, V. S., Athinarayanan, J., & Alshatwi, A. A. (2016). Anticancer activity of an ultrasonic nanoemulsion formulation of *Nigella sativa* L. essential oil on human breast cancer cells. *Ultrasonics Sonochemistry*, *31*, 449–455.

Pez, F., Lopez, A., Kim, M., Wands, J. R., Caron de Fromentel, C., & Merle, P. (2013). Wnt signaling and hepatocarcinogenesis: Molecular targets for the development of innovative anticancer drugs. *Journal of Hepatology*, *59*(5), 1107–1117.

Prescott, L. M. (1995). Doxil offers hope to KS sufferers. *Journal of the International Association of Providers of AIDS Care*, *1*(11), 43–44.

Psahoulia, F. H., Drosopoulos, K. G., Doubravska, L., Andera, L., & Pintzas, A. (2007). Quercetin enhances TRAIL-mediated apoptosis in colon cancer cells by inducing the accumulation of death receptors in lipid rafts. *Molecular Cancer Therapeutics*, *6*(9), 2591–2599.

Pyo, H., Choy, H., Amorino, G. P., Kim, J. S., Cao, Q., Hercules, S. K., & DuBois, R. N. (2001). A selective cyclooxygenase-2 inhibitor, NS-398, enhances the effect of radiation in vitro and in vivo preferentially on the cells that express cyclooxygenase-2. *Clinical Cancer Research*, *7*(10), 2998–3005.

Ramasamy, K., & Agarwal, R. (2008). Multi-targeted therapy of cancer by silymarin. *Cancer Letters*, *269*(2), 352–362.

Rayan, A., Raiyn, J., & Falah, M. (2017). Nature is the best source of anticancer drugs: Indexing natural products for their anticancer bioactivity. *PLoS One*, *12*(11), e0187925.

Raza, H., & John, A. (2005). Green tea polyphenol epigallocatechin-3-gallate differentially modulates oxidative stress in PC12 cell compartments. *Toxicology and Applied Pharmacology*, *207*(3), 212–220.

Rickards, R. W., Rothschild, J. M., Willis, A. C., de Chazal, N. M., Kirk, J., Kirk, K., Saliba, K. J., & Smith, G. D. (1999). Calothrixins A and B, novel pentacyclic metabolites from calothrix Cyanobacteria with potent activity against malaria parasites and human cancer cells. *Tetrahedron*, *55*(47), 13513–13520.

Rifai, Y., Arai, M. A., Koyano, T., Kowithayakorn, T., & Ishibashi, M. (2010). Terpenoids and a flavonoid glycoside from *Acacia pennata* leaves as Hedgehog/GLI-mediated transcriptional inhibitors. *Journal of Natural Products*, *73*(5), 995–997.

Rivera, E. (2003). Liposomal anthracyclines in metastatic breast cancer: Clinical update. *Oncologist*, *8*(90002), 3–9.

Romano, G., Costantini, M., Sansone, C., Lauritano, C., Ruocco, N., & Ianora, A. (2017). Marine microorganisms as a promising and sustainable source of bioactive molecules. *Marine Environmental Research*, *128*, 58–69.

Roy, A., Ahuja, S., & Bharadvaja, N. (2017). A review on medicinal plants against cancer. *Journal of Plant Sciences and Agricultural Research*, *2*, 1008.

Rui, X., Pan, H.-F., Shao, S.-L., & Xu, X.-M. (2017). Anti-tumor and anti-angiogenic effects of fucoidan on prostate cancer: Possible JAK-STAT3 pathway. *BMC Complementary Medicine and Therapies*, *17*(1), 378.

Satomi, Y. (2017). Antitumor and cancer-preventative function of fucoxanthin: A marine carotenoid. *Anticancer Research*, *37*(4), 1557–1562.

Schaub, F. X., Dhankani, V., Berger, A. C., Trivedi, M., Richardson, A. B., Shaw, R., Zhao, W., Zhang, X., Ventura, A., Liu, Y., Ayer, D. E., Hurlin, P. J., Cherniack, A. D., Eisenman, R. N., Aredes, N. D., & Mariamidze, A. (2018). Pan-cancer alterations of the MYC oncogene and its proximal network across the cancer genome atlas. *Cell Systems*, *6*(3), 282–300.e2.

Senthilkumar, K., Manivasagan, P., Venkatesan, J., & Kim, S.-K. (2013). Brown seaweed fucoidan: Biological activity and apoptosis, growth signaling mechanism in cancer. *International Journal of Biological Macromolecules*, *60*, 366–374.

Shankland, K. R., Armitage, J. O., & Hancock, B. W. (2012). Non-Hodgkin lymphoma. *Lancet*, *380*(9844), 848–857.

Sharifi-Rad, J., Ozleyen, A., Boyunegmez Tumer, T., Oluwaseun Adetunji, C., El Omari, N., Balahbib, A., Taheri, Y., Bouyahya, A., Martorell, M., Martins, N., & Cho, W. C. (2019). Natural products and synthetic analogs as a source of antitumor drugs. *Biomolecules*, *9*(11), 679.

Singh, T. D., Meitei, H. T., Sharma, A. L., Robinson, A., Singh, L. S., & Singh, T. R. (2015). Anticancer properties and enhancement of therapeutic potential of cisplatin by leaf extract of *Zanthoxylum Armatum* DC. *Biological Research*, *48*(1), 46.

Skubitz, K. M., & D'Adamo, D. R. (2007). Sarcoma. *Mayo Clinic Proceedings*, *82*(11), 1409–1432.

Smith, S. (2001). Technology evaluation: SGN-15, Seattle Genetics Inc. *Current Opinion in Molecular Therapeutics*, *3*(3), 295–302.

Solowey, E., Lichtenstein, M., Sallon, S., Paavilainen, H., Solowey, E., & Lorberboum-Galski, H. (2014). Evaluating medicinal plants for anticancer activity. *Scientific World Journal*, *2014*, 721402.

Somasundaram, S., Edmund, N. A., Moore, D. T., Small, G. W., Shi, Y. Y., & Orlowski, R. Z. (2002). Dietary curcumin inhibits chemotherapy-induced apoptosis in models of human breast cancer. *Cancer Research*, *62*(13), 3868–3875.

Suganya, A. M., Sanjivkumar, M., Chandran, M. N., Palavesam, A., & Immanuel, G. (2016). Pharmacological importance of sulphated polysaccharide carrageenan from red seaweed *Kappaphycus alvarezii* in comparison with commercial carrageenan. *Biomedicine & Pharmacotherapy*, *84*, 1300–1312.

Suhail, M. M., Wu, W., Cao, A., Mondalek, F. G., Fung, K.-M., Shih, P.-T., Fang, Y.-T., Woolley, C., Young, G., & Lin, H.-K. (2011). *Boswellia sacra* essential oil induces tumor cell-specific apoptosis and suppresses tumor aggressiveness in cultured human breast cancer cells. *BMC Complementary and Alternative Medicine*, *11*(1), 129.

Suhitha, S., Devi, S. K., Gunasekaran, K., Carehome Pakyntein, H., Bhattacharjee, A., & Velmurugan, D. (2015). Phytochemical analyses and activity of herbal medicinal plants of north-east India for anti-diabetic, anti-cancer and anti-tuberculosis and their docking studies. *Current topics in medicinal chemistry*, *15*(1), 21–36.

Takahashi, K., Hosokawa, M., Kasajima, H., Hatanaka, K., Kudo, K., Shimoyama, N., & Miyashita, K. (2015). Anticancer effects of fucoxanthin and fucoxanthinol on colorectal cancer cell lines and colorectal cancer tissues. *Oncology Letters*, *10*(3), 1463–1467.

Tamura, S., Narita, T., Fujii, G., Miyamoto, S., Hamoya, T., Kurokawa, Y., Takahashi, M., Miki, K., Matsuzawa, Y., Komiya, M., Terasaki, M., Yano, T., & Mutoh, M. (2019). Inhibition of NF-Kappa B transcriptional activity enhances fucoxanthinol-induced apoptosis in colorectal cancer cells. *Genes and Environment*, *41*(1), 1.

Tan, L. T. (2007). Bioactive natural products from marine cyanobacteria for drug discovery. *Phytochemistry*, *68*(7), 954–979.

Teicher, B. A., Korbut, T. T., Menon, K., Holden, S. A., & Ara, G. (1994). Cyclooxygenase and lipoxygenase inhibitors as modulators of cancer therapies. *Cancer Chemotherapy and Pharmacology*, *33*(6), 515–522.

Thyagarajan, A., Jedinak, A., Nguyen, H., Terry, C., Baldridge, L. A., Jiang, J., & Sliva, D. (2010). Triterpenes from *Ganoderma lucidum* induce autophagy in colon cancer through the inhibition of P38 Mitogen-Activated Kinase (P38 MAPK). *Nutrition and Cancer*, *62*(5), 630–640.

Ting, P. T., Kasper, R., & Arlette, J. P. (2005). Metastatic basal cell carcinoma: Report of two cases and literature review. *Journal of Cutaneous Medicine and Surgery*, *9*(1), 10–15.

Velmurugan, D., Kutumbarao, N. H. V., Viswanathan, V., & Bhattacharjee, A. (2019) Structure-based drug design with a special emphasis on herbal extracts. In *Challenges and advances in computational chemistry and physics* (pp. 271–305). Cham: Springer International Publishing.

Vignesh, S., Raja, A., & Arthur Jam, R. (2010). Marine drugs: Implication and future studies. *International Journal of. Pharmacology*, *7*(1), 22–30.

Wangsa, K., Sarma, I., Saikia, P., Ananthakrishnan, D., Sarma, H. N., & Velmurugan, D. (2020). Estrogenic effect of *Scoparia dulcis* (linn) extract in mice uterus and in silico molecular docking studies of certain compounds with human estrogen receptors. *Journal of Reproduction & Infertility*, *21*(4), 247–258.

Williams, D. E., Moore, R. E., & Paul, V. J. (1989). The structure of ulithiacyclamide B. antitumor evaluation of cyclic peptides and macrolides from *Lissoclinum patella*. *Journal of Natural Products*, *52*(4), 732–739.

World Health Organization (WHO). (2018). Latest global cancer data: Cancer burden rises to 18.1 million new cases and 9.6 million cancer deaths in 2018. *International Agency for Research on Cancer*, 263.

Wu, X. S., Xie, T., Lin, J., Fan, H. Z., Huang-Fu, H. J., Ni, L. F., & Yan, H. F. (2009). An investigation of the ability of element to pass through the blood-brain barrier and its effect on brain carcinomas. *Journal of Pharmacy and Pharmacology*, *61*, 1653–1656.

Yan, W., Wistuba, I. I., Emmert-Buck, M. R., & Erickson, H. S. (2011). Squamous cell carcinoma—Similarities and differences among anatomical sites. *American Journal of Cancer Research*, 1, 275–300.

Yurgelun, M. B., Kulke, M. H., Fuchs, C. S., Allen, B. A., Uno, H., Hornick, J. L., Ukaegbu, C. I., Brais, L. K., McNamara, P. G., Mayer, R. J., Schrag, D., Meyerhardt, J. A., Ng, K., Kidd, J., Singh, N., Hartman, A.-R., Wenstrup, R. J., & Syngal, S. (2017). Cancer susceptibility gene mutations in individuals with colorectal cancer. *Journal of Clinical Oncology*, *35*(10), 1086–1095.

Zhang, J., Zheng, Z., Wu, M., Zhang, L., Wang, J., Fu, W., Xu, N., Zhao, Z., Lao, Y., & Xu, H. (2019). The natural compound neobractatin inhibits tumor metastasis by up regulating the RNA-binding-protein MBNL2. *Cell Death and Disease*, *10*(8), 554.

Zhang, W., Lan, Y., Huang, Q., & Hua, Z. (2013). Galangin induces B16F10 melanoma cell apoptosis via mitochondrial pathway and sustained activation of P38 MAPK. *Cytotechnology*, *65*(3), 447–455.

Zhang, Y., Zhou, T., Wang, H., Cui, Z., Cheng, F., & Wang, K. P. (2016). Structural characterization and in vitro antitumor activity of an acidic polysaccharide from *Angelica sinensis* (Oliv.) Diels. *Carbohydrate Polymers*, *147*, 401–408.

Zhou, G.-X., Ding, X.-L., Huang, J.-F., Zhang, H., Wu, S.-B., Cheng, J.-P., & Wei, Q. (2008). Apoptosis of human pancreatic cancer cells induced by triptolide. *World Journal of Gastroenterology*, *14*(10), 1504–1509.

Zhu, Y., & Liao, L. (2015). Applications of nanoparticles for anticancer drug delivery: A review. *Journal of Nanoscience and Nanotechnology*, *15*(7), 4753–4773.

Zhuang, C., Itoh, H., Mizuno, T., & Ito, H. (1995). Antitumor active fucoidan from the brown seaweed, Umitoranoo (*Sargassum thunbergii*). *Bioscience, Biotechnology, and Biochemistry*, *59*(4), 563–567.

https://doi.org/10.1142/9789811254796_0011

11 Missense Mutations in Fumarate Hydratase Leading to Cancer: Molecular Modeling and Molecular Dynamics Simulations of the Mutants

S. Subasri[†], Santosh Kumar Chaudhary[‡], Manish Kesharwani[†], K. Sekar[§] and D. Velmurugan[*,¶]

[†]*Centre of Advanced Studies in Crystallography and Biophysics, University of Madras, Chennai 600 025, India*
[‡]*Department of Physics, Indian Institute of Science, Bangalore 560012, India*
[§]*Department of Computational and Data Sciences, Indian Institute of Science, Bangalore 560012, India*
[¶]*Office of the Dean Sponsored Research, Publications and Collaborations, AMET University, Kanathur, ECR Road, Chennai, P.C.-603 112*

Abstract

Mutations in fumarase hydratase (FH) which affect the hydrogen bond interactions with active site residues lead to multiple cutaneous and uterine leiomyomatosis and hereditary leiomyomatosis and renal cell cancer(RCC). R233 mutation is reported as the most commonly described FH mutation and it has been associated with RCC. This negative dominant mutation might affect the

*Corresponding author: e-mail: shirai2011@gmail.com

active site without affecting the overall three-dimensional structure, or could exhibit effects on the overall structure resulting in misfolding. Modeling studies carried out with R233H mutation showed the loss of interaction with E355. Also, the K230R mutation leads to the loss of interaction with E355. E355K mutation is found to lead to the loss of interaction with K230 and R233. Molecular dynamics simulations studies show that the mutation in R233 to H233 causes loss of structural integrity in the active site of FH structure.

1. Introduction

FH gene encodes for fumarate hydratase or fumarase (EC: 4.2.1.2) is a housekeeping gene which encodes the Kreb's cycle proteins involved in the fundamental process of energy production and can act as tumor suppressor (King *et al.*, 2006). There are three forms of fumarases, namely, fumarase A, B, and C (Fum C). Depending on its relative subunit arrangement, metal requirement, and thermal stability, each fumarase has been classified as either class I or class II. Fum C belongs to the class II-type fumarases, which are iron-independent, thermally stable, and tetrameric enzymes of 200 kDa, harboring three distinct segments of amino acids with significant homology. There are two types of fumarase found within human tissues, cytosolic and mitochondrial, and both share sequence identity to Fum C from *Escherichia coli* (Woods *et al.*, 1986). Whereas the mitochondrial enzyme is a part of the TCA cycle, the cytosolic form is thought to be involved in amino acid metabolism. Through amino acid sequence homology, fumarase is found to belong to a family of enzymes that includes aspartase, arginosuccinatelyase, adinylosuccinatlyase, and δ-crystalline (Stone *et al.*, 1993; Williams *et al.*, 1992; Woods *et al.*, 1988). The catalytic reaction scheme for conversion of fumarate to malate by fumarase is well known (Weaver *et al.*, 1997). The first class II fumarase enzyme to be solved was Fum C and its active site was shown to harbor many of the amino acids within the three highly conserved regions (Weaver *et al.*, 1995). In particular, homology

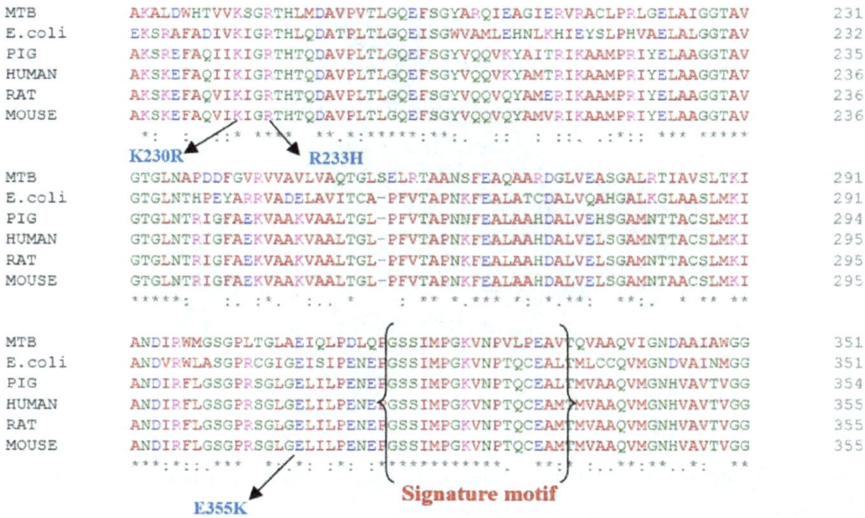

Fig. 1 A portion of the multiple sequence alignment of various fumarate hydratases from different sources.

between Gly 317 through Glu 331 within the third region has provided a signature sequence motif, which defines not only the class II fumarase family, but also the other superfamily of proteins. The signature sequence (GSSxMPxKxNPxxxE) lying between Gly 317 and Glu 331 has provided a means to establish an evolutionary link between a broad superfamily of proteins (**Fig. 1**). Although the family members share high sequence identity within the signature motif region, other segments are less well conserved (Estévez *et al.*, 2002).

The FH protein was found to be highly conserved (47.3% identical, 18.2% conserved, and 9.0% similar). The higher levels of conservation correspond to residues that formed the enzyme's active site or activation site or those that were involved in protein loops with important roles in folding and tertiary structure (Tomlinson *et al.*, 2002). The FH enzyme functions as a homotetramer, consisting of four identical subunits of 50 kDa. Each subunit consists of three domains: An N-terminal domain (residues 49–185), a large central α-helical domain (residues 186–441), and C-terminal domain (residues 442–510). In the tetrameric fumarase, the

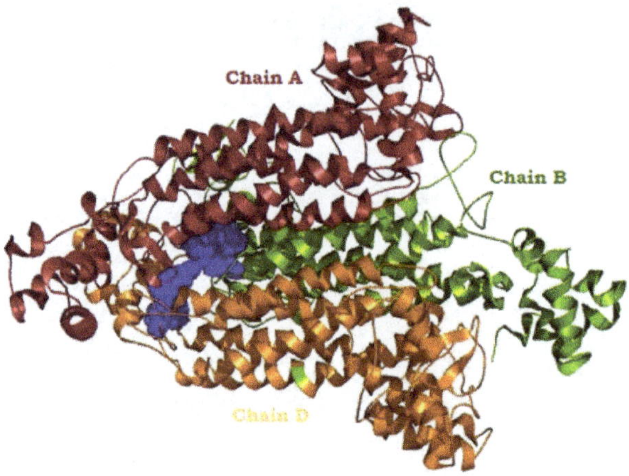

Fig. 2 The active site formed by three subunits of fumarate hydratase (highlighted in blue color).

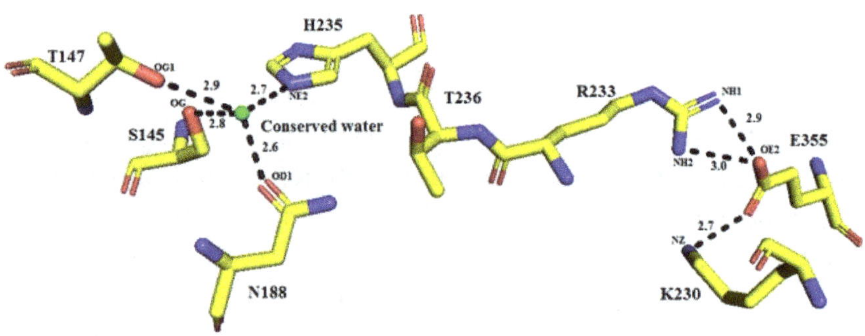

Fig. 3 Conserved water coordinations with active site residues stabilized by the interaction of R233, K230, and E355 residues. It is indicated in sphere shape with green color. The distances (in Å) with atom name are also labeled.

"active site" is formed by the three segments, one from each of the three subunits, as shown in **Fig. 2**. The highly conserved water molecule is present in the active site and it is located in a deep pit on the surface (Subasri *et al.*, 2017), as shown in **Fig. 3**.

Germline mutations in the fumarase (FH) gene are associated with two distinct types. Homozygous FH mutation can cause the FH deficiency (OMIM 606812) characterized by growth and developmental delay and severe neurological impairment, whereas heterozygous FH mutations are known to be involved in the autosomal dominant syndrome of multiple cutaneous and uterine leiomyomata (MCUL) or Reed syndrome (Tomlinson *et al.*, 2002). Missense mutations occurred mostly at evolutionarily conserved residues. Affected individuals develop benign smooth muscle tumors of the skin and females develop fibroids of the uterus. The loss of heterozygosity leads to the loss of the wild-type allele in cutaneous, uterine and renal tumors and the enzyme activity of FH is low or absent in tumors from individuals with leiomyomas. When coexisting with an aggressive form of renal cell carcinoma (papillary renal type II cancer or renal collecting duct cancer), it is also known as hereditary leiomyomatosis and renal cell cancer (HLRCC) (OMIM 605839) (Pithukpakorn *et al.*, 2006). There are many case studies which reported that the mutation on the FH can cause MCUL and HLRCC (Alam *et al.*, 2005; Kuwada *et al.*, 2014; Tolvanen *et al.*, 2012; Toro *et al.*, 2003). Both are frequently present with metastatic disease before the age of 50 and are associated with high mortality rate. Table 1 shows the selective mutations observed in the human fumarase gene and association to MCUL, RCC, and HLRCC diseases (Picaud *et al.*, 2011).

Deficiency or mutation in FH activity causes an impaired energy production by interrupting the flow of metabolites through the Kreb's cycle. Biochemical studies have shown that FH-deficient cells and tumors accumulate fumarate and succinate, while SDH-deficient tumors mainly accumulate succinate (Isaacs *et al.*, 2005). Accumulation of these metabolic intermediates may affect other biochemical processes in the cell and considerable evidence indicates that the inhibition of hypoxia-inducible factor (HIF) prolyl-hydroxylase leads to the overexpression of the transcription factor, HIF1α, resulting in accumulation of HIF. With increased HIF1α levels, HIF target genes such as VEGF and GLUT1 are transcriptionally activated, providing increased vasculature and glucose transport for this glucose-dependent FH-deficient tumor (Selak *et al.*, 2005).

Table 1 Various missense mutations resulting in MCUL, RCC, and HLRCC diseases.

Mutation site	Conservation	Localization	Phenotype
R101P	Semi-conserved	Surface	HLRCC
N107T	Conserved	Active site	MCUL
A117P	Semi-conserved	Near active site	MCUL
L132S	Semi-conserved	Surface	HLRCC
H135R	Semi-conserved	Surface	MCUL
Q142K	Conserved	Near active site	MCUL
S158I	Semi-conserved	Near active site	MCUL
R160G	Conserved	Surface	MCUL
P174R	Not conserved	Active site	MCUL
H180R	Semi-conserved	Active site	MCUL
Q185R	Conserved	Active site	MCUL
S187L	Conserved	Active site	MCUL
N188S	Conserved	Active site	MCUL
P192L	Conserved	Active site	MCUL
M195T	Conserved	In core helice	MCUL
H196R	Conserved	In core helice	RCC
K230R	Conserved	Subunit stabilization	MCUL
R233C	Conserved	Active site	MCUL, HLRCC
R233H	Conserved	Active site	MCUL, HLRCC
R233L	Conserved	Active site	MCUL
G282V	Conserved	Active site	MCUL
P192L	Conserved	Active site	MCUL
M195T	Conserved	In core helice	MCUL
N310Y	Conserved	Surface	MCUL
H318L	Semi-conserved	Surface	HLRCC
V322D	Conserved	In core helice	MCUL
C333Y	Semi-conserved	In core helice	MCUL
L335P	Conserved	In core helice	MCUL
N340K	Semi-conserved	In core helice	MCUL
E355K	Conserved	Subunit stabilization	MCUL

(Continued)

Table 1 (*Continued*)

Mutation site	Conservation	Localization	Phenotype
N361K	Conserved	Active site	HLRCC
S365G	Conserved	Active site	MCUL
S366N	Conserved	Active site	MCUL
M368T	Conserved	Active site	MCUL
N373S	Conserved	Active site	HLRCC
A385D	Not-conserved	Active site	MCUL
V394L	Not-conserved	In core helice	MCUL
G397R	Semi-conserved	In core helice	MCUL
S419P	Conserved	In core helice	MCUL
Q439P	Not-conserved	Surface	HLRCC
Y465C	Semi-conserved	Surface	MCUL
L507P	Semi-conserved	Surface near opening active site	MCUL

Abbreviations: HLRCC: Hereditary leiomyomatosis and renal cell cancer; MCUL: Multiple cutaneous and uterine leiomyomatosis; RCC: Renal cell carcinoma. Amino acid numbering is based on the mitochondrial FH.

One of the most commonly described FH mutation is R233 and it has been associated with RCC and among the base substitutions reported, the c.569G>A transversion is the most frequent (Alam *et al.*, 2005; Toro *et al.*, 2003) and gives rise to the arginine to histidine amino acid change. This residue is located near the catalytic site and adjacent to the K230; both residues are involved in the charge–charge interaction with E355, thought to greatly stabilize one of the active sites (Alam *et al.*, 2003). The dominant negative action of the R233H mutation has recently been demonstrated to occur in patients suffering from RCC (Lorenzato *et al.*, 2008). This negative dominant mutation might affect the active site without affecting the overall structure, or could exhibit effects on the overall structure resulting in misfolding. Modeling studies of three mutant forms of FH (R233H, K230R, and E355K) are carried out and further molecular dynamics (MD) simulations studies have also been carried out for the above cases to understand the conformational changes due to single point mutation of human FH structure.

2. Materials and Methods

2.1. Target Preparation

The crystal structure of human fumarate hydratase at the resolution of 1.95 Å (PDB ID-3E04; Toro *et al.*, 2003) was downloaded from Protein Data Bank (PDB). The protein was prepared by removing water molecules, stabilizing the charges and fixing the missing residues and side chains by the prime module (Schrödinger, 2009). Energy minimization of the protein was carried out using protein preparation wizard, where addition of H atoms, adjusting bond order, and further energy minimization were carried out using optimized potentials for liquid simulations (OPLS) 2005 force field (Jorgensen *et al.*, 1983) with root mean square deviation (RMSD) of not more than 0.3 Å. The respective residues (K230, R233, and E355) were mutated and the energy was minimized.

2.2. MD Simulations

MD simulations were carried out for wild-type FH and single mutant structures (R233H, K230R, and E355K) with (NAnoscale MD) NAMD (Phillips *et al.*, 2005), and trajectories were analyzed using Amber 12 (Case *et al.*, 2005) to determine the conformational changes upon mutation. Crystal structure of human fumarate hydratase was systematically prepared by using tleap module of Amber 12 suit. Molecular mechanics force field ff99sb (Lindorff-Larsen *et al.*, 2010) Amber was used to parameterize amino acids of protein; antechamber module was used to obtain the charges of ligand and were parameterized by using generalized amber force field for system preparation and simulations (Duan *et al.*, 2003; Ponder & Case, 2003). The protein was solvated in a cubic TIP3P (Mark & Nilsson, 2001) box of three-point charged water molecule at 10 Å marginal radius. Following the solvation, charge neutralization was carried out by the addition of Na^+ and Cl^- ions. Initially, the solvent molecules were relaxed while all the solute atoms and calcium ion were harmonically restrained to their original position with a force constant of 100 kcal/mol Å^2. The water molecules were relaxed by 5000 steps of steepest descent algorithm and 2000 cycles of conjugate gradient algorithm. Finally, minimization was carried out for 2500 iterations by conjugate gradient without restraints for the whole box. The structure was analyzed for its stability and potential energy after the completion of the run.

Before the simulations, the system was equilibrated in three phases with 2 fs time integration step. Berendsen temperature coupling method (Berendsen *et al.*, 1984) was used to regulate the temperature and pressure at 300 K and 1 atm, respectively, inside the box with time constant of 2 ps in first phase. Electrostatic interactions were computed using the Particle Mesh Ewald method (Cheatham *et al.*, 1995). In the second phase, isotropic position scaling and constant pressure were provided to the system. In these two stages, all non-solvent atoms were restrained. Finally, equilibration was extended at constant temperature and pressure without restraints. Consequently, simulations were performed in explicit solvent environment using NPT ensemble with 1 ps integration time step. SHAKE algorithm (Ryckaert *et al.*, 1977) was used to constrain the bonds involving hydrogen atoms. The initial velocities were assigned from a Maxwell distribution at a given temperature. Finally, MD simulations for 50 ns each were carried out using CRAY supercomputer, at Indian Institute of Science, Bangalore. Potential energy of each system was validated by equilibration and simulations processes. The simulated trajectory files were saved at every picosecond for analysis. Trajectories were used for the analysis of RMSD, root mean square residual fluctuation (RMSF), radius of gyration (Rg), and distance calculations.

3. Results and Discussion

In Fumarate Hydratase crystal structure, R233 is located near the catalytic site and adjacent to the K230; both residues are involved in the charge–charge interaction with E355, thought to greatly stabilize one of the active sites. **Figure 4a** shows the involvement of K230 and R233 residues in charge–charge interaction with E355.

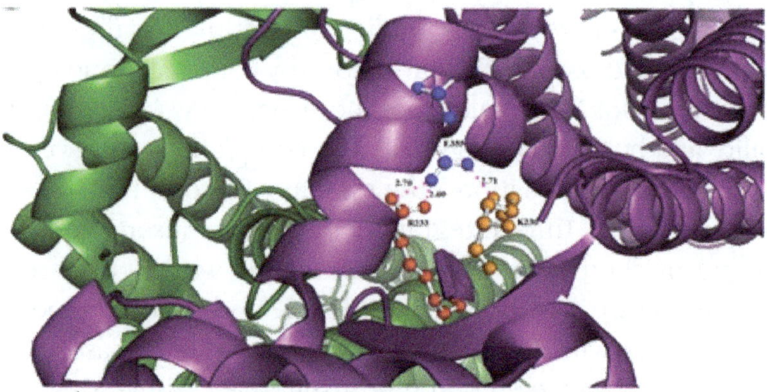

(a)

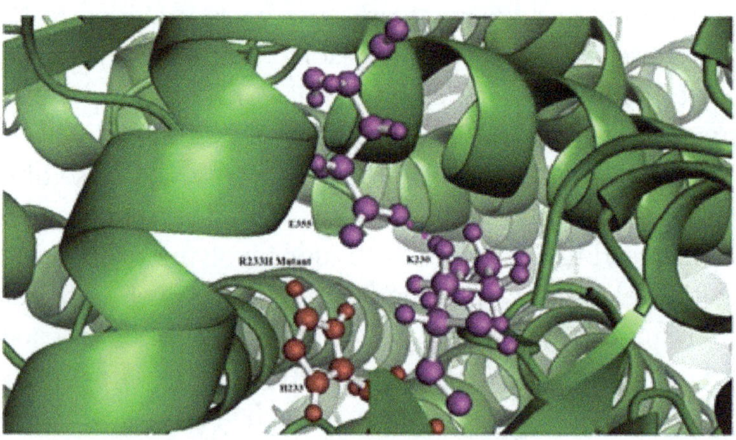

(b)

Fig. 4 (a) Active site stabilizing region. The residues K230 (orange) and R233 (red) are involved in the interaction with E355 (blue) at a distance of 2.7 Å. (b) R233H mutant FH mutant (maroon) leads to the loss of E355 (purple) interaction. The side chains of K230, R233, and E355 are shown as ball and stick model for a clear representation.

FH structure energy was minimized and the potential energy was −3,72,169 kcal/mol. In this chapter, FH mutant structures such as R233H, K230R, and E355K were modeled by mutating the respective residues in wild-type crystal structure of fumarate hydratase using Schrödinger suit followed by energy minimization using OPLS 2005 force field. Energetically optimized mutant structures were analyzed and compared with wild-type FH.

In the initial analysis, the mutation of R233 residue to His led to the loss of interaction with E355 as shown in **Fig. 4b**. But it maintains the interaction with K230 residue. K230R mutation leads to the loss of interaction with E355 (**Fig. 5a**) and R233 residue maintains its interaction with E355. E355K mutation is found to lead to the loss of interaction with both K230 and R233 residues (**Fig 5b**). Final potential energy was found to be −3,70,964 kcal/mol when R233 is mutated to His which is less stable than the other two mutants suggesting that R233 residue is important for stabilizing the active site by interacting with K230 and E355. E355K mutant has the potential energy of −3,71,424 kcal/mol which is less compared with R233H mutant and more compared with K230R. The potential energy of K230R mutant was −3,72,170 kcal/mol which is similar to wild-type FH suggesting stable conformation.

RMSD was calculated for the residues around 12 Å radius from the active site of the wild-type and the three mutants. The superposition of the wild-type and R233H mutant FH is shown in **Fig. 6a**, and the RMSD is found to be 1.28 Å. The superposition of the wild-type and K230R FH mutant is shown in **Fig. 6b**, and the RMSD is found to be 1.04 Å. When superposing the two mutant structures (R233H and K230R) RMSD is 1.1 Å, suggesting less deviation. When superposing the wild-type and E355K mutant FH structures (**Fig. 6c**), the RMSD is found to be 0.44 Å. The superposition of the two mutants R233H and E355K showed an RMSD of 0.25 Å, and that of E355K and K230R showed an RMSD of 0.22 Å suggesting less deviation (Table 2). Furthermore, to confirm the above phenomenon, MD simulations studies were carried out.

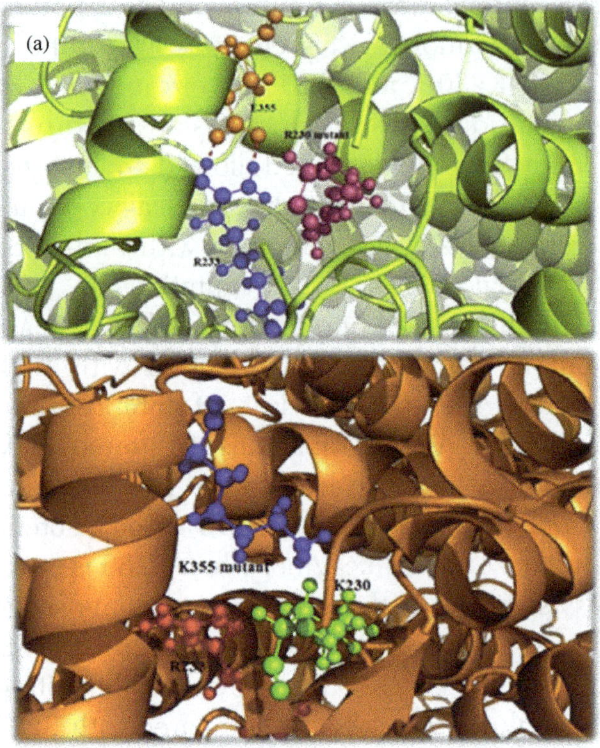

(b)

Fig. 5 (a) K230R mutant (pink) leads to the loss of E355 (orange) interaction. (b) E355K mutant (blue) leads to the loss of K230 (green) and R233 (red) interactions. The side chains of K230, R233, and E355 are shown as ball and stick model for a clear representation.

Table 2 RMSD for the wild-type and mutant FH structures after MD simulations.

Protein	RMSD (Ǎ)
Wild vs R233H mutant	1.28
Wild vs K230R mutant	1.04
Wild vs E355K mutant	1.12

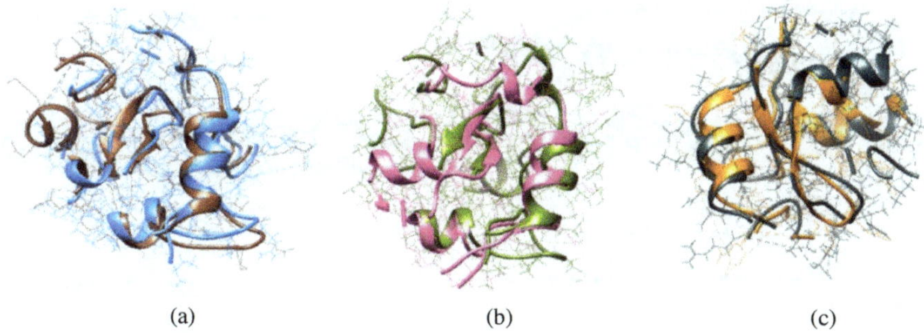

Fig. 6 Superposition of (a) wild-type FH (brown) and R233H mutant FH (blue), (b) wild-type FH (Pink) and K230R mutant FH (green), and (c) wild-type FH (orange) and E355K mutant FH (dark gray).

3.1. MD Simulations of Wild-type FH and Three Mutant Forms of FH

MD simulations were carried out for the wild-type FH and the three mutant FH structures for calculating the RMSD and RMSF. Rg calculation was also carried out to understand the conformational changes that have occurred in all the forms of mutants and wild-type FH structure. Distances for pair of atoms (R233, K230, and E355) between the two residues were calculated to inspect the stability of the structure as a function of simulation time. The stability of each system was confirmed through reasonable RMS fluctuations in kinetic and total energies and correlation between potential energy and temperature.

3.2. Conformational Stability Analysis of Wild-type and Mutant forms of FH

The conformational changes in human FH with respect to the single mutations were examined using RMSD. RMSD was calculated and represented for each subunit in all the three forms of the

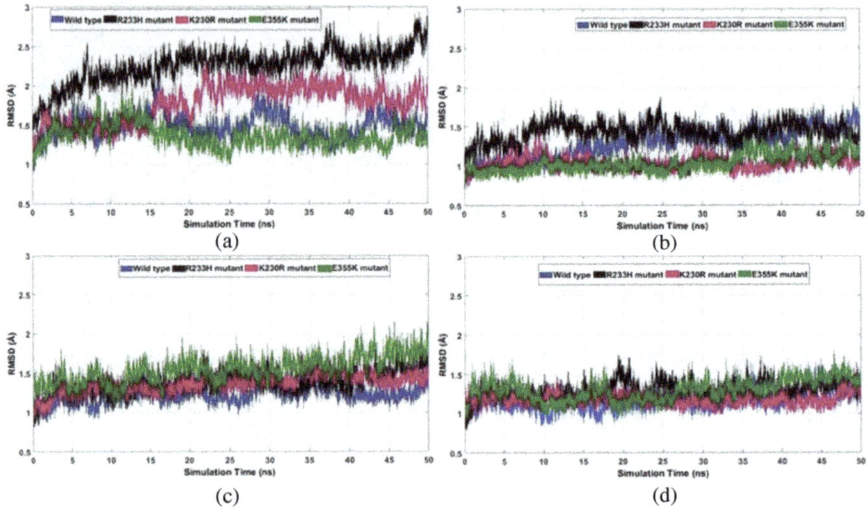

Fig. 7 Variation of RMSD of the backbone atoms of fumarate hydratases with simulations time: RMSD of (a) subunit A, (b) subunit B, (c) subunit C, and (d) subunit D.

mutant and the wild-type FH. In A chain, R233H mutant deviates more initially and at the end of simulations it results in final backbone RMSD of 2.0–2.8 Å, greater than that of the other two mutants. Beyond 18 ns, K230R mutant starts to have more RMSD than the wild-type and E355K mutant.

Wild-type and E355K mutant structures of FH deviate less and it indicates that these systems attained steady state at the end of each simulation as shown in **Fig. 7a**. Beyond 15 ns simulations, E355K mutant FH structure has less RMSD (better than the wild type) up to the end of simulations. **Figure 7b** shows the RMSD for B chain corresponding to wild type and the three FH mutants. It can be seen from the figure that the RMSD variation is maximum for E355K mutant. The deviation of R233H and K230R mutants more or less vary in the same fashion and this variation is lesser than that of E355K mutant and greater than that of the wild type. Variation of RMSD shows that the wild type has the least variation compared to all the three mutants. In subunit C,

R233H mutant deviates more than the other two mutants and the wild type also deviates more than the K230R and E355K mutants, which results in the back bone RMSD of 2.0 Å at the end of simulations as shown in **Fig. 7c**.

In subunit D, variation of RMSD in E355K mutant resembles a wave motion and has maximum followed minimum and again maximum and minimum and so on. E355K mutant loses its stability and deviates more than the R233H FH mutant at the end of simulations. R233H mutant has more variations in RMSD than the K230R mutant and the wild type. Wild type and K230R mutant maintain more or less the same variation as shown in **Fig. 7d**. The comparison of RMSD for the overall FH structure is shown in **Fig. 8a**. The variation of R233H mutant is more compared to wild type and the other two mutants, and R233H mutant structure loses its conformational stability. Even though the RMSD for K230R is lesser than E355K mutant up to 20 ns, beyond that RMSD variation of K230R is more than that of E355K mutant up to 35 ns and there after it is on par with the E355K mutant.

Conformational analysis of MD simulations shows the compactness of the systems through calculation of Rg as shown in **Fig. 8b**. Rg signifies the moment of inertia of atoms from their center of mass. It indicates that the wild type and K230R mutant retained compactness than the other three mutants. As shown in the figure, E355K and R233H mutants are found to have more deviation confirming that there is a major effect on the protein folding in FH structure due to point mutations.

The conformational stability of all the fumarate hydratases was characterized by their respective RMSF values by calculating the fluctuation of Cα atoms (around its average position) for each residue. The larger RMSF value indicates more flexibility while the smaller RMSF values suggest more stable/constrained region.

As discussed in the introduction, active site is formed with three subunits (subunit A, B, and D), RMSF was calculated only for the residues around 12Å radius from the active site in the three

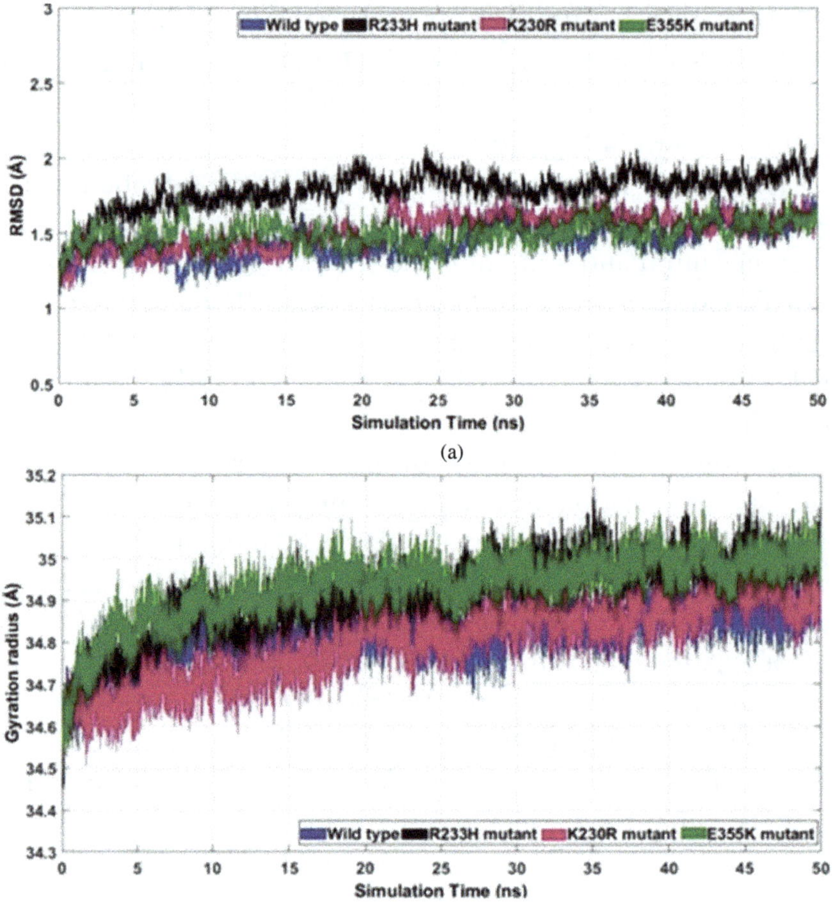

(a)

(b)

Fig. 8 (a) Variation of RMSD of the backbone atoms of overall FH structures with simulations time. (b) Variation of radius of gyration for FH structures with simulations time.

subunits. The active site residues are 145, 147, and 188 from subunit A, 362–368 and 372–375 from subunit B, and H235 from subunit D. **Figure 9a** depicts RMSF of the residues of subunit A and it shows that R233H mutant fluctuates more than the E355K and K230R mutants. Around residue 275, E355K mutant is found to have more RMSF. Wild-type FH is found to be more stable than all mutants and maintains less fluctuation. Residues 145, 147, and

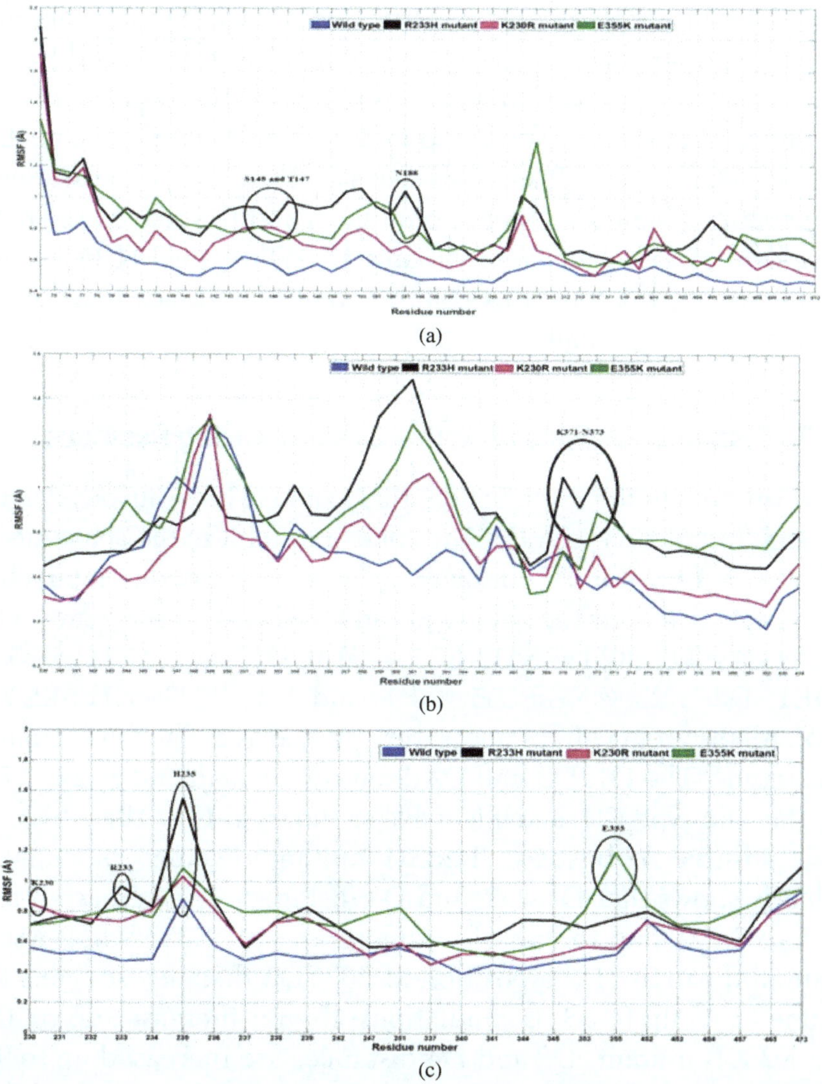

Fig. 9 Residual fluctuations around 12 Å radius from the active site in three subunits of fumarate hydratase: RMSF of (a) subunit A residues, (b) subunit B residues, and (c) subunit D residues.

188 fluctuate more in all forms of mutants, particularly in R233H mutant. In subunit B, R233H mutant fluctuates more in the region 365–368 and in 372–375 confirming that conformational changes have occurred. RMSF of wild-type FH and the three FH mutants

are shown in **Fig. 9b and c** shows RMSF of D subunit, the residues 233, 230, 235, and 355 fluctuate more in R233H and E355K mutants than in the K230R mutant. But, at the position of 355, more fluctuation was found up to 1.35 Å in E355K mutant than the R233H mutant. It suggests that E355K mutation causes more fluctuations than the other two mutants and this may cause more conformational changes in subunit D. Wild-type FH still maintains less fluctuations; this confirms that it becomes more stable than the three mutants.

3.3. Distance Analysis of Active Site Stabilizing Residues

As discussed in the introduction, R233 and K230 are involved in the charge interaction with E355 residue and stabilize the active site as shown in **Fig. 4a**. The distances of each non-bonded interaction were calculated for the wild-type and three mutant structures. Distances are D1: R233@NH2-E355@OE2, D2: R233@NH1-E355@OE1, D3: K230@NZ-E355@OE1, and D4: R233@NH2-K230@NZ. All the atom pair distances were plotted as a function of simulations time. The D1, D2, and D3 distances are in the range 2.6–4.5 Å in the wild-type FH, and it is stable as shown in **Fig. 10a**.

Figure 10b shows R233H mutant distance plot and it clearly shows that D1, D2, and D4 distances are increased from 4.5 to 7.5 Å due to loss of interactions with E355 when Arg is mutated to His at the position of 233. D3 distance remains the same (3 Å) up to 38 ns simulations; then it increases up to 4 Å. In K230R mutant, D3 and D4 distances are increased up to 9 Å due to mutation, D1 and D2 distances remain less (2.8 and 5 Å) and are shown in **Fig. 10c**. D1, D2, and D3 distances increased in E355K mutant up to 12.5, 11.8, and 8.8 Å, respectively, due to mutation of Glu to Lys at 355 positions. Distance plot indicates that there was loss of interactions due to mutations. Mutation of E355K confirms the unfavorable nature of the active site region

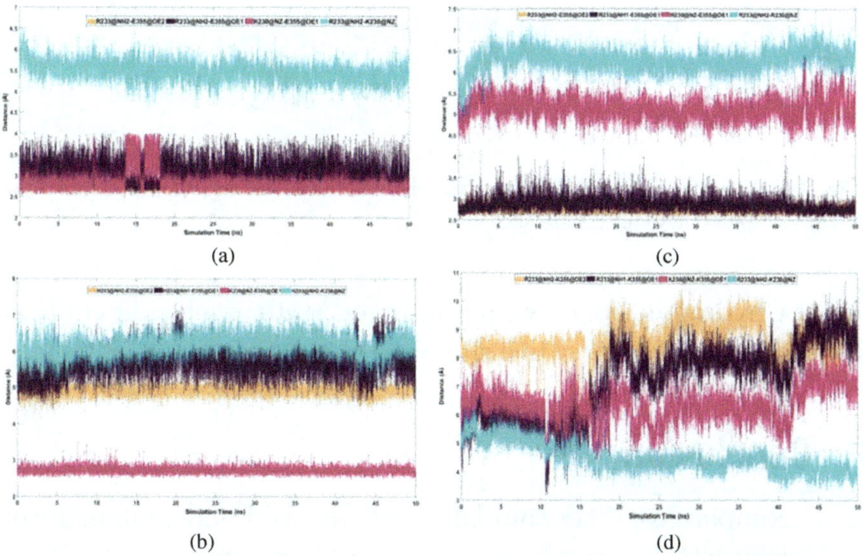

Fig. 10 Distance plot of FH structure during simulations time: (a) Wild-type FH, (b) R233H mutant of FH, (c) K230R mutant of FH, and (d) E355K mutant of FH.

due to breaking of the hydrogen bonds with K230 and R233 as shown in **Fig. 10d**.

As discussed in the introduction, the three residues R233, K230, and E355 are facilitating to stabilize the active site of FH by having the charge–charge interactions (**Fig. 3**). Due to single point mutation on these three residues, the active site is destabilized as shown in **Fig. 11**. In the case of R233H, distances of conserved water with T147, N188, and H235 residues increased to 4.7, 5.0, and 4.0 Å, respectively, as shown in **Fig. 11a**. In K230R mutation, distance of water with N188 and H235 residues is also increased to 4.3 and 4.5 Å, respectively, as shown in **Fig. 11b**. Two other coordinations (S145 and T147) are maintained as the same. **Figure 11c** shows E355K mutation; the distance of conserved water with N188 and H235 residues is 4.4 and 4.5 Å, respectively, but S145 distance is decreased to 1.9 Å. The result shows that the

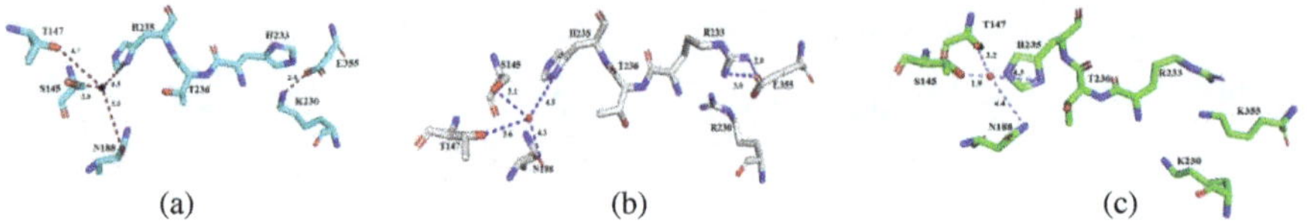

Fig. 11 Destabilization of the active site due to mutations: (a) R233H mutation, (b) K230R mutation, and (c) E355K mutation.

loss of hydrogen bonds with conserved water molecule confirms the destabilization of active site of FH.

4. Conclusion

This comparative MD simulation of the wild and mutant forms of human FH reveal their common and distinctive structural features. The results of MD simulations clearly indicate that R233H mutant structure is the least stable, and it undergoes conformational changes compared with that of the wild-type structure which has the best stability and the other two mutant structures which are less stable. Clinical studies indicate that among the patients with MCUL/HLRCC, R233H mutant was observed commonly. This correlation signifies that the breaking of the stability of the wild-type structure by the mutation of R233 (Arg) to His cause's loss of structural integrity at the active site. This mutation affects the conversion of fumarate to malate leading to the accumulation of fumarate which is the main cause of MCUL and HLRCC. Further experimental analysis is needed for the confirmation of the above phenomenon as the clinical data come from a smaller number of patients.

The MD simulations suggest that E355K mutation causes more fluctuation than the other two mutants R233H and K230R and this may lead to more conformational changes in subunit D. The wild-type mutant has the least fluctuation suggesting its more stable nature. RMSD calculations for the wild-type FH with each of the three mutants show that in case of K230R mutant, it has the least value and the maximum value for R233H mutant. Water hydrogen bonds with active site residues before and after mutation show that out of four water hydrogen bonds in the wild type, 2–3 hydrogen bonds are lost in the case of mutants.

References

Alam, N., Rowan, A., Wortham, N., Pollard, P., Mitchell, M., Tyrer, J., Adams, S. J., *et al.* (2003). Genetic and functional analyses of FH mutations in multiple cutaneous and uterine leiomyomatosis, hereditary leiomyomatosis and renal cancer, and fumarate hydratase deficiency. *Human Molecular Genetics*, *12*(11), 1241–1252.

Alam, N. A., Olpin, S., Rowan, A., Kelsell, D., Leigh, I. M., Tomlinson, I. P., & Weaver, T. (2005). Missense mutations in fumarate hydratase in multiple cutaneous and uterine leiomyomatosis and renal cell cancer. *The Journal of Molecular Diagnostics*, *7*(4), 437–443.

Berendsen, H. J., Postma, J. V., Van Gunsteren, W. F., DiNola, A., & Haak, J. (1984). Molecular dynamics with coupling to an external bath. *The Journal of Chemical Physics*, *81*(8), 3684–3690.

Case, D. A., Cheatham, T. E., Darden, T., Gohlke, H., Luo, R., Merz, K. M., & Woods, R. J. (2005). The Amber biomolecular simulations programs. *Journal of Computational Chemistry*, *26*(16), 1668–1688.

Cheatham, T. I., Miller, J., Fox, T., Darden, T., & Kollman, P. (1995). Molecular dynamics simulations on solvated biomolecular systems: The particle mesh Ewald method leads to stable trajectories of DNA, RNA, and proteins. *Journal of the American Chemical Society*, *117*(14), 4193–4194.

Duan, Y., Wu, C., Chowdhury, S., Lee, M. C., Xiong, G., Zhang, W., & Lee, T. A. (2003). Point-charge force field for molecular mechanics simulations of proteins based on condensed-phase quantum mechanical calculations. *Journal of Computational Chemistry*, *24*(16), 1999–2012.

Estévez, M., Skarda, J., Spencer, J., Banaszak, L., & Weaver, T. M. (2002). X-ray crystallographic and kinetic correlation of a clinically observed human fumarase mutation *Protein Science*, *11*(6), 1552–1557.

Isaacs, J. S., Jung, Y. J., Mole, D. R., Lee, S., Torres-Cabala, C., Chung, Y.-L., & Toro, J. (2005). HIF overexpression correlates with biallelic loss of fumarate hydratase in renal cancer: Novel role of fumarate in regulation of HIF stability. *Cancer Cell*, *8*(2), 143–153.

Jorgensen, W. L., Chandrasekhar, J., Madura, J. D., Impey, R. W., & Klein, M. L. (1983). Comparison of simple potential functions for simulating liquid water. *The Journal of Chemical Physics*, *79*(2), 926–935.

King, A., Selak, M., & Gottlieb, E. (2006). Succinate dehydrogenase and fumarate hydratase: Linking mitochondrial dysfunction and cancer. *Oncogene*, *25*(34), 4675–4682.

Kuwada, M., Chihara, Y., Lou, Y., Torimoto, K., Kagebayashi, Y., Tamura, K., & Samma, S. (2014). Novel missense mutation in the FH gene in familial renal cell cancer patients lacking cutaneous leiomyomas. *BMC Research Notes*, *7*(1), 203–208.

Lindorff-Larsen, K., Piana, S., Palmo, K., Maragakis, P., Klepeis, J. L., Dror, R. O., & Shaw, D. E. (2010). Improved side-chain torsion potentials for the Amber ff99SB protein force field. *Proteins*, *78*(8), 1950–1958.

Lorenzato, A., Olivero, M., Perro, M., Brière, J. J., Rustin, P., & Renzo, M. F. D. A. (2009). Cancer-predisposing "hot spot" mutation of the fumarase gene creates a dominant negative protein. *International Journal of Cancer*, *122*(4), 947–951.

Mark, P., & Nilsson, L. (2001). Structure and dynamics of the TIP3P, SPC, and SPC/E water models at 298 K. *Journal of Physical Chemistry A*, *105*(43), 9954–9960.

Phillips, J. C, Braun, R., Wang, W., Gumbart, J., Tajkhorshid, E., Villa, E., & Schulten, K. (2005). Scalable molecular dynamics with NAMD. *Journal of Computational Chemistry*, *26*(16), 1781–1802.

Picaud, S., Kavanagh, K. L., Yue, W. W., Lee, W. H., Muller-Knapp, S., Gileadi, O., & Oppermann, U. (2011). Structural basis of fumarate hydratase deficiency. *Journal of Inherited Metabolic Disease*, *34*(3), 671–676.

Pithukpakorn, M., Wei, M.-H., Toure, O., Steinbach, P. J., Glenn, G. M., Zbar, B., & Toro, J. R. (2006). Fumarate hydratase enzyme activity in lymphoblastoid cells and fibroblasts of individuals in families with hereditary leiomyomatosis and renal cell cancer. *Journal of Medical Genetics*, *43*(9), 755–762.

Ponder, J. W., & Case, D. A. (2003). Force fields for protein simulations. *Advances in Protein Chemistry*, *66*, 27–85.

Ryckaert, J.-P., Ciccotti, G., & Berendsen, H. J. (1977). Numerical integration of the Cartesian equations of motion of a system with constraints: Molecular dynamics of n-alkanes. *Journal of Computational Physics*, *23*(3), 327–341.

Selak, M. A., Armour, S. M., MacKenzie, E. D., Boulahbel, H., Watson, D. G., Mansfield, K. D., & Gottlieb, E. (2005). Succinate links TCA cycle dysfunction to oncogenesis by inhibiting HIF-α prolyl hydroxylase. *Cancer Cell*, *7*(1), 77–85.

Schrödinger, L. (2009). *Schrödinger Suite 2009*. New York, NY: Schrödinger, LLC.

Stone, R. L., Zalkin, H., & Dixon, J. E. (1993). Expression, purification, and kinetic characterization of recombinant human adenylosuccinate lyase. *Journal of Biological Chemistry*, *268*(26), 19710–19716.

Subasri, S., Chaudhary, S. K., Sekar, K., Manish K., & Velmurugan, D. (2017). Molecular docking and molecular dynamics simulations of fumarate hydratase and its mutant H235N complexed with pyromellitic acid and citrate. *Journal of Bioinformatics and Computational Biology*, *15*(6), 1750026.

Tolvanen, J., Uimari, O., Ryynänen, M., Aaltonen, L. A., & Vahteristo, P. (2012). Strong family history of uterine leiomyomatosis warrants fumarate hydratase mutation screening. *Human Reproduction*, *27*(6), 1865–1869.

Tomlinson, I. P., Alam, N. A., Rowan, A. J., Barclay, E., Jaeger, E. E., Kelsell, D., & Rahman, S. (2002). Germline mutations in FH predispose to dominantly inherited uterine fibroids, skin leiomyomata and papillary renal cell cancer. *Nature Genetics*, *30*(4), 406–410.

Toro, J. R., Nickerson, M. L., Wei, M.-H., Warren, M. B., Glenn, G. M., Turner, M. L., & Sharma, N. (2003). Mutations in the fumarate hydratase gene cause hereditary leiomyomatosis and renal cell cancer in families in North America. *The American Journal of Human Genetics*, *73*(1), 95–106.

Weaver, T., Lees, M., & Banaszak, L. (1997). Mutations of fumarase that distinguish between the active site and a nearby dicarboxylic acid binding site. *Protein Science*, *6*(4), 834–842.

Weaver, T., Levitt, D., Donnelly, M., Stevens, P. W., & Banaszak, L. (1995). The multisubunit active site of fumarase C from *Escherichia coli*. *Nature Structural & Molecular Biology*, *2*(8), 654–662.

Williams, S. E., Woolridge, E. M., Ransom, S. C., Landro, J. A., Babbitt, P. C., & Kozarich, J. W. (1992). 3-Carboxy-cis, cis-muconate lactonizing enzyme from *Pseudomonas putida* is homologous to the class II fumarase family: A new reaction in the evolution of a mechanistic motif. *Biochemistry*, *31*(40), 9768–9776.

Woods, S. A., Miles, J. S., & Guest, J. R. (1988). Sequence homologies between argininosuccinase, aspartase and fumarase: A family of structurally-related enzymes. *FEMS Microbiology Letters*, 51(2–3), 181–186.

Woods, S. A., Miles, J. S., Roberts, R. E., & Guest, J. R. (1986). Structural and functional relationships between fumarase and aspartase. Nucleotide sequences of the fumarase (fum C) and aspartase (asp A) genes of *Escherichia coli* K12. *Biochemical Journal*, *237*(2), 547–557.

https://doi.org/10.1142/9789811254796_0012

12 Analysis of the Secondary Metabolites of *Indigofera Aspalathoides* DC Oil to Control Various Human Ailments

Allwyn Vyas Gopalakrishnan[†], Nagasathiya Krishnan[†], Pinki Kumari Singh[†], Velmurugan Devadasan[‡], Rangasamy Kandasamy[§] and Pachaiappan Raman[*,†]

[†]*Department of Biotechnology, School of Bioengineering, SRM Institute of Science and Technology, Kattankulathur, Chennai 603203, Tamil Nadu, India*
[‡]*Office of the Dean Sponsored Research, Publications and Collaborations, AMET University, Kanathur, ECR Road, Chennai, P.C.-603 112*
[§]*Kongana Vedic Science Academy and Herbal Research Trust, Kavalapatti, Palani 624621, Tamil Nadu, India*

Abstract

About 60% of the world population, the rural population of the developing countries, including the developed countries where there is a domination of modern medicines, uses alternative medicines. Siddha is one among the primary medicinal systems in South India, particularly in Tamil Nadu. Other than emergency

*Corresponding author: e-mail: pachaiar@srmist.edu.in

situations, this system is capable of combating all forms of diseases and is appropriate for the treatment of psoriasis, sexually transmitted diseases, urinary tract infections, liver and gastrointestinal disorders, general weakness, postpartum anemia, diarrhea, inflammation or tumor, and general fever. Thailam is an oil preparation in Siddha medicinal system. Some thailams are prepared in a special process called pudam process. This type of oil is termed as kuzhi thailam. In the present study, Sivanar vembu (*Indigofera aspalathoides* DC) kuzhi thailam which is being used in the treatment of chronic weeping eczema, psoriasis, leprosy, insect bites, leukoderma, boils, and infected wounds, is subjected to GC-MS and LC-MS analyses to investigate its bioactive constituents. This oil was obtained only from *I. aspalathoides* DC. The marketed oil in this name contains three herbs, two herbs in addition to the one used here. The GC-MS analysis revealed that many of the bioactive compounds present in the Sivanar vembu kuzhi thailam are fatty acids. The LC-MS analysis confirms the presence of diterpenes and flavanones. It can be concluded that the reported fatty acids have antibacterial, anti-inflammatory, and immunomodulatory activities, which can validate the significant use of this thailam for various skin diseases. As far as our knowledge is concerned this is the first report about the investigation of bioactive compounds present in the Sivanar vembu (*I. aspalathoides* DC) kuzhi thailam.

1. Introduction

Modern synthetic and chemical medicines are often explored with caution, since they have side effects and the gain of interest in traditional herbs is growing, as they do not exhibit any side effects and are ecofriendly and natural. Therefore, people still choose plant-based natural remedies over synthetic medicines in many parts of the world (Konappa *et al.*, 2020). However, the claim that natural products are safe is a global misconception due to the fact that the evidence indicates otherwise. Since a product is "natural," it does not guarantee that the product is safe. Despite the limited evidence that the herbal products affect adversely less likely than the conventional drugs, the occurrence of side effects by the usage of herbal drugs typically affects a very limited number of people in a milder way (George, 2011).

About 60% of the world population uses alternative medicines which includes the rural population of the developing countries and also some of the developed countries where there is a domination of modern medicines. The history of Indian healthcare system was described in the ancient literature like "Rig Veda" and "Atharvana Veda," which dates back to 5000 years BC. Later, back in the 10th century BC, the use of plants in the healthcare system was highlighted in the literature like "Charaka Samhita" and "Sushruta Samhita." The Indian subcontinent has the largest repository of medicinal plants where 20,000 plants have been recorded. Only about 7,500 plants are used by traditional practitioners for various diseases (Krupa *et al.*, 2019; Pandey *et al.*, 2013). The folk and traditional medicines use around 25,000 ingenious plant-derived formulations, and about 1.5 million practitioners use this healthcare medicinal system in India (Pandey *et al.*, 2008). It is clear that the market for traditional medicines is significantly high. With an annual growth of 14%, the herbal market in India is worth 10 billion rupees and India exports billion rupees worth of herbal products. World Health Organization projected that the current 62-billion-dollar global herbal market will grow up to 5 trillion dollars in 2050. India and China produce more than 70% of the global diversity (Bhardwaj *et al.*, 2018).

1.1. The Siddha System of Medicines

India is renowned for its conventional drug system, which includes Ayurveda, Siddha, and Unani. Siddha is one among the primary medicinal systems in South India, particularly in Tamil Nadu. It is believed that the Siddha system was established in earlier civilization by 18 siddhars, a class of Tamil sages, (Agasthiar, Tirumular, and Bogar being the important ones). Siddha medical system resembles Ayurveda in several respects; it has its own theory and definition, a comprehensive approach, and way of living therapies (Sen & Chakraborty, 2017).

The Materia Medica system of Siddha involves plant extracts, metals/minerals, marine products, and animal products. This system is primarily based upon the relationship between the cosmos and the human body, connecting five fundamental elements such as air, fire, water, earth, and space. Herbs play a significant role in therapeutic applications in both the Ayurvedic and Siddha medicine systems. The use of herb and mineral combinations with arsenic, copper, gold, iron, mercury, and sulfur is extensively described in the siddha system of medicines. Other than emergency situations, this system is capable of combating all forms of diseases, and is appropriate for the treatment of psoriasis, STD, UTIs, liver and gastrointestinal disorders, general weakness, postpartum anemia, diarrhea, inflammation or tumor and general fever, and so on (Yadav *et al.*, 2012). The Siddha medicinal system seeks to establish a person's good health and an inextinguishable prosperous balance of physical, emotional, cultural, and spiritual well-being to facilitate longevity (Parasuraman & Perumal, 2020; Shukla & Saraf, 2011).

1.1.1. *The concept of disease etiology in the Siddha system of medicines*

The humors in the Siddha system of medicines are based on three aspects: "Vatham," "Pitham," and "Kabham," which are involved in development, maintenance, and destruction of physical and emotional health of the human. As long as these humors stay in the ratio of 4:2:1, as they exist, the human body remains in a stable condition; should any disorder happens to this equilibrium, the body enters into a state of disease or death. The "Vatham" represents air and space elements, and is responsible for the motion of mind and the body. It is claimed that "Vatham" controls the motor and sensory activities of the body. The fire element of the body is represented by "Pitham" which controls the chest and abdominal regions and it is involved in the preservation of health maintenance of the normal physiology and body heat. The elements earth and water form "Kabham" dominating neck areas and the head. The strength of the body, endurance, body build, and movements of the joints are responsibilities of this humor. Climatic conditions, environmental factors, food style, physical activities, as well as stress influence the disruption of the above-mentioned equilibrium. In the Siddha system of medicines, the health and curing diseases are highly dependent on diet and lifestyle. There is a list of do's and don'ts in diet to be followed to overcome the diseases, termed as pathya and apathya (Karunamoorthi *et al.*, 2012). For example, as in Ayurveda, the Siddha also evidently advices the patients suffering from various diseases such as psoriasis, vitiligo, eczema, urticaria, anemia, duodenal ulcer, irritable bowel syndrome, and rheumatoid arthritis, to avoid fish. This is due to the fact that the Siddha and Ayurvedic scholars might have had knowledge about the histamine content in the fish. Reduction of histamine content is one of the treatment strategies as the histamine plays an important role in causing or triggering all of the above-mentioned diseases (Aruna *et al.*, 2019).

1.1.2. *Diagnosis in the Siddha system of medicines*

In any system of medicine, diagnosis of the disease is a crucial step before combinations of treatments. In Siddha system of medicines, the diagnosis is based on observation of eight vital factors known as "ashta sthana pariksha," namely, pulse readings, inspection of tongue, sensation of touch, assessment of voice, body color, inspection of eyes, feces, and urine (Guguloth *et al.*, 2017). Examination of the urine is a major diagnostic method in this system. As in all the systems of medicines, in Siddha the frothing of the urine, turbidity, quantity, color, and smell are assessed (Parasuraman & Perumal, 2020; Thas, 2008). Apart from these common urine assessments, another test is also performed in Siddha, the surface tension and spread test of oil in urine. A drop of gingelly oil is put on to the urine in a basin and the color pattern, way of spreading is noted. The mixing, sinking, the rapid spread of the oil into smaller drops, formation of patterns of sword or spear, all indicate a bad prognosis (Guguloth *et al.*, 2017).

1.1.3. *Medication and preparation in the Siddha system of medicines*

The medicines used in Siddha are differentiated according to their taste, characteristics, potency, class, and action. Siddha medicine can be categorized according to the mode of administration as internal medicines and external medicines. The internal medicines which are taken internally via oral administration are again categorized into other 32 on mode of preparation, forms, shelf life, and so on. The external medicines are also categorized into 32, applied as ear, eye, and nasal drops and special leech application procedures (Shukla & Saraf, 2011). Some particular preparatory methods of drugs and therapeutic approaches are the finest and exclusive in the Siddha system of medicines. Siddha literature contains numerous formulations, only very few are recorded and many others are classical and still remain as ancient palm scripts. The mode of treatments and formulations are precise in the Siddha system and are open to modification according to the environmental conditions, lifestyle, body condition, and constituents of an individual. These formulations are natural and contain active ingredients, inert fibers, and residues. In this way they are not extracting the active ingredients and are not drawn to the notion of using drugs as chemicals. In this way the toxins in the drugs can be trapped by fibers and debris and excreted by the system (Rajkumar & Lekha, 2016).

There are six main types of formulations of medical preparations in the Siddha system of medicines. They are as follows:

1. Bhasmam
2. Churnam

3. Kashayam
4. Lehyam
5. Ghritam
6. Thailam

The **bhasmam** or ashes are prepared by conversion of metal and gem into ashes. The herbal extract and metal or gem are homogenized and are calcined to convert the mixture into ashes. This process is a type of converting a material or substance into biocompatible known as bhasmikaran. The objectives of these processes are to purify the drug from toxic substances, modification of any physical undesirable attributes of the drug, and to enhance the therapeutic effect of the drug.

The **churnam** is basically a powder, prepared by making a fine powder out of dried roots or herbs. Only one ingredient is present in a simple churnam and compound churnam will have multiple ingredients. The freshness, careful combination of genuine herbs gives a complete efficacy of churnam.

The **kashayam** is a decoction of multiple herbal plant extracts prepared by boiling in an earthen pot and then evaporated to obtain a concentrate. This concentrate is then strained through sterile cloth before use. The kashayam boosts the immunity of a body and helps in expulsion of digestive wastes.

The **lehyam** is a very concentrated herbal combination with a sugary medium which can be sugar itself, honey, and jaggery in water. It is used for treating respiratory illness and disturbances in digestion. The easy absorption of active ingredients of lehyam starts from the mouth itself.

The **ghritam** is a combination of ghee and herbs or its extract. It can be administered internally as well as externally. The dosage of the internal version is established by the efficiency of digestion of a patient. The ghritam can be used as ointment eternally as directed by the physician.

The **thailam** is an oil preparation in combination with medicines and crude extracts. It can be administered both internally and externally as directed by the physician. For external applications, the oil is warmed and massaged gently and rapid for an effective absorption (Parasuraman & Perumal, 2020).

Some thailams are prepared by a special destructive distillation process called pudam process. In this process, the herbs or the herbal combinations are crushed and filled in a sealed earthen pot. Small holes are perforated at the bottom of this earthen pot and kept in a vessel. The whole setup is then kept into a pit dug on the ground. The exposed part of the pot is then covered with cow dung arranged around it and set on fire. After the required time, it is allowed to cool down and the whole setup is dismantled; the oil recovered from the process is collected in the above-mentioned vessel. This kind of oil prepared by the pudam process is termed as **kuzhi thailam** (Sahayam *et al.*, 2020).

In the present study Sivanar vembu kuzhi thailam, a medicated oil from the single herb *Indigofera aspalathoides* DC was selected. Sivanar vembu kuzhi thailam is used in treatment for many skin diseases such as leukoderma, leprosy, chronic weeping eczema, infected wounds, insect bites and boils which can be used both externally and internally. The internal administration should be as directed by a physician; it has to be noted that the commercial sivenar vembu kuzhi thailam from shops contain three herbs including *I. aspalathoides* DC.

1.2. Sivanar Vembu Kuzhi Thailam

Commercial Sivanar vembu kuzhi thailam sold in shops is a medicated oil prepared with combination of three plant parts by the previously mentioned pudam process. The whole herb of *I. aspalathoides* DC, seeds of *Celastrus paniculatus* Willd, and tuber from *Corallocarpus epigaeus* (Rottler) Hook. f. are used in the preparation. And here we will briefly deal with these three herbs and their phytoconstituents.

Indigofera aspalathoides DC belongs to the Fabaceae family (**Fig. 1a**). It is an under shrub with expanded dense branches and

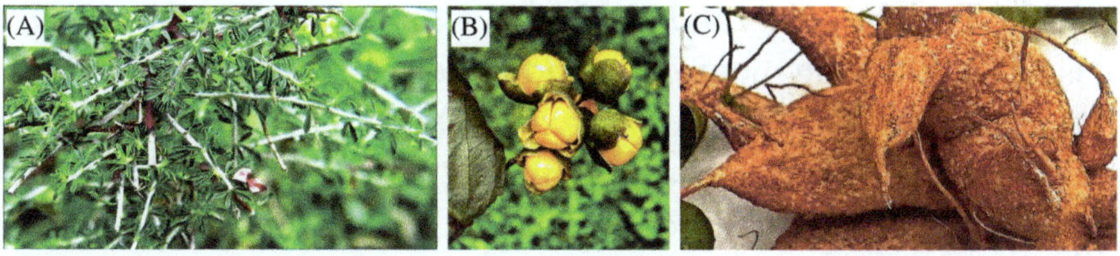

Fig. 1 Plant parts used in Sivanar vembu kuzhi thailam: (a) *Indigofera aspalathoides*, (b) *Celastrus paniculatus*, and (c) *Corallocarpus epigaeus*.

the entire plant is low to the ground (Omprakash *et al.*, 2013). In Ayurveda it is known as Neeli, shivanimba, and so on, and commonly known as Sivanar vembu in Tamil and Siddha medicinal system. The plant has anti-inflammatory, antitumor, and antileprotic activities. It is also used in treatment for psoriasis and erysipelas. For dandruff, burnt plant ashes are used and roots are chewed for toothache and aphthae (Khare, 2007c). The plant is known for its antibacterial and antifungal activities (Ariharan *et al.*, 2015; Bhuvaneswari & Balasundaram, 2006; Elangovan *et al.*, 2014; Kumar *et al.*, 2018; Malini *et al.*, 2019; Mythili *et al.*, 2011; Raju *et al.*, 2013, 2014; Tamilselvi *et al.*, 2011); antioxidant properties (Elangovan *et al.*, 2014; Philips *et al.*, 2010; Ravi *et al.*, 2018); antiproliferative, anti-cancerous, and chemopreventive activities (Gupta *et al.*, 2010; Haldar *et al.*, 2010; Kumar *et al.*, 2012; Mahajan *et al.*, 2016; Paramashivam *et al.*, 2015; Rajkapoor *et al.*, 2005; Sivagnanam *et al.*, 2012); and anti-inflammatory and anti-arthritic properties (Raj *et al.*, 2015; Rajkapoor *et al.*, 2009; Selvam *et al.*, 2004).

Celastrus paniculatus Willd belongs to the family Celastraceae. It is a woody vine with a long stem rooted on the ground. It is known as black oil tree, intellect tree, staff tree, and so on. In Ayurveda it is well known as jyotishmati, kangunikaa, kanguni, katu veeka, and so on (vaaluluvai in Tamil and Siddha). The seed oil is used in various treatments like paralysis, eczema, rheumatism, gout, mental depression, hysteria, memory improvements and so on. The seeds (**Fig. 1b**) are used as emetics, brain tonic, antipyretic, etc (Khare, 2007a). Many biological activities have been reported on the seeds and seed oil of *C. paniculatus*. The seed oil has wound healing, nootropic, and antidepressant activities (Bhagya *et al.*, 2016; Kulkarni *et al.*, 2015; Malik *et al.*, 2017; Maurya & Dwivedi, 2020; Valecha & Dhingra, 2016). The seeds possess biological activities like wound healing, antioxidant, anti-arthritic, hypolipidemic, anti-apoptotic, and also cholinergic activities (Bhanumathy *et al.*, 2010; Kulkarni *et al.*, 2015; Kumar *et al.*, 2015; Malik *et al.*, 2017; Patil *et al.*, 2010).

***Corallocarpus epigaeus* (Rottler) Hook. f.** belongs to the Cucurbitaceae family. It is known as Shukanaasaa, Nahikaa, Katunaahi, and Patala-garuda in the Ayurveda, while in Siddha and Tamil is known as aakasha-garudan. The tuber (**Fig. 1c**) of this plant has been used in later stages of diarrhea (Khare, 2007b). The other biological activities include anthelmintic, antibacterial, antiviral, analgesic, and anti-arthritic (Arbab *et al.*, 2017; Ishnava & Konar, 2020; Priyavardhini *et al.*, 2012; Uthrapathy *et al.*, 2011). The phytochemicals reported from the above three plants are listed in **Tables 1–3**. The diagrammatic representation of comparison of common phytochemicals is shown in **Fig. 2**.

2. Materials and Methods

2.1. Sample Collection

The Sivanar vembu kuzhi thailam was collected from non-institutionally trained traditional Siddha practitioner K. Rangasamy from Palani hills, Tamil Nadu, India. *I. aspalathoides* DC alone was used in the preparation of the thailam for which the results are presented here.

2.2. GC-MS Analysis of Sivanar Vembu Kuzhi Thailam

The detection of compounds in Sivanar vembu kuzhi thailam was carried out on a GC-MS system (7890B GC Connected with 5977A MSD Agilent, USA) using HP 5MS fused silica capillary

Table 1 Reported phytochemicals from the plant *Indigofera aspalathoides*.

Mome inositol	1-Octadecanol
Hexadecanoic acid	4-Heneicosanone
Hexadecanoic acid, ethyl ester	α-Amyrin
n-Heneicosane	n-Octacosanol
Oleic acid	β-Sitosterol
1H-Benzocycloheptane	Salicylic acid
Octadecanoic acid	Erythroxydiol X
Valerenol	Erythroxydiol Y
Labda-8(20), 13(16), 14-triene	β-Sitosterol-3β-d-glucopyranoside
Kauran-16-OL	Indocarpan
Kaur-16-ENE	Mucronulatol
(Rac)-Hesperetin	Hydroxydione
Medicarpin	3-Methyl-2-(2-oxopropyl)furan
Acridine, 9-(*p*-anisidino)	Cyclobutanine, 2,2,3-trimethyl-
Dehydroisoandrosterone acetate	2,4,6,8-Tetramethylundecene
Kauren-19-YL-acetate	α-Cubebene
3-(2,4-Dimethoxyphenyl)-7-chromanol	(Z,Z)-α-Farnesene
Nonadecane	2-Picolylmethylamin
Isopimaradien-3-one	Bicyclosesquiphellandrene
5,7-Dihydroxy-3-(4-hydroxy-2-methoxyphenyl)-3-methoxy-2,3-dihydro-4H-chromen-4-one	Hydrazine, 1,2-dimethyl-
2-(3,4-Dimethoxyphenyl)-3,7-dihydroxy-4H-chromen-4-one	Cyclohexanol, 5-methyl-2-2(1-methylethyl)-, [1s-1a,2a,5a)]-
5,7-Dihydroxy-2-(3,4,5-trimethoxyphenyl)-4-chromanone	8a(2H)-Phenanthrenol, 7-ethenyldodecahydro-1,1,4a,7-tetramethyl-, acetate, [4as-(4aa,4ba,7a,8aa,10aa)]-
4-[2-(3,4-Dimethoxy-phenyl)-ethylamino]1-OXA-Spiro [4,5] DEC-3-EN-2-ONE	3-(2-Hydroxy-3,4-Dimethoxyphenyl)-7-Chromanol

(*Continued*)

Table 1 (*Continued*)

Labda-8(20), 12,14-triene	1-Benzyl-7-methoxy-1,2,3,4-tetrahydro-6-isoquinolinol
14-Isopropyl-3,7,11-Trimethyl-1,3,6,10-Cyclotetradecatetraene	2-(4-Methoxy-2,6-dimethylphenyl)-3-methyl-2H-benzo[g] indazole
Kaur-16-EN-19-OL	Hexatriacontane
Kaur-16-EN-18-OIC acid	Stigmasterol
2-Methoxy-[4-(2-pyridin-4-yl-ethylimino)-methyl]-phenol	Norolean-12-ENE
Dodecanoic acid	7-Cyano-4a, 7-dimethyl-8-(2-oxoethyl) tetradecahydro-2-phenanthrenyl acetate
Tetradecanoic acid	n-Butyl ester of nonadecanoic acid
n-Hexadecadienoic acid	Adrenic acid
9,12-Octadecadienoic acid (Z,Z)	Kaur-16-ene3
Pregnanetriol	

Table 2 Reported phytochemicals from the plant *Celastrus paniculatus*.

Linalool	Phytol acetate
α-Terpinyl acetate	Octadecyl bromide
Nerol acetate	tert-Hexadecanethiol
Iscomene	Octacosane
allo-Aromadendrene	Heptacosane
α-Selinene	17-Pentatriacontene
Calacorene	Squalene
Valerenal	n-Docosane
Spathulenol	Dihydrotestosterone formate-17-benzoate
Caryophyllene oxide	Carpesterol benzoate
Globulol	Maymyrsine
Viridiflorol	2-Benzoyl-3,4-diacetyl-d-galactosan
Humulene epoxide II	Callicarpenal

(*Continued*)

Table 2 (***Continued***)

Andrographolide	Sclareolide
Dihydroisocaryophyllene epoxide	Cycloartenol acetate
trans-Longipinocarveol	Malonic acid
Cubenol	1,7-Octadiene
Cadinol	2,4,6,8-Tetramethyl-1-undecene
iso-Pulegol	9,12,15-Octadecatrienoic acid, 2,3-bis (acetyloxy) propyl ester, (Z,Z,Z)-
trans-Carveol	
Myristyl chloride	Capric acid ethyl ester
Hexahydrofarnesol	Glyphosate, free acid
Fokienol	Hexadecanoic acid ethyl ester
Cepacol	2-Furoic acid
Hystrene	2,6-Piperazinedione, 4-benzoyl-, 2-oxime
Epiglobulol	Prazosin
trans-beta-Copaene	2-Benzoyloxy-1,1,10-trimethyl-6, 9-epidioxy-7-octalin
1-Octadecyne	2-Cyclohexenone,4R-benzamido-5cis, 6trans-dimethoxy-
Phytone	1,3-Phenylene dibenzoate
Bicyclogermacrene	(4-t-Butylphenyl) benzoate
Panasinsene	3-Buten-1-one, 2,2-dimethyl-1-phenyl-
Muurolene	Benzoic acid, phenyl ester
iso-Phytol	Ethanone, 2-(acetyloxy)-1-phenyl-
Hexadecanoic acid	1,3-Phenylene dibenzoate
Deoxyqinghaosu	Benzene acetonitrile, α-oxo-squalene
Oxalic acid, hexadecyl isohexyl ester	Humulane-1,6-dien-3-ol
Valeric acid, 3-pentadecyl ester	α-Sitosterol
Phytol	Pilocarpine
Palmitaldehyde, diallyl acetal	Valeric acid, 2-cyano-2-hydroxy-4-methyl, ethyl ester, benzoate ester
Erucic acid	Octadecanoic acid

Table 3 Reported phytochemicals from the plant *Corallocarpus epigaeus*.

α-Thujene	Aristolene
α-Pinene	α-Guaiene
Camphene	β-Selinene
Sabinene	α-Selinene
β-Pinene	Selina-4(14),7(1l)-diene
Myrcene	Selina-3,7(1l)-diene
β-Cymene	γ-Cadinene
1,8-Cineole	Epiglobulol
Terpinolene	Aromadendrene epoxide
Camphor	Caryophyllene epoxide
Borneol	Isogermacrone epoxide
Terpinen-4-01	Globulol
α-Terpineol	Viridiflorol
Bornyl formate	Viridiflorene epoxide
Terpinen-4-yl acetate	$C_{15}H_{26}O$
α-Terpinyl acetate	Ishwarone
Cyclosativene	Tridecanoic acid, methyl ester
α-Copaene	9,12-Octadecadienoicacid, methyl ester
β-Elemene	9,12-Octadecadienoic acid, (2-phenyl-1,3-dioxolan-4-yl) methyl ester, cis-
α-Gurjunene	Spheroidenone
α-Cedrene	1,1-Cyclobutanedicarboxamide, 2-phenyl-N-N′-bis (1-phenylethyl)-
β-Gurjunene	Cyclopentane propanoic acid, 3,5-bis(acetyloxy)-2-[-(acetyloxy)-3-(methoxyimino)octyl]-, methyl ester
3,7-Guaiadiene	Hexadecenoic acid
Ishwarane	Octadecanoic acid

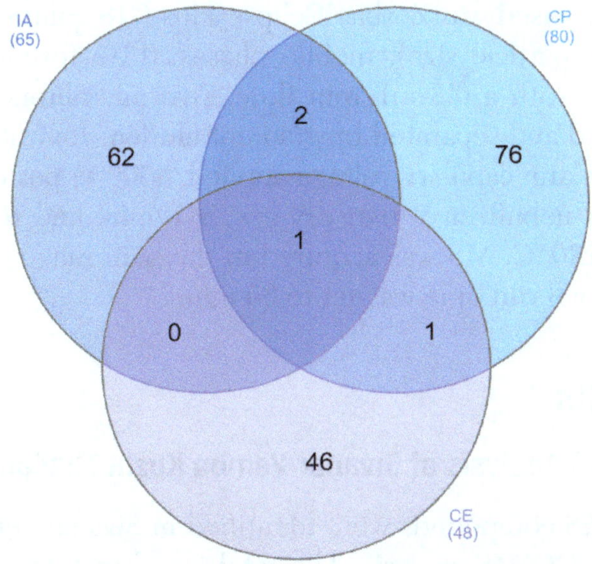

Fig. 2 The diagrammatic representation of reported phytochemicals from the plants. (clockwise) IA — *Indigofera aspalathoides*; CP — *Celastrus paniculatus*; CE — *Corallocarpus epigaeus*. Octadecanoic acid was found to be a common compound in IA, CP, and CE. Hexadecanoic acid and dodecanoic acid were found both in IA and CP; α-Terpinyl acetate is found both in CE and CP. Venn diagram is developed with InteractiVenn (Heberle *et al*., 2015).

column (30 m × 0.25 μm, composed of (5%-phenyl)-methylpolysiloxane) operating in an electron impact mode at 70 eV. The carrier gas employed was 99.999% helium gas at a constant flow of 1 mL/min. One microliter of sample was injected (split ratio of 100:1), at an injector temperature of 250°C and ion source temperature of 280°C. The temperature of the oven was programmed from 50°C to 250°C with an increment of 3°C (isothermal for 15 min). The scan range was set at 50–600 m/z and the total runtime of GC is 96 min. The data obtained were compared with NIST 2011 library.

2.3. LC-MS Analysis of Sivanar Vembu Kuzhi Thailam

The fractions were analyzed using Nexera X2 UPHLC (Shimadzu, Japan) coupled with ESI-qTOF, Impact HD (Bruker, Germany).

The column used was Zorbax Eclipse Plus C18 column (2.6×150 mm, 3 μm particle size), mobile phases: 0.1% formic acid and acetonitrile with a 0.3 mL/min flow. Five microliters of sample was injected and separated by gradient elution. Ionization source parameters are: capillary voltage applied, 4500 V; positive ionization mode; nebulizer, 2 bar; dry gas, 8 L/min; and source temperature, 220 °C. MS was acquired in the scan range of 50–1300 m/z. The total run time was set to 60 min.

3. Results

3.1. GC-MS Analysis of Sivanar Vembu Kuzhi Thailam

A total of 28 compounds were identified in Sivanar vembu kuzhi thailam by GC-MS analysis. The total ion chromatogram of Sivanar vembu kuzhi thailam is shown in **Fig. 3**. Compounds with retention time, chemical structure, formula, and molecular weight are presented in **Table 4**. Ethylbenzene; cyclohexanol; octanoic acid- methyl ester; octanoic acid; benzene, 1,3-bis(1,1-dimethy-

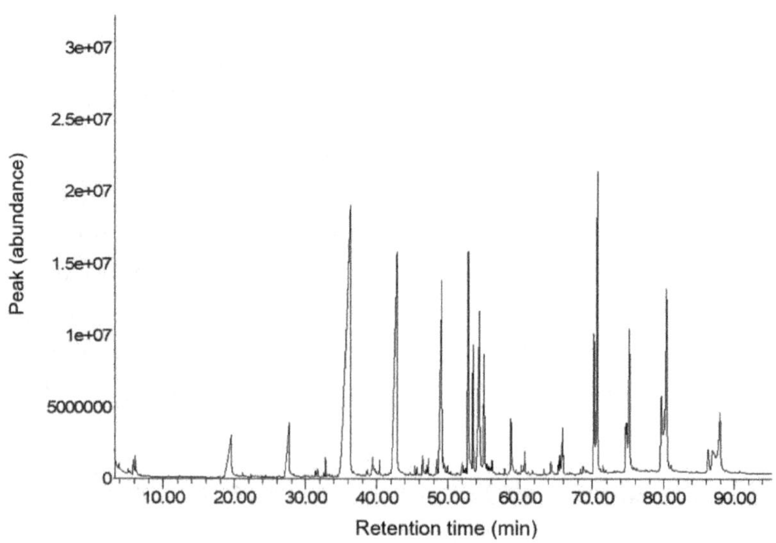

Fig. 3 GC-MS analysis total ion chromatogram of Sivanar vembu kuzhi thailam.

Table 4 Compounds identified from Sivanar vembu kuzhi thailam by GC-MS analysis.

No.	Retention time (min)	Compounds	Formula	Molecular Formula	Chemical Structure	Probability (%)	Peak Area (%)	Biological Activity
1	5.14	Ethylbenzene [Benzene, ethyl-]	C_8H_{10}	106.16	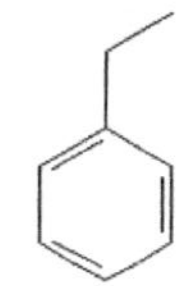	66.3	0.061	Antimicrobial activity (Kalimuthu *et al.*, 2015)
2	5.85	Cyclohexanol [Cyclohexyl alcohol]	$C_6H_{12}O$	100.16	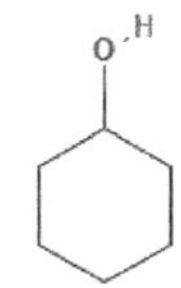	65.4	0.257	Antibacterial activity (Hassan, 2016)
3	15.43	Octanoic acid, methyl ester [Caprylic acid methyl ester]	$C_9H_{18}O_2$	158.24	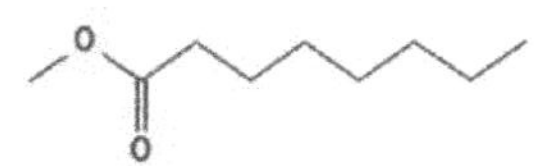	64	0.008	Antibacterial and antifungal activity (Upadhyaya *et al.*, 2015; Yin *et al.*, 2011)
4	19.57	Octanoic acid [ss caprylic acid]	$C_8H_{16}O_2$	144.21	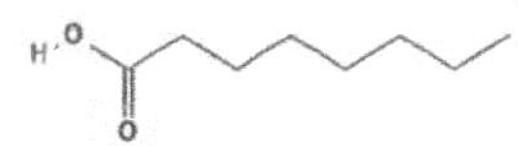	95	3.213	Antibacterial and anti-inflammatory activity (Upadhyaya *et al.*, 2015)
5	21.16	1,3-Ditert-butylbenzene [Benzene, 1,3-bis(1,1-dimethylethyl)-]	$C_{14}H_{22}$	190.32	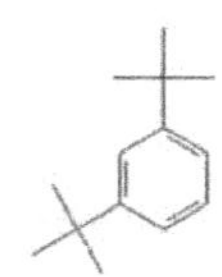	73.8	0.039	Lipid oxidation (Li *et al.*, 2017)

(Continued)

Table 4 (*Continued*)

No.	Retention time (min)	Compounds	Formula	Molecular Formula	Chemical Structure	Probability (%)	Peak Area (%)	Biological Activity
6	22.53	*p*-Ethylguaiacol [2-Methoxy-4-ethylphenol]	$C_9H_{12}O_2$	152.19	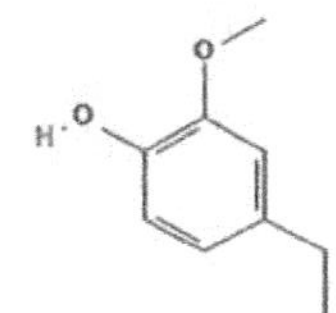	65.6	0.016	Inflammatory and antioxidant activity (Huang *et al.*, 2011)
7	27.68	n-Decanoic acid [n-Capric acid]	$C_{10}H_{20}O_2$	172.26	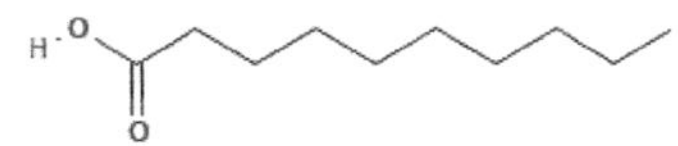	86.9	2.837	Inflammatoryand antioxidant activity (Chang *et al.*, 2016), Anticancer activity (Jóźwiak *et al.*, 2020)
8	31.66	2-Tridecankje [Tridecan-2-one]	$C_{13}H_{26}O$	198.34	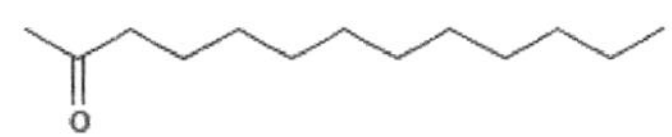	74.2	0.073	Antimalarial activity (Onyeji *et al.*, 2017)
9	32.80	Dodecanoic acid, methyl ester [Methyl dodecanoate]	$C_{13}H_{26}O_2$	214.34	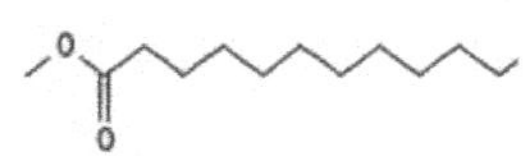	73.4	0.198	Antimicrobial activity (Nitbani *et al.*, 2016)
10	36.28	Dodecanoic acid [ss lauric acid]	$C_{12}H_{24}O_2$	200.32	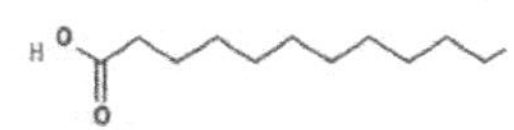	89.3	26.721	Antimicrobial activity (Nakatsuji *et al.*, 2009)
11	40.38	Tetradecanoic acid, methyl ester [Methyl n-tetradecanoate]	$C_{15}H_{30}O_2$	242.4	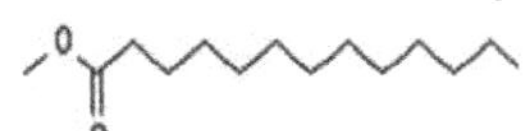	72.7	0.162	Antimicrobial and antioxidant activity (Gideon, 2015)

12	42.83	Tetradecanoic acid [ss myristic acid]	$C_{14}H_{28}O_2$	228.37	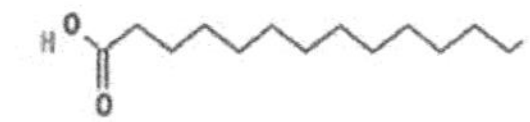	88.2	12.622	Antibacterial activity (Narasimhan *et al.*, 2006) Anticancer activity (Intisar *et al.*, 2013)
13	44.70	Lauric anhydride [Dodecanoic acid, anhydride]	$C_{24}H_{46}O_3$	382.6	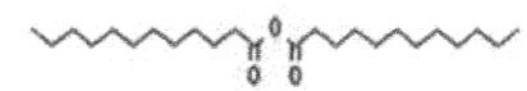	60.8	0.037	Antioxidant activity (Ghani *et al.*, 2018)
14	47.05	7,9-Di-tert-butyl-1-oxaspiro (4,5) deca-6,9-diene-2,8-dione [1-Oxa-spiro[4.5]deca-6,9-diene-2,8-dione, 7,9-di-tert-butyl-]	$C_{17}H_{24}O_3$	276.4	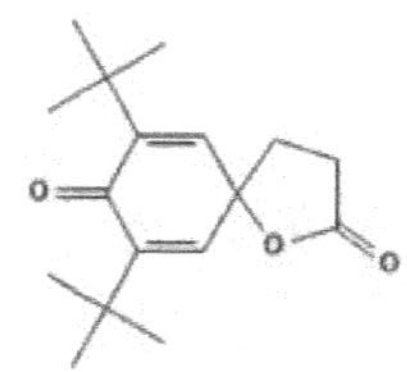	94.5	0.137	Antioxidant activity (Lagacé *et al.*, 2017)
15	47.26	Hexadecenoic acid, methyl ester [n-Hexadecanoic acid methyl ester]	$C_{17}H_{34}O_2$	270.5	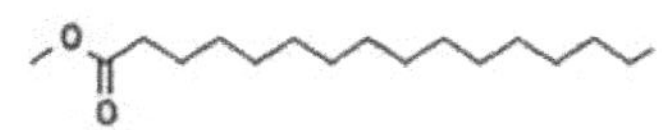	64.9	0.181	Antioxidant activity (Belakhdar *et al.*, 2015)
16	49.14	Hexadecanoic acid [ss palmitic acid]	$C_{16}H_{32}O_2$	256.42	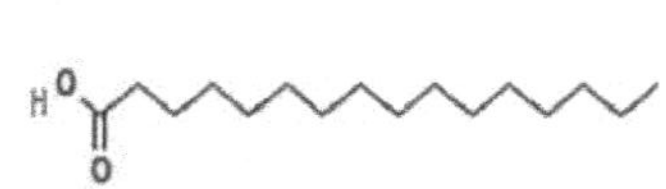	73.5	7.089	Antiinflammatory and antioxidant activity (Aparna *et al.*, 2012)

(*Continued*)

Table 4 (*Continued*)

No.	Retention time (min)	Compounds	Formula	Molecular Formula	Chemical Structure	Probability (%)	Peak Area (%)	Biological Activity
17	52.26	(Z)-Octadec-9-enenitrile [Oleanitrile]	$C_{18}H_{33}N$	263.5	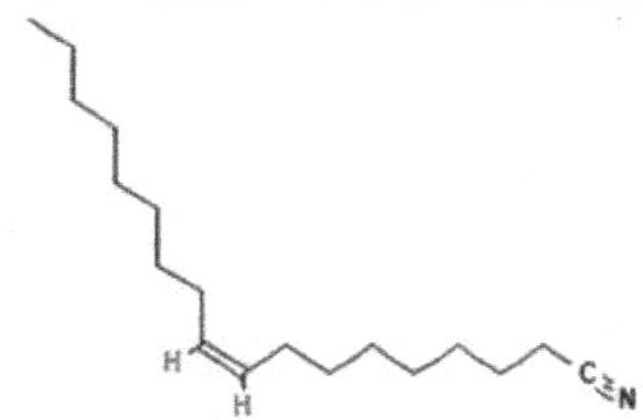	72.6	0.04	Antimicrobial activity (El-Kassas & El-Sheekh, 2016)
18	52.81	2,3-Dihydroxypropyl dodecanoate [α-Monolaurin]	$C_{15}H_{30}O_4$	274.4	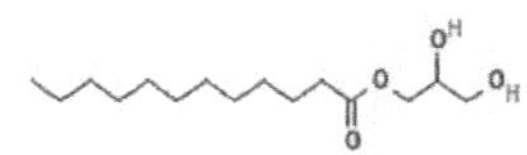	62.7	4.581	Antimicrobial, and anti-inflammatory activity (Li *et al.*, 2009; Schlievert *et al.*, 2019)
19	53.49	Phenol, 4-(3,7-dimethyl-3-ethenylocta-1,6-dienyl)- [Bakuchiol]	$C_{18}H_{24}O$	256.4	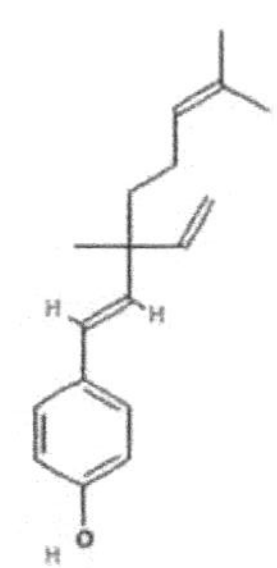	91.1	1.78	Antimicrobial activity (Katsura *et al.*, 2001)

20	54.38	(Z)-11-Octadecenoic acid [cis-Vaccenic acid]	$C_{18}H_{34}O_2$	282.5	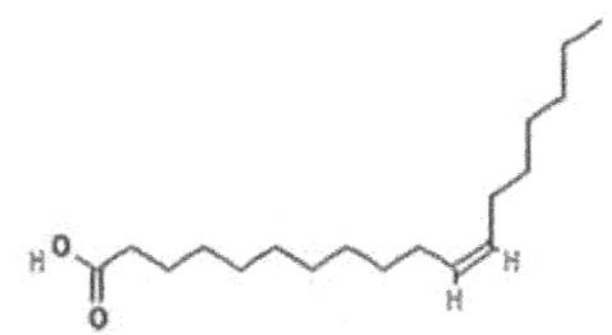	23.7	5.658	Anticancer activity (Song *et al.*, 2019)
21	55.05	Octadecanoic acid [ss stearic acid]	$C_{18}H_{36}O_2$	284.48	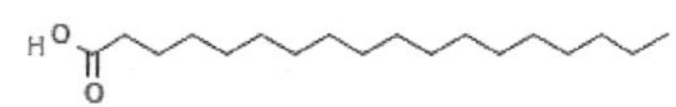	84.9	2.154	Antifungal and antibacterial activity (Kim & Rhee, 2015)
22	55.40	Palmitamide [n-Hexadecanamide]	$C_{16}H_{33}NO$	255.44	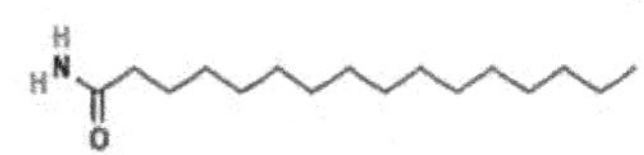	59	0.056	Anticancer activity (El-Garawani *et al.*, 2020)
23	58.72	1,3-Dihydroxypropan-2-yl tetradecanoate [2-Monomyristin]	$C_{17}H_{34}O_4$	302.4	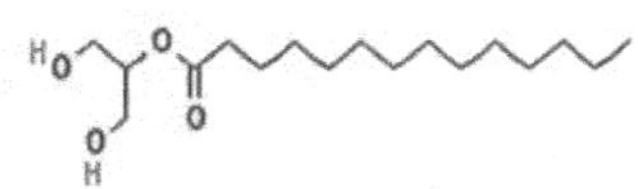	76	1.241	Antibacterial and antifungal activity (Nurmala *et al.*, 2018)
24	61.71	1,3-Diacetyloxypropan-2-yl tetradecanoate [Myristin, 1,3-diaceto-2-]	$C_{21}H_{38}O_6$	386.5	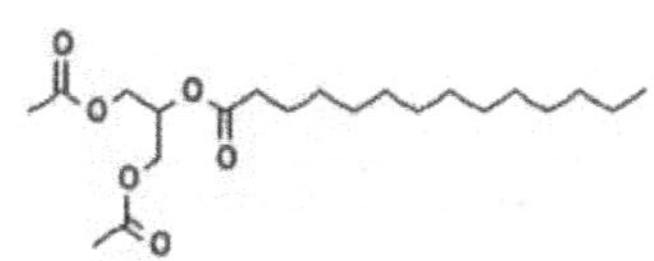	67.2	0.054	–

(*Continued*)

Table 4 (*Continued*)

No.	Retention time (min)	Compounds	Formula	Molecular Formula	Chemical Structure	Probability (%)	Peak Area (%)	Biological Activity
25	63.30	Tricosan-12-one [12-Tricosanone]	$C_{23}H_{46}O$	338.6	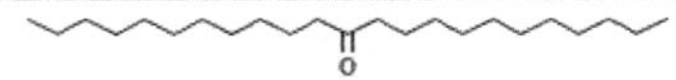	88.7	0.064	–
26	75.12	Butyl dodecanoate [n-Butyl laurate]	$C_{16}H_{32}O_2$	256.42	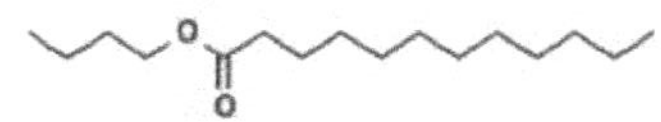	31.9	2.92	–
27	80.33	(2-Dodecanoyloxy-3-hydroxypropyl) dodecanoate [Dodecanoic acid, 1-(hydroxymethyl)-1,2-ethanediyl ester]	$C_{27}H_{52}O_5$	456.7	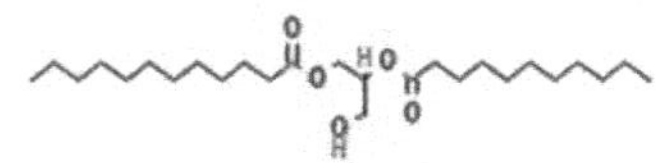	83.2	0.755	Emusifying agent (Yakubu *et al.*, 2017)
28	86.25	2,3-Di(octanoyloxy) propyl octanoate [Glycerol tricaprylate]	$C_{27}H_{50}O_6$	470.7	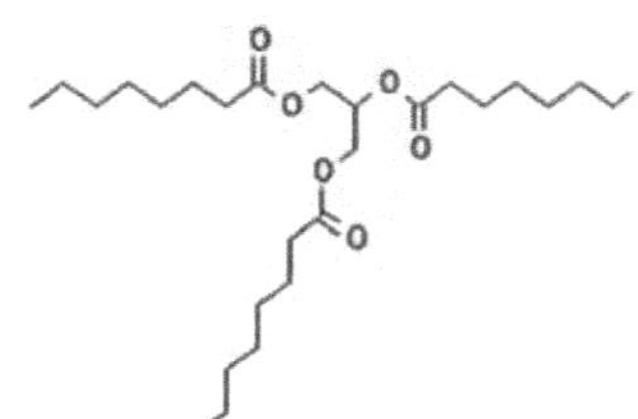	83.6	1.132	Antimicrobial activity (Steinstrasser *et al.*, 2019)

The term "ss" represents the synonym of the bioactive compounds present in the table.

lethyl)-; *p*-ethylguaiacol; n-decanoic acid, 2-tridecankje; lauric acid- methyl ester; dodecanoic acid; myristic acid- methyl ester; myristic acid; lauric anhydride; 7,9-di-tert-butyl-1-oxaspiro (4,5) deca-6,9-diene-2,8-dione; palmitic acid- methyl ester; palmitic acid; oleanitrile; α-monolaurin; phenol, 4-(3,7-dimethyl-3-etheny-locta-1,6-dienyl)-; cis-Vaccenic acid (CVA); stearic acid; palmitamide; 2-monomyristin; myristin, 1,3-diaceto-2-; 12-tricosanone; n-butyl laurate; dodecanoic acid; 1-(hydroxymethyl)-1,2-ethanediyl ester; and glycerol tricaprylate are the 28 compounds detected by GC-MS analysis of the Sivanar vembu kuzhi thailam.

3.2. LC-MS Analysis of Sivanar Vembu Kuzhi Thailam

The LC-MS analysis detected eight compounds. The LC-MS data were acquired by using Bruker Compass DataAnalysis Version 4.4 software and processed in mzMine (Pluskal *et al.*, 2010) mass spectrum was compared with libraries and reference Mass spectrums with the help of Global Natural Products Social Molecular Networking (Wang *et al.*, 2016), an open access website based platform for sharing processed, identified, or extracted raw tandem mass spectrometry data.

LC-MS base peak chromatogram is shown in **Fig. 4**. The compounds identified are tetradecanoic acid, 2,3-dihydroxypropyl

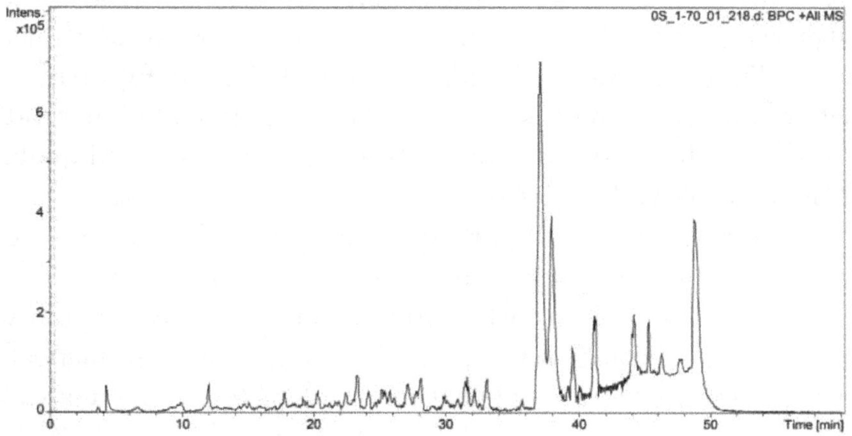

Fig. 4 Base peak chromatogram of Sivanar vembu kuzhi thailam.

ester; ceratodictyol; dibutyl phthalate; (2S)-2-(4-hydroxyphenyl)-7-methoxy-6-(3-methylbut-2-enyl)-2,3-dihydrochromen-4-one; cembrene; monoelaidin; 7-hydroxy-3-[4-hydroxy-3-(3-methylbut-2-enyl) phenyl] chromen-4-one; 3-[3-[(2E)-3,7-dimethylocta-2,6-dienyl]-4-hydroxyphenyl]-7-hydroxychromen-4-one. The retention time, chemical structure, formula, and molecular weight of the identified compounds are shown in **Table 5**.

4. Discussion

Humans have been using herbal plants and medicines for centuries as medications against several diseases and disease conditions like swelling, wounds, skin infections like scabies, eczema, diabetes, jaundice, mental illness, cancer, and countless others, for the reason that the herbal plants are available locally, cheap, and the common misconception that these are devoid of any side effects. The increase for the demand of these herbal medicines also raises the concern of safety, quality, availability, efficacy, and so on, by the health professionals, policy makers, and indeed the general citizens. Therefore, many recent researches are committed to the investigation of the therapeutic effects of herbal medicines documented in the Ayurvedic, Siddha, and other traditional medicinal systems. The most modern methodology in research and analytical techniques are used to investigate and validate the herbal medicines according to the modern drugs standards (Khan & Ahmad, 2019). The preservation of traditional knowledge and future use of natural products can be achieved by the development of the traditional medicinal systems with safety and effectiveness and quality (Mukherjee & Wahile, 2006).

The present study reports the compounds identified by GC-MS and LC-MS analyses of Sivanar vembu kuzhi thailam.

Upon comparison with already reported phytochemicals from individual plants, it was found that lauric acid (systematically dodecanoic acid) and pregnanetriol are detected in the analyzed

Table 5 Compounds identified from Sivanar vembu kuzhi thailam by LC-MS analysis.

S. No.	Retention Time	Compounds	Formula	Molecular Weight	Structure	Peak Area (%)	Biological Activity
1	2.0	2,3-Diacetyloxypropyl octadecenoate [Tetradecanoic acid, 2,3-dihydroxypropyl ester]	$C_{17}H_{34}O_4$	302.44	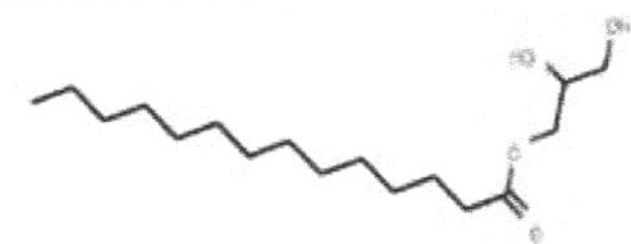	1.16	Anticancer and antioxidant activity
2	4.2	3-[(E)-6-hydroxyhexadec-4-enoxy]propane-1,2-diol [Ceratodictyol]	$C_{19}H_{38}O_4$	330.5	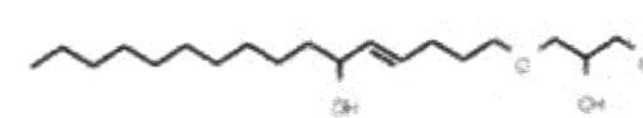	0.24	Anticancer, antioxidant, and antimicrobial activity
3	30.6	Dibutyl benzene-1,2-dicarboxylate [Dibutyl phthalate]	$C_{16}H_{22}O_4$	278.34	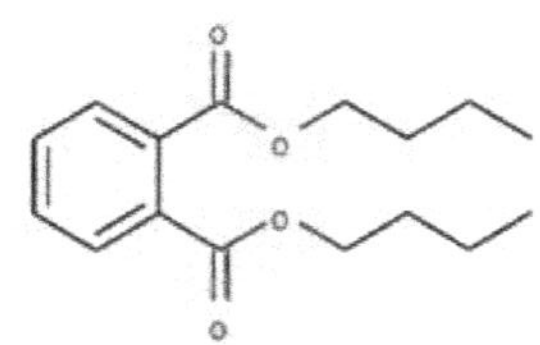	0.33	Anticancer and antimicrobial activity (Roy *et al.*, 2006; Wang *et al.*, 2012)

(*Continued*)

Table 5 (*Continued*)

S. No.	Retention Time	Compounds	Formula	Molecular Weight	Structure	Peak Area (%)	Biological Activity
4	38.0	(2S)-2-(4-hydroxyphenyl)-7-methoxy-6-(3-methylbut-2-enyl)-2,3-dihydrochromen-4-one [Bavachinin]	$C_{21}H_{22}O_4$	338.152	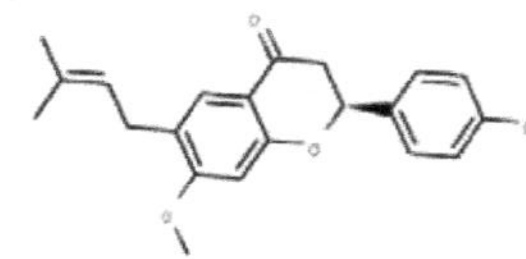	2.82	Antibacterial activity (Chen *et al.*, 2013)
5	40.0	(1E,3Z,6E,10E)-3,7,11-trimethyl-14-propan-2-ylcyclotetradeca-1,3,6,10-tetraene [Cembrene]	$C_{20}H_{32}$	272.25	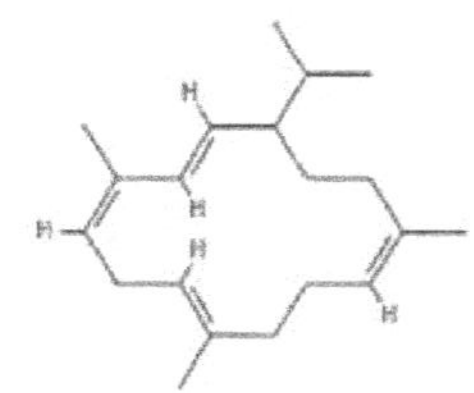	1.12	Anticancer, antimicrobial, and antibacterial activity (Gautam *et al.*, 2014; Hegazy *et al.*, 2017)
6	41.0	2,3-Dihydroxypropyl (E)-octadec-9-enoate [Monoelaidin]	$C_{21}H_{40}O_4$	356.5	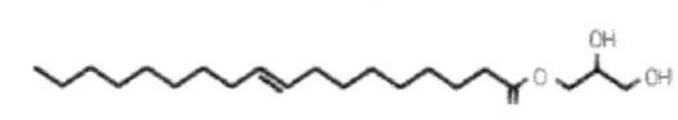	1.28	Antimicrobial and antibacterial activity (Li *et al.*, 2009; Schliever *et al.*, 2019)

7	44.0	7-Hydroxy-3-[4-hydroxy-3-(3-methylbut-2-enyl) phenyl] chromen-4-one		322.121	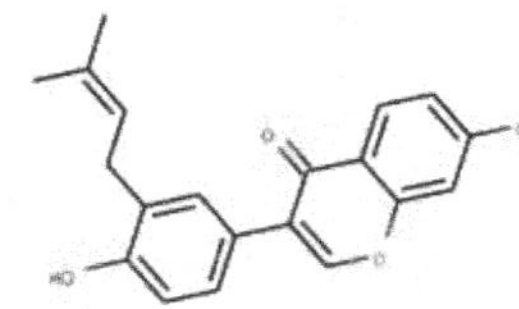	4.02	—
8	48.0	3-[3-[(2E)-3,7-dimethylocta-2,6-dienyl]-4-hydroxyphenyl]-7-hydroxychromen-4-one	$C_{25}H_{26}O_4$	391.19	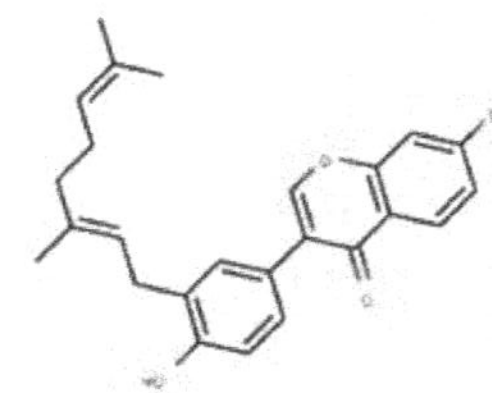	3.43	—

sample as well as in the individual plant *I. aspalathoides* (Abirami & Rajendran, 2011). Caryophyllene, a bicyclic sesquiterpene, has also been reported in the seed extracts of *C. paniculatus* as caryophyllene oxide (Kumar *et al.*, 2014). Both palmitic acid and stearic acid found in *C. paniculatus* seed oil and in the tuber of *C. epigaeus* (Arora & Pandey, 2014; Rana & Das, 2017) are also detected in GC-MS analysis of Sivanar vembu kuzhi thailam sample.

The compounds present both in the kuzhi thailam sample and in the individual plants indicate that these compounds are stable even after a destructive distillation process.

Figure 5 represents the comparison of compounds detected in GC-MS and LC-MS analyses of Sivanar vembu kuzhi thailam

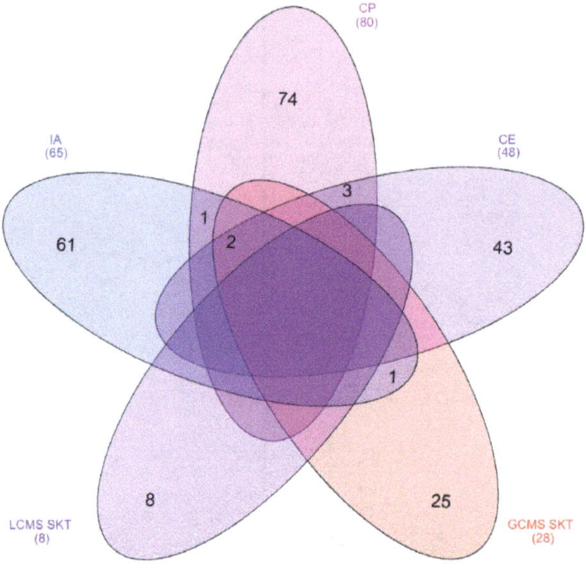

Fig. 5 Diagrammatic representation of comparison of compounds detected in GC-MS and LC-MS analyses of Sivanar vembu kuzhi thailam with reported phytochemicals of individual plants. (clockwise) SKT — Sivanar vembu kuzhi thailam; IA — *Indigofera aspalathoides*; CP — *Celastrus paniculatus*; CE — *Corallocarpus epigaeus*. Octadecanoic and hexadecanoic acids are commonly found in individual plants as well as in the GC-MS analysis of kuzhi thailam sample. Hexadecanoic ethyl ester is common for the IA and CP. And globulol, viridiflorol, and epiglobulol are common for CP and CE. Dodecanoic acid is commonly found between IA and GC-MS. No common compound in our LC-MS was found between our GC-MS and already reviewed report.Venn diagram developed with InteractiVenn (Heberle *et al.*, 2015).

with reported phytochemicals of individual plants. Octadecanoic and hexadecanoic acids are commonly found in individual plants as well as in the GC-MS analysis of kuzhi thailam sample. Hexadecanoic ethyl ester is common for the *Indigofera aspalathoides* and *Celastrus paniculatus*. And globulol, viridiflorol, and epiglobulol are common for *C. paniculatus* and *Corallocarpus epigaeus*. Dodecanoic acid is commonly found between *I. aspalathoides* and GC-MS. No common compound in our LC-MS was found between our GC-MS and already reviewed report.

4.1. Biological Activities of Compounds Identified from Sivanar Vembu Kuzhi Thailam

Octanoic acid or caprylic acid is a medium-chain fatty acid. In a study to eliminate the colonization of *Salmonella enteritidis* which infects the intestines and oviduct leading to the egg contamination in layer hens, it was found that 1% of caprylic acid added with the feed was able to reduce the population of *S. enteritidis* by 14% in egg shells and 10% in yolks in comparison with control birds. The addition of 1% caprylic acid with feed also reduced the bacterial population in cecum and liver compared to the untreated birds (Upadhyaya *et al*., 2015). The study conducted by Kim & Rhee (2015) reported that lower concentrations of caprylic acid in addition with citric acid eliminated the *Escherichia coli* O157:H7 and endogenous microbiota in unpasteurized carrot juice, indicating its synergistic antibacterial property. Zhang *et al*. (2019) reported that caprylic acid can suppress cytokine inflammation and reduce atherosclerosis through the TLR4/NF-κB signaling in apolipoprotein A-deficient mouse, suggesting that caprylic acid can be used in nutrition to fight chronic inflammatory diseases. Another antimicrobial study on meat contamination reports that 3% caprylic acid effectively reduced the shiga-toxin producing *E. coli* in beef products (Cap *et al*., 2019).

p-Ethylguaiacol or 4-ethyl-2-methoxyphenol is a smoke flavoring phenol. In a study investigating the effects of three smoke flavoring phenols, 4-ethyl-2-methoxyphenol (5–20 μM) has been shown as an effective protection against cytotoxicity induced by tert-butyl hydroperoxide. Out of the other phenols subjected to the study, 4-ethyl-2-methoxyphenol has shown highest inhibition on production of radicals and oxidation of biomolecules suggesting that 4-ethyl-2-methoxyphenol has antioxidant and anti-inflammatory properties (Huang *et al.*, 2011).

n-Decanoic acid or capric acid is a C_{10} straight-chain saturated fatty acid with many biological activities. Decanoic acid was found to have anti-inflammatory and antibacterial effects on *Propionibacterium acnes*. Huang *et al.* (2014) reported that the anti-inflammation process by decanoic acid is by phosphorylation of MAP kinases and by inhibiting the activation of NF-κB. In another study by Shen *et al.* (2021), PMAP-23RI, an antimicrobial peptide derived from cathelicidin PMAP-23RI modified with decanoic acid (PMAP-23RIi-Dec), has shown a high bactericidal effect with stability. It was also intriguing that PMAP-23RIi-Dec eradicated biofilm and ameliorated the organ damages caused by *Pseudomonas aeruginosa* GIM1.551 and *Staphylococcus aureus* ATCC25923. The decanoic acid also exhibits antiseizure activity; the MCT diet is prescribed for drug-resistant epilepsy. This diet increases the ketone and decanoic acid levels in blood plasma. In a study by Chang *et al.* (2016), decanoic acid alone has been reported to have the antiseizure activity. They also described the antagonistic activity of decanoic acid on AMPA receptors, thereby decreasing the fast bulk glutamatergic signals, which in turn proves the therapeutic activity in antiseizure. Decanoic acid also inhibits the mTORC1 activity regardless of glucose and insulin levels. mTORC1 or rapamycin 1 is a protein complex that activates the translation process. In disease conditions like cancer and neuro-related diseases the mTORC1 activity is higher. Warren *et al.* (2020) suggests therapeutic properties of decanoic acid in a range of disorders and diseases.

2-Tridecankje or 2-tridecanone is found naturally in wild tomato plant trichomes. Most vector-borne diseases are spread by ticks in the USA; the tick repellent activity of 2-tridecanone was first reported by Kimps *et al.* (2011) which was experimented on two tick species, the lone star tick, *Amblyomma americanum* (L.), and the American dog tick, *Dermacentor variabilis*. 2-Tridecanone also exhibits repellent property toward the *Anopheles gambiae* ss, a mosquito known to be a transmitter of malaria (Innocent *et al.*, 2008).

A study by Manosroi *et al.* (2013) reported that methyl myristate loaded on cationic niosomes can be used for canities treatment, as they have induced melanin at a higher rate in B16F10 melanoma cells, with no cytotoxic activity toward the normal cells.

Dodecanoic acid or lauric acid is one of the major compounds that has a number of biological activities. In a study on colonization of *Campylobacter jejuni* in chicken, it was found that lauric acid effectively limited the infection and decreased excretion of the bacteria (Hankel *et al.*, 2018). Another study by Yang *et al.* (2017) on lauric acid proved it as an antibacterial, it inhibited the growth of *Clostridium difficile* and inflammation of intestines were reduced as well as the severity of diarrhea was also observed to be reduce. Dose-dependent introduction of lauric acid was able to inhibit *S. aureus*, *Bacillus cereus*, *Salmonella typhimurium*, and *E. coli* in the study conducted by Nitbani *et al.* (2016). Lappano *et al.* (2017) elucidated the molecular mechanism of lauric acid inducing pro-apoptotic and antiproliferative effects in endometrial and breast cancer cells. Antibacterial study by Nakatsuji *et al.* (2009) proved that lauric acid inhibits the growth of *P. acnes*. Administration of lauric acid also reduced granulomatous inflammation and swelling of the infection site.

The antibacterial activity of myristic acid or tetradecanoic acid recently revealed that myristic acid with an MIC ranging from 64 to 256 μg/mL inhibited the growth of 13 strains of *Listeria monocytogenes* in milk (Chen *et al.*, 2019). They have also confirmed by transmission electron microscopy and fluorescence that myristic acid affected the cell integrity of the organism at various degrees which led to the death of the cells in a dose dependent manner. In addition to this they have also found that myristic acid can bind with the DNA of the organism which can alter the structure of the DNA. Wada *et al.* (2016) reported that glucose uptake got increased when myristic acid was used. They also reported that upon myristic treatment, the expression of diacylglycerol kinase δ got increased, suggesting that uptake of myristic acid-rich diet can improve maintenance of glucose in type II diabetes. A study by Intisar *et al.* (2013) concluded that myristic acid (400 μg/mL) has a strong cytotoxic effect on human hepatocellular carcinoma cell line (HCCLM3), suggesting its anticancer activity. In another study conducted by Nurmala *et al.* (2018) it was found that the monomyristin has antibacterial activity against *S. aureus*, *A. actinomycetemcomitans*, and *E. coli* and antifungal activity against *Candida albicans* compared with monopalmitin derivatives.

Palmitic acid or n-hexadecanoic acid has anti-inflammatory properties. Aparna *et al.* (2012) reported the inhibitory activity of n-decanoic acid on phospholipase A2. One of the first steps in initiation of inflammation is the release of fatty acids by the action of phospholipase A2, hydrolyzing the ester bonds of membrane phospholipids. This study validates the use of medicated oils rich in palmitic acid on tropical applications for symptoms of rheumatism in the traditional system of medicines in India.

α-Monolaurin or glycerol monolaurate (GML) has a higher degree of antimicrobial property than lauric acid. Schlievert *et al.* (2019) reported that the antimicrobial activity of human milk is due to the presence of GML. GML also provided anti-inflammatory activity in human milk. Upon addition of increasing amounts of GML, bovine milk also exhibited antimicrobial activity but comparatively lesser than human milk. Immunomodulatory activity of GML was reported in a study on transmission of HIV-1 infection (Li *et al.*, 2009). GML has shown an antagonistic effect in production of MIP-3α and other proinflammatory cytokines, thereby inhibiting the mucosal signaling. The innate and inflammatory response toward HSV-1 and SIV are also found to be inhibited, suggesting that GML effectively blocked mucosal transmission of HIV-1 infections.

Yu *et al.* (2005) evaluated the action of methyl esters and their derivatives such as 12-octadecenoic acid methyl ester; (Z,Z)-methyl ester-9,12-octadecadienoic acid, 10-methyl-heptadecanoic acid methyl ester, hexadecanoic acid methyl ester, in controlling of human gastric cancer cell line (SGC-7901).

A recent study by Paramashivam *et al.* (2021) evaluated the indigocarpan belonging to pterocarpan family has antioxidant and anti-proliferative activities in human cancer cell lines via induction of caspase-dependent apoptosis pathway. (Mahajan *et al.* (2016) studied the effect of indigocarpan on cell proliferation using MTT assay. Poonkodi *et al.* (2017) investigated the anticancer property of the dibutyl phthalate compound from the leaves of the *Tridax procumbens*. Rajkapoor *et al.* (2004) evaluated the antitumor activity of the ethanol extract of *I. aspalathoides* against enrich ascites carcinoma in mice.

Roy *et al.* (2006) reported that the dibutyl phthalate or dibutyl benzene-1,2-dicarboxylate has potent antibacterial activity against both Gram-positive and Gram-negative bacteria, as well as unicellular and filamentous fungi, with no acute toxicity. Akpuaka *et al.* (2012) and Shobi *et al.* (2018) reported the antifungal activity of this compound. Beulah *et al.* (2018) investigated that the dibutyl phthalate extracted from the leaf of *Dendrophthoe falcata* has antimicrobial and antifouling property. Wang *et al.* (2012) reported that this compound is also present in *Polyalthia rumphii* which exhibits anticancer activity.

Palmitamide or n-hexadecanamide is one of the primary fatty acids, which has been found to have anticancer property (El-Garawani *et al.*, 2020).

Cembrene or (1E,3Z,6E,10E)-3,7,11-trimethyl-14-propane-2-ylcyclotetradeca-1,3,6,10-tetraene is a 14-membered-ring diterpenoid natural product which exhibits anticancer property, as studied by Hegazy *et al.* (2017) and Gautam *et al.* (2014). Another study by Poma *et al.* (2018) reported the antitumor and pro-oxidant properties of cembrene present in *Glandora rasmarinifolia* essential oil.

The antimicrobial, antioxidant, anticancer, and antifungal properties of the phytoconstituents such as 9-hexadecanoic acid, methyl ester hexadecenoic acid, 9-octadecanoic acid(Z)- methyl ester, and octadecanoic acid, methyl ester have also been reported (Ezekwe & Chikezie, 2017; Tulandi *et al*., 2021).

CVA or (z)-11-octadecanoic acid is naturally occurring in nature, and it is found abundantly in human milk, ruminant fats, and in dairy products. Aimola *et al*. (2016) showed that CVA induced differentiation of K562 JK-1 cells and upregulated the expression of γ-globins. The authors reported that JK-1 and TMbmEPSCs were differentiated directly by CVA and γ-globins expressed in these cells indirectly by CVA. Hydroxyurea is the only Food and Drug Administration-approved medication that can induce γ-globins for ameliorating sickle cell anemia; bone marrow transplant is the only way to clear the disease and this is impossible and cannot be afforded by a large population. Therefore, the findings of the authors suggest CVA's therapeutic ability in treatment of sickle cell anemia. Lipogenesis is a process of generating triglycerides from acetyl CoA, and in a study conducted by Burns *et al*. (2012) the rate of lipogenesis was reduced by supplementing CVA in bovine adipocytes and addition of palmitoleic acid reduced the rate of desaturation. The mitochondrial dysfunction caused by diseases like cancer, neurodegenerative diseases, aging, and so on, can be improved by supplementation of stearic acid to the diet. Senyilmaz *et al*. (2015) reported the pathway of this process where stearic acid improves the mitochondrial functions. Stearic acid and human transferrin receptor 1 (TFR1) are identified as the regulators of mitochondria. JNK signals are inactivated by the stearic acid together with TFR1, which leads to the decreased mitofusin ubiquitination by HUWE1. This promotes the fusion of mitochondria and restoration of functions in mitochondria. The supplementation of stearic acid with a high-protein diet in parkin null Drosophila improved the climbing ability, membrane potential of mitochondria respiration, and so on, as reported by Bajracharya *et al*. (2019).

Based on literature survey, we found that *I. aspalathoides* possess potent antineoplastic, antioxidant, antimicrobial, antifungal, anticancer and antibacterial activities.

5. Conclusion

GC-MS analysis of Sivanar vembu kuzhi thailam reports the presence of biologically active fatty acids. These fatty acids have a number of biological activities, especially anti-inflammatory, anticancer, antibacterial, antifungal, and immunomodulatory activities which can validate Sivanar vembu kuzhi thailam for its topical applications and its significance in the treatment of various skin diseases like chronic weeping eczema, psoriasis, leprosy, insect bites, leukoderma, boils, infected wounds, etc. Literature survey shows that most of the compounds identified from LC-MS-MS analysis showed antibacterial and anticancer activities.

Acknowledgment

The authors greatly acknowledge the SRM management and Department of Biotechnology, School of Bioengineering for providing the instrumentation facilities.

References

Abirami, P., & Rajendran, A. (2011). GC-MS determination of bioactive compounds of *Indigofera aspalathoides*. *Journal of Natural Product and Plant Resources*, *1*(4), 126–130.

Aimola, I. A., Inuwa, H. M., Nok, A. J., Mamman, A. I., & Bieker, J. J. (2016). Cis-vaccenic acid induces differentiation and up-regulates gamma globin synthesis in K562, JK1 and transgenic mice erythroid progenitor stem cells. *European Journal of Pharmacology*, *776*, 9–18.

Akpuaka, A., Ekwenchi, M. M., Dashak, D. A., & Dildar, A. (2012). Gas Chromatography-Mass Spectrometry (GC/MS) analysis of phthalate isolates in n-hexane extract of *Azadirachta indica A. Juss* (Neem) leaves. *Journal of American Science*, *8*(12), 146–155.

Aparna, V., Dileep, K. V., Mandal, P. K., Karthe, P., Sadasivan, C., & Haridas, M. (2012). Anti-inflammatory property of n-hexadecanoic acid: Structural evidence and kinetic assessment. *Chemical Biology and Drug Design*, *80*(3), 434–439.

Arbab, A. H., Parvez, M. K., Al-Dosari, M. S., & Al-Rehaily, A. J. (2017). In vitro evaluation of novel antiviral activities of 60 medicinal plants extracts against hepatitis B virus. *Experimental and Therapeutic Medicine*, *14*(1), 626–634.

Ariharan, V. N., Devi, V. N. M., Parameswaran, N. K., & Prasad, P. N. (2015). Antibacterial activity of Sivanar Vembu (*Indigofera aspalathoides*) against some human pathogenic bacteria. *Journal of Chemical and Pharmaceutical Research*, *7*(3), 937–941.

Arora, N., & Pandey-Rai, S. (2014). GC–MS analysis of the essential oil of *Celastrus paniculatus* Willd. seeds and antioxidant, anti-inflammatory study of its various solvent extracts. *Industrial Crops and Products*, *61*, 345–351.

Aruna, V., Amrythavalli, G. V., & Gayathri, R. (2019). Was histamine toxicity known to Ayurveda and Siddha 5000 years ago? *World News of Natural Sciences. An International Sientific Journal*, *23*.

Bajracharya, R., Bustamante, S., & O Ballard, J. W. (2019). Stearic acid supplementation in high protein to carbohydrate (P:C) ratio diet improves physiological and mitochondrial functions of *Drosophila melanogaster* parkin Null mutants. *The Journals of Gerontology. Series A, Biological Sciences and Medical Sciences*, *74*(10), 1564–1572.

Belakhdar, G., Benjouad, A., & Abdennebi, E. H. (2015). Determination of some bioactive chemical constituents from *Thesium humile* Vahl. *Journal of Materials and Environmental Science*, *6*(10), 2778–2783.

Beulah, G. G., Soris, P. T., & Mohan, V. R. (2018). GC-MS Determination of bioactive compounds of *Dendrophthoe falcata* (LF) Ettingsh: An epiphytic plant. *International Journal of Health Sciences and Research*, *8*, 261–269.

Bhagya, V., Christofer, T., & Shankaranarayana Rao, B. S. (2016). Neuroprotective effect of *Celastrus paniculatus* on chronic stress-induced cognitive impairment. *Indian Journal of Pharmacology*, *48*(6), 687–693.

Bhanumathy, M., Harish, M. S., Shivaprasad, H. N., & Sushma, G. (2010). Nootropic activity of *Celastrus paniculatus* seed. *Pharmaceutical Biology*, *48*(3), 324–327.

Bhardwaj, S., Verma, R., & Gupta, J. (2018). Challenges and future prospects of herbal medicine. *International Research in Medical and Health Science*. https://doi.org/10.36437/irmhs.2018.1.1

Bhuvaneswari, R. A., & Balasundaram, C. (2006). Traditional Indian herbal extracts used in vitro against growth of the pathogenic bacteria – *Aeromonas hydrophila*. *The Israeli Journal of Aquaculture – Bamidgeh*, *58*(2), 89–96.

Burns, T. A., Kadegowda, A. K. G., Duckett, S. K., Pratt, S. L., & Jenkins, T. C. (2012). Palmitoleic (16:1 cis-9) and cis-vaccenic (18:1 cis-11) acid alter lipogenesis in bovine adipocyte cultures. *Lipids*, *47*(12), 1143–1153.

Cap, M., Vaudagna, S., Mozgovoj, M., Soteras, T., Sucari, A., Signorini, M., & Leotta, G. (2019). Inactivation of Shiga toxin-producing *Escherichia coli* in fresh beef by electrolytically-generated hypochlorous acid, peroxyacetic acid, lactic acid and caprylic acid. *Meat Science*, *157*, 107886.

Chang, P., Augustin, K., Boddum, K., Williams, S., Sun, M., Terschak, J. A., Hardege, J. D., Chen, P. E., Walker, M. C., & Williams, R. S. B. (2016). Seizure control by decanoic acid through direct AMPA receptor inhibition. *Brain: A Journal of Neurology*, *139*(Pt 2), 431–443.

Chen, X., Yang, Y., & Zhang, Y. (2013). Isobavachalcone and bavachinin from *Psoraleae fructus* modulate Aβ42 aggregation process through different mechanisms in vitro. *FEBS Letters*, *587*(18), 2930–2935.

Chen, X., Zhao, X., Deng, Y., Bu, X., Ye, H., & Guo, N. (2019). Antimicrobial potential of myristic acid against *Listeria monocytogenes* in milk. *The Journal of Antibiotics*, *72*(5), 298–305.

Elangovan, K., Thanigaivel, S., Shahinbanu, Z., & Murugesan, K. (2014). Phytochemical evaluation, in vitro antioxidant and antibacterial potential of *Indigofera aspalathoides*. *International Journal of Pharmacy and Biological Sciences*, *4*(1), 161–168.

El-Garawani, I. M., El-Sabbagh, S. M., Abbas, N. H., Ahmed, H. S., Eissa, O. A., Abo-Atya, D. M., Khalifa, S. A. M., & El-Seedi, H. R. (2020). A newly isolated strain of *Halomonas* sp. (HA1) exerts anticancer potential via induction of apoptosis and G 2/M arrest in hepatocellular carcinoma (HepG2) cell line. *Scientific Reports*, *10*(1), 1–15.

El-Kassas, H. Y., & El-Sheekh, M. M. (2016). Induction of the synthesis of bioactive compounds of the marine alga *Tetraselmis tetrathele* (West) Butcher grown under salinity stress. *The Egyptian Journal of Aquatic Research*, *42*(4), 385–391.

Ezekwe, S. A., & Chikezie, P. C. (2017). GC–MS analysis of aqueous extract of unripe fruit of *Carica papaya*. *Journal of Nutrition & Food Sciences*, *7*(3), 1–5.

Gautam, N., Mantha, A. K., & Mittal, S. (2014). Essential oils and their constituents as anticancer agents: A mechanistic view. *BioMed Research International*, *2014*.

George, P. (2011). Concerns regarding the safety and toxicity of medicinal plants – An overview. *Journal of Basic and Applied Pharmaceutical Sciences*, *1*(6), 40–44.

Ghani, N. A. A., Channip, A. A., Chok Hwee Hwa, P., Ja'afar, F., Yasin, H. M., & Usman, A. (2018). Physicochemical properties, antioxidant capacities, and metal contents of virgin coconut oil produced by wet and dry processes. *Food Science and Nutrition*, *6*(5), 1298–1306.

Gideon, V. A. (2015). GC-MS analysis of phytochemical components of *Pseudoglochidion anamalayanum* Gamble: An endangered medicinal tree. *Asian Journal of Plant Science and Research*, *5*(12), 36–41.

Guguloth, R., Yadav, C. R., & Vasam, K. (2017). A comparative study of Ayurveda and Siddha system of medicine. *International Journal of Innovative Research in Medical Science*, *2*(9), 1285–1288.

Gupta, M., K.anti Mazumder, U., Haldar, P., Kandar, C. H., Manikandan, L., & Senthil, G. (2010). Anticancer activity of *Indigofera aspalathoides* and *Wedelia calendulaceae* in Swiss Albino mice. *Iranian Journal of Pharmaceutical Research: IJPR*, *6*(2), 141–145.

Haldar, P. K., Bhattacharya, S., Bala, A., Kar, B., Mazumder, U. K., & Dewanjee, S. (2010). Chemopreventive role of *Indigofera aspalathoides* against 20-methylcholanthrene-induced carcinogenesis in mouse. *Toxicological and Environmental Chemistry*, *92*(9), 1749–1763.

Hankel, J., Popp, J., Meemken, D., Zeiger, K., Beyerbach, M., Taube, V., Klein, G., & Visscher, C. (2018). Influence of lauric acid on the susceptibility of chickens to an experimental *Campylobacter jejuni* colonisation. *PLoS One*, *13*(9), e0204483.

Hassan, G. (2016). *Synthesis of abietic and dehydroabietic acid derivatives to target bacterial biofilms* [Master's thesis].

Heberle, H., Meirelles, G. V., da Silva, F. R., Telles, G. P., & Minghim, R. (2015). InteractiVenn: A web-based tool for the analysis of sets through Venn diagrams. *BMC Bioinformatics*, *16*, 169.

Hegazy, M. E. F., Elshamy, A. I., Mohamed, T. A., Hamed, A. R., Ibrahim, M. A., Ohta, S., & Paré, P. W. (2017). Cembrene diterpenoids with ether linkages from *Sarcophyton ehrenbergi*: An anti-proliferation and molecular-docking assessment. *Marine Drugs*, *15*(6), 192.

Huang, M.-H., Chang, L.-W., Sung, W.-C., Vong, W.-J., & Wang, B.-S. (2011). Protective effects of three smoke flavouring phenols on oxidative damage and nitric oxide production. *Food Chemistry*, *126*(4), 1655–1661.

Huang, W.-C., Tsai, T.-H., Chuang, L.-T., Li, Y.-Y., Zouboulis, C. C., & Tsai, P.-J. (2014). Anti-bacterial and anti-inflammatory properties of capric acid against *Propionibacterium acnes*: A comparative study with lauric acid. *Journal of Dermatological Science*, *73*(3), 232–240.

Innocent, E., Gikonyo, N. K., & Nkunya, M. H. H. (2008). Repellency property of long chain aliphatic methyl ketones against *Anopheles gambiae* s.s. *Tanzania. Journal of Health Research*, *10*(1), 50–54.

Intisar, A., Zhang, L., Luo, H., Kiazolu, J. B., Zhang, R., & Zhang, W. (2013). Anticancer constituents and cytotoxic activity of methanol-water extract of *Polygonum bis-*

torta L. *African Journal of Traditional, Complementary and Alternative Medicines*, *10*(1), 53–59.

Ishnava, K. B., & Konar, P. S. (2020). In vitro anthelmintic activity and phytochemical characterization of *Corallocarpus epigaeus* (Rottler) Hook. f. tuber from ethyl acetate extracts. *Bulletin of the National Research Centre*, *44*(1), 33.

Jóźwiak, M., Filipowska, A., Fiorino, F., & Struga, M. (2020). Anticancer activities of fatty acids and their heterocyclic derivatives. *European Journal of Pharmacology*, *871*, 172937.

Kalimuthu, P., Heider, J., Knack, D., & Bernhardt, P. V. (2015). Electrocatalytic hydrocarbon hydroxylation by ethylbenzene dehydrogenase from *Aromatoleum aromaticum*. *The Journal of Physical Chemistry B*, *119*(8), 3456–3463. https://doi.org/10.1021/jp512562k

Karunamoorthi, K., Jegajeevanram, K., Xavier, J., Vijayalakshmi, J., & Melita, L. (2012). Tamil traditional medicinal system – Siddha: An indigenous health practice in the international perspectives. *CELLMED*, *2*(2), 12.1–12.11.

Katsura, H., Tsukiyama, R. I., Suzuki, A., & Kobayashi, M. (2001). In vitro antimicrobial activities of bakuchiol against oral microorganisms. *Antimicrobial Agents and Chemotherapy*, *45*(11), 3009–3013. https://doi.org/10.1128/AAC.45.11.3009-3013.2001

Khan, M. S. A., & Ahmad, I. (2019). Herbal medicine: Current trends and future prospects. In *New look to phytomedicine* (pp. 3–13). Elsevier.

Khare, C. P. (2007a). *Celastrus paniculatus* Willd. in *Indian medicinal plants* (pp. 1–1). New York, NY: Springer.

Khare, C. P. (2007b). *Corallocarpus epigaeus* Benth. ex Hook. f. In *Indian medicinal plants* (pp. 1–1). New York, NY: Springer.

Khare, C. P. (2007c). *Indigofera aspalathoides* Vahl ex DC. In C. P. Khare (Ed.), *Indian medicinal plants: An illustrated dictionary* (p. 1). New York: Springer.

Kim, S. A., & Rhee, M. S. (2015). Synergistic antimicrobial activity of caprylic acid in combination with citric acid against both *Escherichia coli* O157:H7 and indigenous microflora in carrot juice. *Food Microbiology*, *49*, 166–172.

Kimps, N. W., Bissinger, B. W., Apperson, C. S., Sonenshine, D. E., & Roe, R. M. (2011). First report of the repellency of 2-tridecanone against ticks. *Medical and Veterinary Entomology*, *25*(2), 202–208.

Konappa, N., Udayashankar, A. C., Krishnamurthy, S., Pradeep, C. K., Chowdappa, S., & Jogaiah, S. (2020). GC-MS analysis of phytoconstituents from *Amomum nilgiricum* and molecular docking interactions of bioactive serverogenin acetate with target proteins. *Scientific Reports*, *10*(1), 16438.

Krupa, J., Sureshkumar, J., Silambarasan, R., Priyadarshini, K., & Ayyanar, M. (2019). Integration of traditional herbal medicines among the indigenous communities in Thiruvarur District of Tamil Nadu, India. *Journal of Ayurveda and Integrative Medicine*, *10*(1), 32–37.

Kulkarni, Y. A., Agarwal, S., & Garud, M. S. (2015). Effect of Jyotishmati (*Celastrus paniculatus*) seeds in animal models of pain and inflammation. *Journal of Ayurveda and Integrative Medicine*, *6*(2), 82–88.

Kumar, K. H., Venuprasad, M. P., Jayashree, G. V., Rachitha, P., Krupashree, K., Pal, A., & Khanum, F. (2015). *Celastrus paniculatus* Willd. mitigates t-BHP induced oxidative and apoptotic damage in C2C12 murine muscle cells. *Cytotechnology*, *67*(6), 955–967.

Kumar K. H., Venuprasad M. P., Pal, A., & Khanum, F. (2014). Phytochemical analysis and exercise enhancing effects of hydroalcoholic extract of *Celastrus paniculatus* Willd. *Industrial Crops and Products*, *55*, 217–224.

Kumar, S. S., Rao, M. R. K., & Balasubramanian, M. P. (2012). Antiproliferative role of *Indigofera aspalathoides* on 20 methylcholanthrene induced fibrosarcoma in rats. *Asian Pacific Journal of Tropical Biomedicine*, *2*(12), 966–974.

Kumar, T. T., Salique, S. M., Ilyas, M. H. M., Thajuddin, N., Panneerselvam, A., Padusha, M. K. S. A., & Jahangir, H. S. (2018). Phytochemical screening and antimicrobial studies in leaf extracts of *Indigofera aspalathoides* (Vahl.). *Pharmacognosy Journal*, *10*(6). http://phcogj.com/article/719

Lagacé, L., Charron, C., & Sadiki, M. (2017). Analysis of plastic residues in maple sap and syrup collected from tubing systems sanitized with isopropyl alcohol. *Heliyon*, *3*(5), e00306.

Lappano, R., Sebastiani, A., Cirillo, F., Rigiracciolo, D. C., Galli, G. R., Curcio, R., Malaguarnera, R., Belfiore, A., Cappello, A. R., & Maggiolini, M. (2017). The lauric acid-activated signaling prompts apoptosis in cancer cells. *Cell Death Discovery*, *3*, 17063.

Li, C., He, L., Jin, G., Ma, S., Wu, W., & Gai, L. (2017). Effect of different irradiation dose treatment on the lipid oxidation, instrumental color and volatiles of fresh pork and their changes during storage. *Meat Science*, 128, 68–76.

Li, Q., Estes, J. D., Schlievert, P. M., Duan, L., Brosnahan, A. J., Southern, P. J., Reilly, C. S., Peterson, M. L., Schultz-Darken, N., Brunner, K. G., Nephew, K. R., Pambuccian, S., Lifson, J. D., Carlis, J. V., & Haase, A. T. (2009). Glycerol monolaurate prevents mucosal SIV transmission. *Nature*, *458*(7241), 1034–1038.

Mahajan, P., Gnana Oli, R., Jachak, S. M., Bharate, S. B., & Chaudhuri, B. (2016). Antioxidant and antiproliferative activity of indigocarpan, a pterocarpan from *Indigofera aspalathoides*. *The Journal of Pharmacy and Pharmacology*, *68*(10), 1331–1339.

Malik, J., Karan, M., & Dogra, R. (2017). Ameliorating effect of *Celastrus paniculatus* standardized extract and its fractions on 3-nitropropionic acid induced neuronal damage in rats: Possible antioxidant mechanism. *Pharmaceutical Biology*, *55*(1), 980–990.

Malini, M., Kumar, J. P., Kumar, R. D., & Joshy, V. A. (2019). Phytochemical analysis and evaluation of antioxidant and antimicrobial activity of *Phyllanthus emblica*, *Phaseolus vulgari*, and *Indigofera aspalathoides* – A step toward alternative cure for cancer. *Drug Invention Today*, *12*(8).

Manosroi, A., Chaikul, P., Abe, M., Manosroi, W., & Manosroi, J. (2013). Melanogenesis of methyl myristate loaded niosomes in B16F10 melanoma cells. *Journal of Biomedical Nanotechnology*, 9(4), 626–638.

Maurya, H., & Dwivedi, V. (2020). Wound healing potential of *Celastrus paniculatus* seed oil in rat model. *International Research Journal of Pharmacology*, *2*, 1–8. https://scirange.com/fulltext/irjp.2020.1.8

Mukherjee, P. K., & Wahile, A. (2006). Integrated approaches towards drug development from Ayurveda and other Indian system of medicines. *Journal of Ethnopharmacology*, *103*(1), 25–35.

Mythili, S., Sathiavelu, A., & Sridharan, T. B. (2011). Antimicrobial activity of selected Indian folk medicinal plants. *Journal of Pharmacy Research*, *4*(6), 1894–1898.

Nakatsuji, T., Kao, M. C., Fang, J. Y., Zouboulis, C. C., Zhang, L., Gallo, R. L., & Huang, C. M. (2009). Antimicrobial property of lauric acid against *Propionibacterium acnes*: Its therapeutic potential for inflammatory acne vulgaris. *Journal of Investigative Dermatology*, *129*(10), 2480–2488.

Narasimhan, B., Mourya, V., & Dhake, A. (2006). Design, synthesis, antibacterial, and QSAR studies of myristic acid derivatives. *Bioorganic and Medicinal Chemistry Letters*, *16*(11), 3023–3029.

Nitbani, F. O., Jumina, Siswanta, D., & Solikhah, E. N. (2016). Isolation and antibacterial activity test of lauric acid from crude coconut oil (*Cocos nucifera* L.). *Procedia Chemistry*, *18*, 132–140.

Nurmala, A., Fitria, A., Pranowo, D., Sholikhah, E. N., Kurniawan, Y. S., & Kuswandi, B. (2018). Monomyristin and monopalmitin derivatives: Synthesis and evaluation as potential antibacterial and antifungal agents. *Molecules*, *23*(12), 3141.

Omprakash, K. K., Chandran, G. S., & Velpandian, V. (2013). *Indigofera aspalathoides* Vahl ex. Dc.(sivanar vembu): A phyto pharmacological review. *International Journal of Pharmaceutical Sciences and Research*, *4*(10), 3775.

Onyeji, C. O., Igbinoba, S. I., Olayiwola, G., & Adehin, A. (2017). Insight into clinically effective herbal antimalarial products: Effects on drug metabolizing enzymes and p-glycoprotein. *African Journal of Pharmacy and Pharmacology*, *11*(48), 591–613.

Pandey, M. M., Rastogi, S., & Rawat, A. K. (2008). Indian herbal drug for general healthcare: An overview. *The Internet Journal of Alternative Medicine*, 6(1), 3.

Pandey, M. M., Rastogi, S., & Rawat, A. K. S. (2013). Indian traditional Ayurvedic system of medicine and nutritional supplementation. *Evidence-Based Complementary and Alternative Medicine: eCAM*, *2013*, 376327.

Paramashivam, S. K., Elayaperumal, K., bhagavan Natarajan, B., Devi Ramamoorthy, M., Balasubramanian, S., & Dhiraviam, K. N. (2015). In silico pharmacokinetic and molecular docking studies of small molecules derived from *Indigofera aspalathoides* Vahl targeting receptor tyrosine kinases. *Bioinformation*, *11*(2), 73.

Paramashivam, S., & Dhiraviam, K. N. (2021). Computational insights into the identification of a potent matrix metalloproteinase inhibitor from *Indigofera aspalathoides* to control cancer metastasis. *3 Biotech*, *11*(5), 1–19.

Parasuraman, S., & Perumal, P. (2020). Siddha, an indigenous medical system of peninsular India. In S. Sen, & R. Chakraborty (Eds.), *Herbal medicine in India: Indigenous knowledge, practice, innovation and its value* (pp. 9–21). Springer Singapore.

Patil, R. H., Prakash, K., & Maheshwari, V. L. (2010). Hypolipidemic effect of *Celastrus paniculatus* in experimentally induced hypercholesterolemic Wistar rats. *Indian Journal of Clinical Biochemistry: IJCB*, *25*(4), 405–410.

Philips, A., Philip, S., Arul, V., Padmakeerthiga, B., Renju, V., Santha, S., & Sethupathy, S. (2010). Free radical scavenging activity of leaf extracts of *Indigofera aspalathoides* – An in vitro analysis. *Journal of Pharmaceutical Sciences and Research*, *2*(6), 322–328.

Pluskal, T., Castillo, S., Villar-Briones, A., & Oresic, M. (2010). MZmine 2: Modular framework for processing, visualizing, and analyzing mass spectrometry-based molecular profile data. *BMC Bioinformatics*, *11*, 395.

Poma, P., Labbozzetta, M., Notarbartolo, M., Bruno, M., Maggio, A., Rosselli, S., Sajeva, M., & Zito, P. (2018). Chemical composition, in vitro antitumor and pro-oxidant activities of *Glandora rosmarinifolia* (Boraginaceae) essential oil. *PLoS One*, *13*(5), e0196947. https://doi.org/10.1371/journal.pone.0196947

Poonkodi, K., Jayapriya, V., Sujitha, K., Jeevitha, R., & Megha, P. (2017). In-vitro anticancer activity and essential oil composition of *Tridax procumbens* (L.). *American Journal of PharmTech Research*, 7(2), 366–371.

Priyavardhini, S., Vasantha, K., TresinaSoris, P., & Mohan, V. R. (2012). Efficacy of phytochemical and antibacterial activity of *Corallocarpus epigaeus* Hook. f. *International Journal of PharmTech Research*, *4*, 35–43.

Raj, V. B. A., Kumar, K. L. S., & Kumar, S. S. (2015). Traditional Indian medicinal plants as a potential anti-inflammatory phytomedicine for psoriasis control. *Journal of Pharmacognosy and Phytochemistry*, *4*(3), 118–122.

Rajkapoor, B., Jayakar, B., & Murugesh, N. (2004). Antitumor activity of *Indigofera aspalathoides* on Ehrlich ascites carcinoma in mice. *Indian Journal of Pharmacology*, *36*(1), 38.

Rajkapoor, B., Kavimani, S., Ravichandiran, V., Sekhar, K., Kumar, R. S., Kumar, M. R., Pradeepkumar, M., Einstein, J. W., & Kumar, E. P. (2009). Effect of *Indigofera aspalathoides* on complete Freund's adjuvant-induced arthritis in rats. *Pharmaceutical Biology*, *47*(6), 553–557.

Rajkapoor, B., Murugesh, N., Chodon, D., & Sakthisekaran, D. (2005). Chemoprevention of N-nitrosodiethylamine induced phenobarbitol promoted liver tumors in rat by extract of *Indigofera aspalathoides*. *Biological and Pharmaceutical Bulletin*, *28*(2), 364–366.

Rajkumar, S., & Lekha, G. S. (2016). Basic principles in Siddha pharmaceutical science – An overview. *IOSR Journal of Pharmacy and Biological Sciences*, *11*(6), 43–48.

Raju, G., Maridass, M., & Subash, N. (2014). Immunostimulatory effect of *Indigofera aspalathoides* extract supplemented with basal diets on *Macrobrachium rosenbergii* (de Man, 1879) against *Vibrio harveyi*. *International Journal of Biological Technology*, *5*(2), 1–14.

Raju, G., Subash, N., & Maridass, M. (2013). GC-MS analysis of chemical constituents and antibacterial activity of *Indigofera aspalathoids* DC stem. *Nature of Pharmaceutical Technology*, *3*(2), 1–5.

Rana, V. S., & Das, M. (2017). Fatty acid and non-fatty acid components of the seed oil of *Celastrus paniculatus* Willd. *International Journal of Fruit Science*, *17*(4), 407–414.

Ravi, A., Khan, S., Suklabaidya, M., Priyadurairaj, Sudarsanan, P. S., & Chandrasekar, K. (2018). Antioxidant activity and in silico analysis of *Centella asiatica* and *Indigofera aspalathoides* in psoriasis. *Biomedical and Pharmacology Journal*, *11*(3), 1403–1412.

Roy, R. N., Laskar, S., & Sen, S. K. (2006). Dibutyl phthalate, the bioactive compound produced by *Streptomyces albidoflavus* 321.2. *Microbiological Research*, *161*(2), 121–126.

Sahayam, S., Chellappan, D., Sriram, S., Rajalakshmi, P., & Brindha, P. (2020). Acute toxicity profiles of Siddha medicine Sivanar vembu kuzhi thailam on rats. *Biomedical and Pharmacology Journal*, *13*(3), 1137–1143.

Schlievert, P. M., Kilgore, S. H., Seo, K. S., & Leung, D. Y. M. (2019). Glycerol monolaurate contributes to the antimicrobial and anti-inflammatory activity of human milk. *Scientific Reports*, *9*(1), 14550.

Selvam, C., Jachak, S. M., Gnana Oli, R., Thilagavathi, R., Chakraborti, A. K., & Bhutani, K. K. (2004). A new cyclooxygenase (COX) inhibitory pterocarpan from *Indigofera aspalathoides*: Structure elucidation and determination of binding orientations in the active sites of the enzyme by molecular docking. *Tetrahedron Letters*, *45*(22), 4311–4314.

Sen, S., & Chakraborty, R. (2017). Revival, modernization and integration of Indian traditional herbal medicine in clinical practice: Importance, challenges and future. *African Journal of Traditional, Complementary, and Alternative Medicines: AJT-CAM/African Networks on Ethnomedicines*, *7*(2), 234–244.

Senyilmaz, D., Virtue, S., Xu, X., Tan, C. Y., Griffin, J. L., Miller, A. K., Vidal-Puig, A., & Teleman, A. A. (2015). Regulation of mitochondrial morphology and function by stearoylation of TFR1. *Nature*, *525*(7567), 124–128.

Shen, T., Chen, L., Liu, Y., Shi, S., Liu, Z., Cai, K., Liao, C., & Wang, C. (2021). Decanoic acid modification enhances the antibacterial activity of PMAP-23RI-Dec. *European Journal of Pharmaceutical Sciences: Official Journal of the European Federation for Pharmaceutical Sciences*, *157*, 105609.

Shobi, T. M., & Viswanathan, M. G. (2018). Antibacterial activity of di-butyl phthalate isolated from *Begonia malabarica*. *Journal of Applied Biotechnology and Bioengineering*, *5*(2), 97–100.

Shukla, S., & Saraf, S. (2011). Fundamental aspect and basic concept of siddha medicines. *Systematic Reviews in Pharmacy*, *2*(1), 48.

Sivagnanam, S. K., Rao, M. R. K., & Balasubramanian, M. P. (2012). Chemotherapeutic efficacy of *Indigofera aspalathoides* on 20-methylcholanthrene-induced fibrosarcoma in rats. *ISRN Pharmacology*, *2012*, 134356.

Song, J., Wang, Y., Fan, X., Wu, H., Han, J., Yang, M., Lu, L., & Nie, G. (2019). Trans-vaccenic acid inhibits proliferation and induces apoptosis of human nasopharyngeal carcinoma cells via a mitochondrial-mediated apoptosis pathway. *Lipids in Health and Disease*, *18*(1), 1–9.

Steinstrasser, G. C., Gioielli, L. A., & Vitolo, M. (2019). Evaluation of caprylins by thin layer chromatography. *World Journal of Pharmacy and Pharmaceutical Sciences*, *8*(6), 103–114.

Tamilselvi, N., Dhamotharan, R., Krishnamoorthy, P., Arumugam, P., & Sagathevan, E. (2011). Antifungal Activity of *Indigofera aspalathoides* (Shivanar Vembu) Vahl ex Dc. http://armatsbioteklab.in/publications2/3.pdf

Thas, J. J. (2008). Siddha Medicine—Background and principles and the application for skin diseases. *Clinics in Dermatology*, *26*(1), 62–78.

Tulandi, S. M., Tanzil, L., & Ulfa, D. M. (2021). Analysis of bioactive compounds from methanol extract of *Diadema setosum* sea urchin gonads using gas chromatography–mass spectrometry. *Research Journal of Pharmacy and Technology*, *14*(3), 1629–1634.

Upadhyaya, I., Upadhyay, A., Yin, H.-B., Nair, M. S., Bhattaram, V. K., Karumathil, D., Kollanoor-Johny, A., Khan, M. I., Darre, M. J., Curtis, P. A., & Venkitanarayanan, K. (2015). Reducing colonization and eggborne transmission of *Salmonella enteritidis* in layer chickens by in-feed supplementation of caprylic acid. *Foodborne Pathogens and Disease*, *12*(7), 591–597.

Uthrapathy, S., Shabi, M. M., Krishnamoorthy, G., Ravindhran, D., Rajamanickam, V. G., & Dubey, G. P. (2011). Analgesic and anti-arthritic effect of *Corallocarpus epigaeus*. *Acta Bioquímica Clínica Latinoamericana*, *45*(4), 749–756.

Valecha, R., & Dhingra, D. (2016). Behavioral and biochemical evidences for antidepressant-like activity of *Celastrus Paniculatus* seed oil in mice. *Basic and Clinical Neuroscience*, *7*(1), 49–56.

Wada, Y., Sakiyama, S., Sakai, H., & Sakane, F. (2016). Myristic acid enhances diacylglycerol kinase ⊠-dependent glucose uptake in myotubes. *Lipids*, *51*(8), 897–903.

Wang, M., Carver, J. J., Phelan, V. V., Sanchez, L. M., Garg, N., Peng, Y., Nguyen, D. D., Watrous, J., Kapono, C. A., Luzzatto-Knaan, T., Porto, C., Bouslimani, A., Melnik, A. V., Meehan, M. J., Liu, W.-T., Crüsemann, M., Boudreau, P. D., Esquenazi, E., Sandoval-Calderón, M., … Bandeira, N. (2016). Sharing and community curation of mass spectrometry data with Global Natural Products Social Molecular Networking. *Nature Biotechnology*, *34*(8), 828–837.

Wang, T., Yuan, Y., Wang, J., Han, C., & Chen, G. (2012). Anticancer activities of constituents from the stem of *Polyalthia rumphii*. *Pakistan Journal of Pharmaceutical Sciences*, *25*(2).

Warren, E. C., Dooves, S., Lugarà, E., Damstra-Oddy, J., Schaf, J., Heine, V. M., Walker, M. C., & Williams, R. S. B. (2020). Decanoic acid inhibits mTORC1 activity independent of glucose and insulin signaling. *Proceedings of the National Academy of Sciences of the United States of America*, *117*(38), 23617–23625.

Yadav, V., Jayalakshmi, S., & Singla, R. K. (2012). Traditional systems of medicine- now and forever. https://www.webmedcentral.com/article_view/3299

Yakubu, E. O., Otitoju, O., & Onwuka, J. (2017). Gas chromatography-mass spectrometry (GC-MS) analysis of aqueous extract of *Daniellia oliveri* stem bark. *Pharmaceutica Analytica Acta*, *8*(11), 1–8.

Yang, H.-T., Chen, J.-W., Rathod, J., Jiang, Y.-Z., Tsai, P.-J., Hung, Y.-P., Ko, W.-C., Paredes-Sabja, D., & Huang, I.-H. (2017). Lauric acid is an inhibitor of *Clostridium difficile* growth in vitro and reduces inflammation in a mouse infection model. *Frontiers in Microbiology*, *8*, 2635.

Yin, Y., Bi, Y., Chen, S., Li, Y., Wang, Y., Ge, Y., Ding, B., Li, Y., & Zhang, Z. (2011). Chemical composition and antifungal activity of cuticular wax isolated from Asian pear fruit (cv. Pingguoli). *Scientia Horticulturae*, *129*(4), 577–582.

Yu, F. R., Lian, X. Z., Guo, H. Y., McGuire, P. M., Li, R. D., Wang, R., & Yu, F. H. (2005). Isolation and characterization of methyl esters and derivatives from *Euphorbia kansui* (Euphorbiaceae) and their inhibitory effects on the human SGC-7901 cells. *Journal of Pharmacy & Pharmaceutical Sciences*, *8*(3), 528–535.

Zhang, X., Xue, C., Xu, Q., Zhang, Y., Li, H., Li, F., Liu, Y., & Guo, C. (2019). Caprylic acid suppresses inflammation via TLR4/NF-κB signaling and improves atherosclerosis in ApoE-deficient mice. *Nutrition and Metabolism*, *16*, 40.

https://doi.org/10.1142/9789811254796_bmatter

Index

Lightning Source UK Ltd.
Milton Keynes UK
UKHW022139191022
410723UK00003B/34

9 789811 254789